Oxford American Handbook of
Endocrinology and Diabetes

About the Oxford American Handbooks in Medicine

The Oxford American Handbooks are pocket clinical books, providing practical guidance in quick reference, note form. Titles cover major medical specialties or cross-specialty topics and are aimed at students, residents, internists, family physicians, and practicing physicians within specific disciplines.

Their reputation is built on including the best clinical information, complemented by hints, tips, and advice from the authors. Each one is carefully reviewed by senior subject experts, residents, and students to ensure that content reflects the reality of day-to-day medical practice.

Key series features

- Written in short chunks, each topic is covered in a two-page spread to enable readers to find information quickly. They are also perfect for test preparation and gaining a quick overview of a subject without scanning through unnecessary pages.
- Content is evidence based and complemented by the expertise and judgment of experienced authors.
- The Handbooks provide a humanistic approach to medicine—it's more than just treatment by numbers.
- A "friend in your pocket," the Handbooks offer honest, reliable guidance about the difficulties of practicing medicine and provide coverage of both the practice and art of medicine.
- For quick reference, useful "everyday" information is included on the inside covers.

Published and Forthcoming Oxford American Handbooks

Oxford American Handbook of Clinical Medicine
Oxford American Handbook of Anesthesiology
Oxford American Handbook of Cardiology
Oxford American Handbook of Clinical Dentistry
Oxford American Handbook of Clinical Diagnosis
Oxford American Handbook of Clinical Examination and Practical Skills
Oxford American Handbook of Clinical Pharmacy
Oxford American Handbook of Critical Care
Oxford American Handbook of Emergency Medicine
Oxford American Handbook of Endocrinology and Diabetes
Oxford American Handbook of Gastroenterology and Hepatology
Oxford American Handbook of Geriatric Medicine
Oxford American Handbook of Nephrology and Hypertension
Oxford American Handbook of Neurology
Oxford American Handbook of Obstetrics and Gynecology
Oxford American Handbook of Oncology
Oxford American Handbook of Ophthalmology
Oxford American Handbook of Otolaryngology
Oxford American Handbook of Pediatrics
Oxford American Handbook of Physical Medicine and Rehabilitation
Oxford American Handbook of Psychiatry
Oxford American Handbook of Pulmonary Medicine
Oxford American Handbook of Rheumatology
Oxford American Handbook of Sports Medicine
Oxford American Handbook of Surgery
Oxford American Handbook of Urology

Oxford American Handbook of **Endocrinology and Diabetes**

Edited by

Boris Draznin, MD, PhD

Director, Adult Diabetes Program
Professor of Medicine
Division of Endocrinology, Metabolism and Diabetes
University of Colorado School of Medicine
Aurora, Colorado

Sol Epstein, MD

Professor of Medicine and Geriatrics
Mount Sinai School of Medicine
New York, NY

with

Helen E. Turner
John A.H. Wass

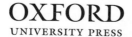

OXFORD
UNIVERSITY PRESS

OXFORD
UNIVERSITY PRESS

Oxford University Press, Inc. publishes works that further
Oxford University's objective of excellence
in research, scholarship and education.

Oxford New York

Auckland Cape Town Dar es Salaam Hong Kong Karachi
Kuala Lumpur Madrid Melbourne Mexico City Nairobi
New Delhi Shanghai Taipei Toronto

With offices in

Argentina Austria Brazil Chile Czech Republic France Greece
Guatemala Hungary Italy Japan Poland Portugal
Singapore South Korea Switzerland Thailand Turkey Ukraine Vietnam

Published by Oxford University Press Inc.
198 Madison Avenue, New York, New York 10016

www.oup.com

Oxford is a registered trade mark of Oxford University Press

First published 2011
UK version published: 2009

Library of Congress Cataloging-in-Publication Data

Oxford American handbook of endocrinology and diabetes / edited by
Boris Draznin ... [et al.].
p. ; cm.
Handbook of endocrinology and diabetes
Includes bibliographical references and index.
ISBN 978-0-19-537428-5
1. Endocrinology—Handbooks, manuals, etc.   2. Diabetes—Handbooks, manuals,
etc. I. Draznin, Boris.   II. Title: Handbook of endocrinology and diabetes.
[DNLM: 1. Endocrine System Diseases—Handbooks.   2. Diabetes
Mellitus—Handbooks. WK 39]
RC649.O94 2011
616.4—dc22
2010050977

10 9 8 7 6 5 4 3

Printed in the United States of America
on acid-free paper

Preface

In this era of rapid electronic transfer of medical information, the question is often posed: "Do we need textbooks anymore, as by the time they are printed much of the information is outdated?" This question is best answered by this publication, which offers the reader current, practical, clinical evidence–based information that will benefit patients with endocrine and metabolic disease. This handbook is not meant to be a fully comprehensive tome but to act as a quick and easily accessible source of information.

While we have endeavored to include material that is as current as possible, the many advances occurring in the field of endocrinology and diabetes made this a daunting task. This meant including emerging advances in translational research, molecular biology, genomics, diagnostic tests, and therapies without sacrificing clinical presentations.

Our expert colleagues, to whom we as co-editors are eternally indebted and who are too numerous to mention individually, have devoted a considerable amount of time to ensuring the provision of the most relevant information in a very readable fashion. They accepted their assignments with grace and a willingness to participate, which made our task as editors so much easier. We are certain that the reader will enjoy this U.S. version of the *Oxford Handbook of Endocrinology and Diabetes* and apply this to their clinical practice.

We thank the authors of the original British edition, Helen E. Turner and John A.H. Wass. We also thank the editorial staff of the Oxford University Press for their professional assistance.

Boris Draznin and Sol Epstein

Contents

Contributors

Marc-Andre Cornier, MD
Associate Professor of Medicine
Division of Endocrinology,
  Metabolism and Diabetes
University of Colorado School of
  Medicine
Aurora, CO
Part: Miscellaneous
  Endocrinology

**Emily Gallagher, MB,
BCh, BAO**
Division of Endocrinology,
  Diabetes, and Bone Disease
Mount Sinai School of Medicine
New York, NY
Part: Neuroendocrine Disorders

Dina Green, MD
Assistant Professor of Medicine
Division of Endocrinology,
  Diabetes, and Bone Disease
Mount Sinai School of Medicine
New York, NY
Parts: Thyroid, Neuroendocrine
  Disorders, Lipids and
  Hyperlipidemia

Janice M. Kerr, MD
Assistant Professor
Division of Endocrinology,
  Metabolism and Diabetes
University of Colorado Denver/
  Anschutz Medical Campus
Aurora, CO
Part: Pituitary

Caroline Messer, MD
Division of Endocrinology,
  Diabetes, and Bone Disease
Mount Sinai School of Medicine
New York, NY
Part: Thyroid

Kristen Nadeau, MS, MD
Assistant Professor of Pediatrics
Division of Pediatric
  Endocrinology
University of Colorado School
  of Medicine
Aurora, CO
Part: Pediatric Endocrinology

Rachel Pessah, MD
Division of Endocrinology,
  Diabetes, and Bone Disease
Mount Sinai School of Medicine
New York, NY
Part: Thyroid

E. Chester Ridgway, MD
Professor of Medicine
Senior Associate Dean for
  Academic Affairs
Vice Chairman: Department
  of Medicine
University of Colorado School
  of Medicine
Aurora, CO
Part: Laboratory Endocrinology

Barrie Weinstein, MD
Division of Endocrinology,
  Diabetes, and Bone Disease
Mount Sinai School of Medicine
New York, NY
Part: Lipids and Hyperlipidemia

Margaret E. Wierman, MD
Chief of Endocrinology, Denver
  VAMC
Professor of Medicine, Physiology
  and Biophysics
University of Colorado School
  of Medicine
Aurora, CO
Part: Reproductive Endocrinology

Detailed contents

Part 1 Thyroid

Part 2 Pituitary

Part 4 Reproductive endocrinology

Part 5 Endocrine disorders of pregnancy

Part 7 Pediatric endocrinology

Part 8 Neuroendocrine disorders

Part 9 Inherited endocrine syndromes and multiple endocrine neoplasia (MEN)

Part 10 Miscellaneous endocrinology

Part 12 Lipids and hyperlipidemia

Part 13 Laboratory endocrinology

Symbols and abbreviations

↑	increased/ing
↓	decreased/ing
→	no change/normal
♂	male
♀	female
5-FU	5-fluorouracil
ACE	angiotensin-converting enzyme
ACTH	adrenocorticotropic hormone
AD	autosomal dominant
ADA	American Diabetes Association
ADH	antidiuretic hormone
ADHH	autosomal dominant hypocalcemic hypercalciuria
AF	atrial fibrillation
AGE	advanced glycation end-products
AHA	American Heart Association
AIH	amiodarone-induced hypothyroidism
AIT	amiodarone-induced thyrotoxicosis
AITD	autoimmune thyroid disease
ALP	alkaline phosphatase
ALT	alanine transaminase
AMH	anti-Müllerian hormone
ANCA	antineutrophil cytoplasmic antibody
ANP	atrial natriuretic peptide
APE	autoimmune polyglandular syndrome
APECED	autoimmune polyendocrinopthy, candidiasis and epidermal dystrophy
APS	autoimmune polyglandular syndrome
ART	assisted reproductive techniques
AST	aspartate transaminase
ATA	American Thyroid Association
ATD	antithyroid drug
ATP	Adult Treatment Panel
AVP	arginine vasopressin
bid	*bis die* (twice a day)
BMD	bone mineral density
BMI	body mass index
BNP	B-type natriuretic peptide

BP	blood pressure
CaE	calcium excretion
CAH	congenital adrenal hyperplasia
CBC	complete blood count
CBG	cortisol-binding globulin
CD	Cushing's disease
CHF	congestive heart failure
CHD	coronary heart disease
CK	creatinine kinase
CKD	chronic kidney disease
CMV	cytomegalovirus
CNS	central nervous system
CPA	cyproterone acetate
CPK	creatine phosphokinase
CRF	chronic renal failure
CRH	corticotropin-releasing hormone
CSF	cerebrospinal fluid
CSII	continuous subcutaneous insulin infusion
CST	cortrosyn stimulating test
CSW	cerebral salt wasting syndrome
CT	computed tomography
CTLA-4	cytotoxic T-lymphocyte antigen 4
CVD	cardiovascular disease
CVP	central venous pressure
DA	dopamine agonist
DCCT	Diabetes Control and Complications Trial
DDAVP	desamino-D-arginine vasopressin
DEX	dexamethasone
DHEA	dihydroepiandrosterone
DHEAS	DHEA sulfate
DHT	dihydrotestosterone
DI	diabetes insipidus
DIDMOAD	**d**iabetes **i**nsipidus, **DM**, **o**ptic **a**trophy + sensorineural **d**eafness (Wolfram's syndrome)
dL	deciliter
DM	diabetes mellitus
DOC	deoxycortisterone
DSD	disorders of sex development
DST	dexamethasone suppression test
DTC	differentiated thyroid carcinoma
DVT	deep vein thrombosis

DXA	dual energy X-ray absorptiometry
EBRT	external beam radiation therapy
ED	erectile dysfunction
EE2	ethinylestradiol
ENT	ear, nose, throat
ESR	erythrocyte sedimentation rate
ESRF	end-stage renal failure
ESS	empty sella syndrome
ETDRS	Early Treatment of Diabetic Retinopathy Study
FAI	free androgen index
FBC	full blood count
FCHL	familial combined hyperlipidemia
FDB	familial defective apolipoprotein B-100
FDG	[18F]fluorodeoxyglucose
FFM	fat free mass
FH	familial hypercholesterolemia
FHH	familial hypocalciuric hypercalcemia
FIHP	familial isolated hyperparathyroidism
FMTC	familial medullary thyroid carcinoma
FNAC	fine needle aspiration cytology
FSH	follicle stimulating hormone
FT_4	free T_4
FTC	follicular thyroid carcinoma
g	gram(s)
GAD	glutamic acid decarboxylase
GC	glucocorticoids
GCT	germ cell tumor
GFR	glomerular filtation rate
GH	growth hormone
GHBH	growth hormone–binding hormone
GHD	growth hormone deficiency
GHRH	growth hormone–releasing hormone
GI	gastrointestinal
GIFT	gamete intrafallopian transfer
GIP	gastric inhibitory peptide
GLP-1	glucogen-like polypeptide 1
GNRH	gonadotropin-releasing hormone
GRA	glucocorticoid remedial aldosteronism
GRTH	generalized resistance to thyroid hormone
h	hour(s)
HAART	highly active antiretroviral therapy

HC	hydrocortisone
hCG	human chorionic gonadotrophin
HDL	high-density lipoprotein
HERS	Heart and Estrogen-Progestin Replacement Study
5HIAA	5-hydroxyindole acetic acid
HLA	human leukocyte antigen
hMG	human menopausal gonadotropin
HMG CoA	3-hydroxy-3-methylglutaryl coenzyme A
HNF	hepatic nuclear factor
HP	hypothalamus–pituitary
HPA	hypothalmic–pituitary–adrenal (axis)
HPT-JP	hyperparathyroidism–jaw tumor syndrome
HPV	human papillomavirus
HRT	hormone replacement therapy
HSG	hysterosalpingography
HZV	herpes zoster virus
ICSI	intracytoplasmic sperm injection
ID	intradermal
IDDM	insulin-dependent diabetes mellitus (type 1)
IDL	intermediate-density lipoprotein
IFG	impaired fasting hyperglycemia
IGF-1	insulin-like growth factor 1
IGFPT	insulin-like growth factor binding protein
IGT	impaired glucose tolerance
IHD	ischemic heart disease
IHH	idiopathic hypogonadotrophic hypogonadism
IM	intramuscular
IPSS	inferior petrosal sinus sampling
IRMA	intraretinal microvascular abnormalities
ITT	insulin tolerance test
IU	international units
IUD	intrauterine device
IUGR	intrauterine growth retardation
IUI	intrauterine insemination
IV	intravenous
IVF	in vitro fertilization
KS	Kaposi sarcoma
L	liter(s)
LCAT	lecithin:cholesterol acyltransferase
LCCSCT	large-cell calcifying Sertoli cell tumor
LDL	low-density lipoprotein

LFT	liver function test
LH	luteinizing hormone
LHRH	luteinizing hormone–releasing hormone
MC	mineralocorticoid
mcg	microgram(s)
MEN	multiple endocrine neoplasia
MHC	major histocompatibility complex
MI	myocardial infarct
MIBG	123iodine-metaiodobenzylguanidine
MIS	Müllerian inhibitory substance
mL	milliliter(s)
MODY	maturity-onset diabetes of the young
MPH	mid-parental height
MRI	magnetic resonance imaging
MRSA	methicillin-resistant *Staphylococcus aureus*
MTC	medullary thyroid cancer
NASH	nonalcoholic steatohepatitis
NF	neurofibromatosis
NFA	nonfunctioning pituitary adenoma
NG	nasogastric
NGF	nerve growth factor
NICE	National Institute for Health and Clinical Excellence
NICH	non–islet cell hypoglycemia
NIDDM	non–insulin-dependent diabetes mellitus (type 2)
NOF	National Osteoporosis Foundation
NSAID	nonsteroidal anti-inflammatory drug
NVD	new vessels on the disc (diabetic retinopathy)
NVE	new vessels elsewhere (diabetic retinopathy)
OCP	oral contraceptive pill
od	*omni die* (once a day)
OGTT	oral glucose tolerance test
25OHD	25-hydroxy vitamin D
17OHP	17-hydroxyprogesterone
OHSS	ovarian hyperstimulation syndrome
PAI	platelet activator inhibitor
PCOS	polycystic ovary syndrome
PCT	postcoital test
PDE	phosphodiesterase
PET	positron emission spectrography
PHP	primary hyperparathyroidism

PI	protease inhibitor
PID	pelvic inflammatory disease
PIH	pregnancy-induced hypertension
PMC	papillary microcarcinoma of the thyroid
PNMT	phenylethanolamine-*N*-methyl transferase
PO	*per os* (by mouth)
POEMS	progressive polyneuropathy, organomegaly, endocrinopathy, monoclonal gammopathy, and skin changes
POF	premature ovarian failure
POI	premature ovary insufficiency
POMC	pro-opiomelanocortin
POP	progesterone-only pill
PP	pancreatic polypeptide
PRA	plasma renin activity
PRH	postprandial reactive hypoglycemia
PPI	proton pump inhibitor
PRL	prolactin
PRTH	pituitary resistance to thyroid hormones
PSA	prostatic-specific antigen
PTC	papillary thyroid carcinoma
PTH	parathyroid hormone
PTHrP	parathyroid hormone–related peptide
PTU	propylthiouracil
q	every (q2h: every 2 hours)
QoL	quality of life
RAI	radioactive iodine therapy
RCAD	renal cysts and diabetes
RCC	Rathke's cleft cyst
RFA	radiofrequency ablation
rhGH	recombinant human GH
rT_3	reverse T_3
RTH	thyroid hormone resistance
SC	subcutaneous
SCII	subcutaneous insulin infusion
SD	standard deviation
SERM	selective estrogen replacement modulator
SGA	small for gestational age
SHBG	sex hormone binding globulin
SLE	systemic lupus erythematosus
SRS	single-fraction radiosurgery

SSRI	selective serotonin reuptake inhibitor
T	testosterone
$t^{\frac{1}{2}}$	half-life
T_3	tri-iodothyronine
T_4	thyroxine
TB	tuberculosis
TBG	thyroxine-binding globulin; thyroid-binding globulin
TBI	traumatic brain injury
TBPA	T_4-binding prealbumin
TC	total cholesterol
TCA	tricyclic antidepressant
TFT	thyroid function test
Tg	thyroglobulin
TG	triglycerides
TGF	transforming growth factor
tid	three times a day
TNF	tumor necrosis factor
TPO	thyroid peroxidase
TPP	thyrotoxic periodic paralysis
TR	thyroid hormone receptor
TRH	thyrotropin-releasing hormone
TSAb	TSH-stimulating antibodies
TSH	thyroid-stimulating hormone
TSH-RAB	TSH receptor antibodies
TSS	transsphenoidal surgery
TTR	transthyretin
U&Es	urea and electolytes
UFC	urinary free cortisol
UKPDS	UK Prospective Diabetes Study
US	ultrasound
VEGF	vascular endothelial growth factor
VHL	von Hippel–Lindau disease
VIP	vasoactive intestinal peptide
VLDL	very high–density lipoprotein
VMA	vanillylmandelic acid
WBS	whole body scan
WHI	Women's Health Initiative
WHO	World Health Organization
XRT	radiotherapy
ZE	Zollinger Ellison syndrome

Part 1

Thyroid

Caroline Messer, Rachel Pessah, and Dina Green

Anatomy and physiology of the thyroid

Anatomy

The thyroid gland comprises
- A midline isthmus lying horizontally just below the cricoid cartilage.
- Two lateral lobes that extend upward over the lower half of the thyroid cartilage.

The gland lies deep to the strap muscles of the neck, enclosed in the pretracheal fascia, which anchors it to the trachea, so that the thyroid moves up on swallowing.

Histology
Fibrous septa divide the gland into pseudolobules. *Pseudolobules* are composed of vesicles called *follicles* or *acini*, surrounded by a capillary network. The follicle walls are lined by cuboidal epithelium.

The lumen is filled with a proteinaceous colloid, which contains the unique protein thyroglobulin. The peptide sequences of thyroxine (T_4) and tri-iodothyronine (T_3) are synthesized and stored as a component of thyroglobulin.

Development
The thyroid develops from the endoderm of the floor of the pharynx with some contribution from the lateral pharyngeal pouches. Descent of the midline thyroid anlage gives rise to the thyroglossal duct, which extends from the foramen caecum near the base of the tongue to the isthmus of the thyroid.

During development, the posterior aspect of the thyroid becomes associated with the parathyroid gland and the parafollicular C cells, derived from the ultimobranchial body, which become incorporated into its substance. The C cells are the source of calcitonin and give rise to medullary thyroid carcinoma when they undergo malignant transformation.

The fetal thyroid begins to concentrate and organify iodine at about 10–12 weeks gestation.

Maternal thyrotropin-releasing hormone (TRH) readily crosses the placenta; maternal thyroid-stimulating (TSH) and T_4 do not.

T_4 from the fetal thyroid is the major thyroid hormone available to the fetus. The fetal hypothalamic–pituitary–thyroid axis is a functional unit distinct from that of the mother—active at 18–20 weeks.

Thyroid examination

Inspection

- Look at the neck from the front. If a goiter (enlarged thyroid gland) is present, the patient should be asked to swallow a mouthful of water. The thyroid moves up with swallowing.
- Watch for appearance of any nodule not visible before swallowing; e.g., in an elderly patient with kyphosis, the thyroid may be partially retrosternal.

Palpation

- Is the thyroid gland tender to touch?
- With the index and middle fingers feel below the thyroid cartilage where the isthmus of the thyroid gland lies over the trachea.
- Palpate the two lobes of the thyroid, which extend laterally behind the sternocleidomastoid muscle.
- Ask the patient to swallow again while you continue to palpate the thyroid.
- Assess size: soft, firm, or hard? Assess *texture*: nodular or diffusely enlarged? Assess whether it *moves* readily on swallowing.
- Palpate along the medial edge of the sternocleidomastoid muscle on either side to look for a pyramidal lobe.
- Palpate for lymph nodes in the neck.

Percussion

- Percuss upper mediastinum for retrosternal goiter.

Auscultation

- Auscultate to identify bruits, consistent with Graves' disease.
- Occasionally, inspiratory stridor can be heard with a large or retrosternal goiter causing tracheal compression (📖 see Pemberton's sign, p. 45).

Assess thyroid status

- Observe for signs of thyroid disease—exophthalmos, proptosis, thyroid acropachy, pretibial myxedema, hyperactivity, restlessness, or immobility and disinterest.
- Take pulse; note the presence or absence of tachycardia, bradycardia, or atrial fibrillation.
- Feel palms—assess if they are warm and sweaty or cold.
- Look for tremor in outstretched hands.
- Examine eyes for exophthalmos (forward protrusion of the eyes—proptosis), lid retraction, sclera visible above cornea, lid lag, conjunctival injection or edema (cheimosis), periorbital edema, or loss of full-range movement.

Physiology

Thyroid hormone contains iodine. Iodine enters the thyroid in the form of inorganic or ionic iodide, which is organized by the thyroid peroxidase enzyme at the cell–colloid interface. Subsequent reactions result in the formation of iodothyronines.

The thyroid is the only source of T_4. The thyroid secretes 20% of circulating T_3; the remainder is generated in extraglandular tissues by the conversion of T_4 to T_3 by deiodinases (largely in the liver and kidneys).

Synthesis of the thyroid hormones can be inhibited by a variety of agents termed *goitrogens*.

- Perchlorate and thiocyanate inhibit iodide transport.
- Thioureas and mercaptoimidazole inhibit the initial oxidation of iodide and coupling of iodothyronines.
- In large doses, iodine blocks organic binding and coupling reactions.
- Lithium has several inhibitory effects on intrathyroidal iodine metabolism.

In the blood, T_4 and T_3 are almost entirely bound to plasma proteins. T_4 is bound in ↓ order of affinity to T_4-binding globulin (TBG), transthyretin (TTR), and albumin. T_3 is bound 10–20 times less avidly by TBG and not significantly by TTR.

Only the free or unbound hormone is available to tissues. The metabolic state correlates more closely with the free than the total hormone concentration in the plasma. The relatively weak binding of T_3 accounts for its more rapid onset and offset of action.

Table 1.1 summarizes states associated with primary alterations in the concentration of TBG. When there is primarily an alteration in the concentration of thyroid hormones, the concentration of TBG changes minimally (Table 1.2).

The concentration of free hormones does not necessarily vary directly with that of the total hormones; e.g., while the total T_4 level rises in pregnancy, the free T_4 (FT_4) level remains normal.

Table 1.1 Disordered thyroid hormone–protein interactions

	Serum total T_4 and T_3	Free T_4 and T_3
Primary abnormality in TBG		
↑ Concentration	↑	Normal
↓ Concentration	↓	Normal
Primary disorder of thyroid function		
Hyperthyroidism	↑	↑
Hypothyroidism	↓	↓

Table 1.2 Circumstances associated with altered concentration of TBG

↑ TBG	↓ TBG
Pregnancy	Androgens
Newborn state	Large doses of glucocorticoids; Cushing's syndrome
OCP and other sources of estrogens	Chronic liver disease
Tamoxifen	Severe systemic illness
Hepatitis A; chronic active hepatitis	Active acromegaly
Biliary cirrhosis	Nephrotic syndrome
Acute intermittent porphyria	Genetically determined
Genetically determined	Drugs, e.g., phenytoin

OCP, oral contraceptive pill.

The levels of thyroid hormone in the blood are tightly controlled by feedback mechanisms involved in the hypothalamic–pituitary–thyroid axis.

- TSH secreted by the pituitary stimulates the thyroid to secrete principally T_4 and also T_3. TRH stimulates the synthesis and secretion of TSH. T_4 and T_3 inhibit TSH synthesis and secretion directly.
- T_4 and T_3 are bound to TBG, TTR, and albumin. The remaining free hormones inhibit synthesis and release of TRH and TSH to influence growth and metabolism.
- T_4 is converted peripherally to the metabolically active T_3 or the inactive reverse T_3 (rT_3).
- T_4 and T_3 are metabolized in the liver by conjugation with glucuronate and sulfate. Enzyme inducers such as phenobarbital, carbamazepine, and phenytoin increase the metabolic clearance of the hormones without decreasing the proportion of free hormone in the blood.

Molecular action of thyroid hormone

T_3 is the active form of thyroid hormone. It binds to thyroid hormone receptors (TRs), of which there are several isoforms and which are members of the nuclear hormone receptor superfamily. TR/T_3 complexes elicit action by binding to response elements in the DNA of gene promoters.

Recruitment of co-activators alters the chromatin configuration, allowing gene transcription to proceed, whereas co-repressors cause the opposite effect.

Abnormalities of development

Remnants of the thyroglossal duct may be found in any position along the course of the tract of its descent:

- In the tongue, it is referred to as *lingual thyroid*.
- *Thyroglossal cysts* may be visible as midline swellings in the neck.

- *Thyroglossal fistula* develops as an opening in the middle of the neck.
- Thyroglossal nodules *or*
- The *pyramidal lobe*, a structure contiguous with the thyroid isthmus, which extends upward.

The gland can descend too far down to reach the anterior mediastinum.

Congenital hypothyroidism results from failure of the thyroid to develop (agenesis). More commonly, however, congenital hypothyroidism reflects enzyme defects impairing hormone synthesis.

Thyroid investigations

Tests of hormone concentration

Highly specific and sensitive chemiluminescent and radioimmunoassays are used to measure serum T_4 and T_3 concentrations. Free hormone concentrations usually correlate better with the metabolic state than do total hormone concentrations because they are unaffected by changes in binding protein concentration or affinity.

Tests of homeostatic control

See Table 2.1.

Serum TSH concentration is used as first line in the diagnosis of primary hypothyroidism and hyperthyroidism. The test is misleading in patients with secondary thyroid dysfunction reflecting hypothalamic or pituitary disease.

The TRH stimulation test, which can be used to assess the functional state of the TSH secretory mechanism, is now rarely used to diagnose primary thyroid disease, since it has been superseded by sensitive TSH assays. Its main use is in the differential diagnosis of elevated TSH in the setting of elevated thyroid hormone levels and in the differential diagnosis of resistance to thyroid hormone and a TSH-secreting pituitary adenoma (Table 2.3).

In interpreting results of thyroid function tests (TFTs), the effects of drugs that the patient might be on should be considered. Table 2.2 lists the influence of drugs on TFTs. Table 2.3 gives some examples of a typical TFT panel.

Box 2.1 Thyroid hormone resistance (RTH)

- This syndrome is characterized by reduced responsiveness to elevated circulating levels of free T_4 and free T_3, normal or elevated serum TSH, and intact TSH responsiveness to TRH. Clinical features apart from goiter are usually absent but may include short stature, hyperactivity disorders, and attention deficits with mental or learning disabilities.
- The etiology is a mutation in the thyroid hormone receptor.
- Differential diagnosis includes TSH-secreting pituitary tumor.
- Most cases require no treatment. If therapy is needed, β-adrenergic blockers may be used to ameliorate the tissue effects of raised thyroid hormone levels.

Table 2.1 Thyroid hormone concentrations in thyroid: various abnormalities

Condition	TSH	Free T$_4$	Free T$_3$
Primary hyperthyroidism	Undetectable	↑↑	↑
T$_3$ toxicosis	Undetectable	Normal	↑↑
Subclinical hyperthyroidism	↓	Normal	Normal
Secondary hyperthyroidism (TSHoma)	↑ or normal	↑	↑
Thyroid hormone resistance	↑ or normal	↑	↑
Primary hypothyroidism	↑	↓	↓ or normal
Subclinical hypothyroidism	↑	Normal	Normal
Secondary hypothyroidism	↓ or normal	↓	↓ or normal

Table 2.2 Influence of drugs on thyroid function tests

Metabolic process	↑	↓
TSH secretion	Amiodarone (transiently increases: normalizes after 2–3 months) Sertraline St John's wort	Glucocorticoids, dopamine agonists, phenytoin, dopamine
T$_4$ synthesis/release	Iodide	Iodide, lithium
Binding proteins	Estrogen, clofibrate, heroin	Glucocorticoids, androgens, phenytoin, carbamazepine
T$_4$ metabolism	Anticonvulsants; rifampin	
Inhibition of T$_4$ binding to TBG (TSH normal)		Salicylates, furosemide, mefenamic acid

Table 2.3 Atypical thyroid function tests

Test	Possible cause
Suppressed TSH and elevated free T_3, normal free T_4	T_3 toxicosis (approximately 5% of thyrotoxicosis)
Suppressed TSH and normal free T_4 and free T_3	Subclinical thyrotoxicosis Recovery from thyrotoxicosis Excess thyroxine replacement Sick euthyroidism
Detectable TSH and elevated free T_4 and free T_3	TSH-secreting pituitary tumor Thyroid hormone resistance Heterophile antibodies leading to spurious measurements of free T_4 and free T_3
Elevated free T_4 and low–normal free T_3, normal TSH	Amiodarone

Antibody screen

High titers of antithyroid peroxidase (anti-TPO) antibodies or antithyroglobulin antibodies are found in patients with autoimmune thyroid disease (Hashimoto's thyroiditis, Graves' disease, and, sometimes, euthyroid individuals). 📖 See Table 2.4.

The American Thyroid Association recommends that adults be screened for thyroid dysfunction with serum TSH measurement, beginning at age 35 years and every 5 years thereafter.[1]

Screening for thyroid disease[2]

The following categories of patients are at risk for thyroid disease and screening should be considered:

- Patients with atrial fibrillation or hyperlipidemia
- Periodic (within every 6 months) assessment in patients receiving medications such as amiodarone hydrochloride and lithium carbonate.
- Annual check of thyroid function in annual review of diabetic patients
- Women with type 1 diabetes in the first trimester of pregnancy and post-delivery (3-fold increase in incidence of postpartum thyroid dysfunction in such patients)
- Women with a past history of postpartum thyroiditis
- Previous thyroid dysfunction or goiter
- History of surgery or radiotherapy affecting the thyroid gland
- Vitiligo
- Pernicious anemia
- Consider annual check of thyroid function in people with Down syndrome, Turner syndrome, and primary adrenal insufficiency (Addison's disease) in light of the high prevalence of hypothyroidism in such patients.
- Women with thyroid autoantibodies have 8× risk of developing hypothyroidism over 20 years compared to antibody-negative controls
- Women with thyroid autoantibodies and isolated elevated TSH have 38× risk of developing hypothyroidism, with 4% annual risk of overt hypothyroidism.

Table 2.4 Antithyroid antibodies and thyroid disease

Condition	Anti-TPO	Antithyroglobulin	TSH receptor antibody
Graves' disease	70–80%	30–50%	70–100% (stimulating)
Autoimmune hypothyroidism	95%	60%	10–20% (blocking)

Note: TSH receptor antibodies may be stimulatory or inhibitory. Heterophile antibodies present in patient sera may cause abnormal interference, causing abnormally low or high values of free T_4 and free T_3, and can be removed with absorption tubes.

1 Ladenson PW, et al. (2000). American Thyroid Association Guidelines for detection of thyroid dysfunction. *Arch Intern Med* 160:1573–1575.
2 Tunbridge WM, Vanderpump MP (2000). Population screening for autoimmune thyroid disease. *Endocrinol Metab Clin North Am* 29(2):239–253.

Scintiscanning

This scanning enables localization of sites of accumulation of radioiodine or sodium pertechnetate [$_{99m}$Tc], which gives information about the activity of the iodine trap (Table 2.5). This can be used

- To define areas of hyper- or hypofunction within the thyroid (Table 2.6). It can be useful to differentiate among causes of thyrotoxicosis (i.e., Graves' disease vs. toxic nodular goiter vs. thyroiditis).
- Provide information about the size and shape of the thyroid gland (detect retrosternal goiter; ectopic thyroid tissue).

The scan may be altered by

- Agents that influence thyroid uptake: high-iodine foods and supplements, such as kelp (seaweed)
- Drugs containing iodine, such as amiodarone
- Recent use of radiographic contrast dyes, which can potentially interfere with the interpretation of the scan

Table 2.5 Radioisotope scans

	^{123} Iodine	^{99} Technitium pertechnetate
Half-life	Short	Short
Advantage	Low emission of radiation. Has higher energy photons, hence useful for imaging a toxic goiter with a substernal component	Maximum thyroid uptake within 30 min of administration. Can be used in breast-feeding women (discontinue feeding for 24 hours)
Disadvantage		Technetium is only trapped by the thyroid without being organified.
Use	Functional assessment of the thyroid	Rapid scanning

Table 2.6 Radionuclide scanning (scintigram) in thyroid disease

Condition	Scan appearance
Graves' hyperthyroidism	Enlarged gland Intense and homogeneous radionucleotide uptake
Thyroiditis (e.g., de Quervain syndrome)	Low or absent uptake
Toxic nodule	A solitary area of high uptake with suppression of extranodular tissue
Thyrotoxicosis factitia	Depressed thyroid uptake
Thyroid cancer	Successful ^{131}I uptake by tumor tissue requires an adequate level of TSH, achieved by stopping T_3 replacement 10 days before scanning, withholding levothyroxine until TSH is >30 uU/mL, or giving recombinant TSH injection.

Ultrasound (US) scanning

Ultrasound provides an accurate indication of thyroid size and is useful for differentiating cystic nodules from solid ones, but it cannot be used to distinguish between benign and malignant disease definitively. Please see the Revised American Thyroid Association Management Guidelines for Patients with Thyroid Nodules and Differentiated Thyroid Cancer (2009) for further details.

Diagnostic features

- Microcalcification within nodules favors the diagnosis of malignancy; microcalcifications <2 mm in diameter are observed in ~60% of malignant nodules, but in <2% of benign lesions.
- Calcification is a prominent feature of medullary carcinoma of the thyroid.
- US can detect whether a nodule is solitary or part of a multinodular process.
- Irregular nodule capsule is more common in malignancy.

Uses

- Sequential scanning can be employed to assess changes in size of thyroid over time.
- Assess neck lymph nodes in thyroid cancer patients

Note: Neither scintigraphy nor US is routinely indicated in a patient with goiter.

Fine needle aspiration (FNAC) cytology

FNAC is now considered the most accurate test for diagnosis of thyroid nodules. It is performed in an outpatient setting.

One to two aspirations are drawn with a 23- to 27-gauge needle, inserted into different sites of each nodule; aspiration is carried out at different sites for each nodule. Cytological findings are *satisfactory* or *diagnostic* in approximately 85% of specimens and *nondiagnostic* in the remainder.

In experienced hands, FNAC is an excellent diagnostic technique, as shown in Table 2.7.

Repeat FNAC after 3–6 months further reduces the proportion of false negatives. FNAC cannot be used to differentiate between benign and malignant follicular neoplasm.

Surgical excision of a follicular neoplasm is always indicated.

📖 See Table 2.8 for diagnostic categories from FNAC.

Table 2.7 Diagnostic features of FNAC

Feature	Range (%)	Mean value (%)
Accuracy	85–100	95
Specificity	72–100	92
Sensitivity	65–98	83
False negative	1–11	5

Table 2.8 Diagnostic categories for FNA

1.	Nondiagnostic
2.	Malignant
3.	Indeterminate/Suspicious for neoplasm
4.	Benign

Taken from American Thyroid Association Management Guidelines for Patients with Thyroid Nodules in Differentiation Thyroid Cancer

Computed tomography (CT)

CT is useful in evaluation of retrosternal and retrotracheal extension of an enlarged thyroid.

Compression of the trachea and displacement of the major vessels can be identified with CT of the superior mediastinum.

CT can demonstrate the extent of intrathoracic extension of thyroid malignancy and infiltration of adjacent structures, such as the carotid artery, internal jugular vein, trachea, esophagus, and regional lymph nodes.

Use of CT imaging with iodine-containing radiocontrast dye interferes with further radioiodine imaging and treatment for at least 6 weeks. Urinary iodine testing can be useful to help determine when further radioiodine imaging and treatment can be performed.

Additional laboratory investigations

Hematological tests

Long-standing thyrotoxicosis may be associated with a *normochromic anemia* and, occasionally, *mild neutropenia, lymphocytosis*, and, rarely, *thrombocytopenia*.

In hypothyroidism, a macrocytosis is typical, although concurrent vitamin B_{12} deficiency should be considered.

There may also be a *microcytic anemia* due to menorrhagia and impaired iron utilization.

Biochemical tests

Alkaline phosphatase may be elevated in thyrotoxicosis.

Mild *hypercalcemia* may occur in thyrotoxicosis and reflects ↑ bone resorption. *Hypercalciuria* is more common.

In a hypothyroid patient, *hyponatremia* may be due to an inability to suppress antidiuretic hormone (ADH) and/or reduced renal tubular water loss, resulting in retention of ingested water. Less commonly, it may be due to coexisting cortisol deficiency.

In hypothyroidism, *creatine kinase* is often raised and the lipid profile altered with ↑ low-density lipoprotein (LDL) cholesterol.

Endocrine tests

In untreated hypothyroidism, there may be inadequate responses to provocative testing of the hypothalamic–pituitary–adrenal (HPA) axis. In hypothyroidism, serum prolactin may be elevated as a result of ↑ TRH.

In thyrotoxicosis there is an increase in *sex hormone binding globulin* (SHBG) and a complex interaction with sex steroid hormone metabolism, resulting in changes in the levels of androgens and estrogens. The net physiological result is an increase in estrogenic activity, with gynecomastia and a decrease in libido and erectile dysfunction in males.

Sick euthyroid syndrome (non-thyroidal illness syndrome)

- Biochemistry:
  - Low T_4 and T_3
  - Inappropriately normal/suppressed TSH
- Tissue thyroid hormone concentrations are very low.
- Clinical context—starvation
  - Severe illness, e.g., severe infections, renal failure, cardiac failure, liver failure, end-stage malignancy
- Thyroxine replacement is not indicated because there is no clear evidence that treatment is effective.

Atypical clinical situations

- Thyrotoxicosis factitia
  - No thyroid enlargement
  - Elevated free T$_4$ and suppressed TSH
  - Depressed thyroid uptake on scintigraphy
  - Low thyroglobulin differentiates from thyroiditis (which shows depressed uptake on scintigraphy but ↑ thyroglobulin) and all other causes of elevated thyroid hormones.
- *Struma ovarii* (ovarian teratoma containing hyperfunctioning thyroid tissue)
  - No thyroid enlargement
  - Depressed thyroid uptake on scintigraphy
  - A body scan after radioiodine confirms diagnosis.
- *Trophoblast tumors:* human chorionic gonadotropin (hCG) has structural homology with TSH and leads to thyroid gland stimulation, and usually mild thyrotoxicosis.
- *Hyperemesis gravidarum:* Thyroid function tests may be abnormal with a suppressed TSH (📖 see Chapter 3, p. 31, and Chapter 62, p. 348).
- *Choriocarcinoma of the testes* may be associated with gynecomastia and thyrotoxicosis—measure hCG.

Thyrotoxicosis

Etiology

Epidemiology

Graves' autoimmune thyroid disease is 5× more common in women than in men. Annual incidence is 0.5 cases per 1000.

Definition of thyrotoxicosis and hyperthyroidism

The term *thyrotoxicosis* denotes the clinical, physiological, and biochemical findings that result when the tissues are exposed to excess thyroid hormone. It can arise in a variety of ways (Table 3.1). It is essential to establish a specific diagnosis as this determines therapy choices and provides important information for the patient regarding prognosis.

The term *hyperthyroidism* should be used to denote conditions in which hyperfunction of the thyroid leads to thyrotoxicosis.

Genetics of autoimmune thyroid disease (AITD)

AITD consists of Graves' disease, Hashimoto's thyroiditis, atrophic autoimmune hypothyroidism, postpartum thyroiditis, and thyroid-associated ophthalmopathy—conditions that appear to share a common genetic predisposition. There is a female preponderance.

Twin studies show a concordance for Graves' disease and autoimmune hypothyroidism in monozygotic compared to dizygotic twins.

It is estimated that genetic factors account for 79% of the susceptibility for Graves' disease. Sibling studies indicate that sisters and children of women with Graves' disease have a 5–8% risk of developing Graves' disease or autoimmune hypothyroidism.

On the background of a genetic predisposition, environmental factors are thought to contribute to the development of disease. A number of interacting susceptibility genes are thought to play a role in the development of disease.

Cytotoxic T-lymphocyte antigen 4 (CTLA-4) is associated with Graves' disease in Caucasian populations. Specifically, the CT60 allele has a prevalence of 60% in the general population, but is also the allele most highly associated with Graves' disease, indicating the complex nature of genetic susceptibility and interplay of environmental factors.

Association of major histocompatibility complex (MHC) loci with Graves' disease has been demonstrated in some populations, but not others. HLA-DR3 is associated with Graves' disease in whites. HLA-DQA1*0501 is associated in some populations, especially for men. However, the overall contribution of MHC genes to Graves' disease has been estimated to be only 10–20% of the inherited susceptibility.

Table 3.1 Classification of the etiologies of thyrotoxicosis

Associated with hyperthyroidism	
Excessive thyroid stimulation	Graves' disease, Hashitoxicosis
	Pituitary thyrotrope adenoma
	Pituitary thyroid hormone resistance syndrome (excess TSH)
	Trophoblastic tumors producing hCG with thyrotrophic activity
Thyroid nodules with autonomous function	Toxic solitary nodule, toxic multinodular goiter
	Thyroid cancer (rare occurrence)

Not associated with hyperthyroidism	
Thyroid inflammation	Silent and postpartum thyroiditis, subacute (de Quervain's) thyroiditis
	Drug-induced thyroiditis (amiodarone)
Exogenous thyroid hormones	Overtreatment with thyroid hormone
	Thyrotoxicosis factitia (thyroxine use in nonthyroidal disease)
Ectopic thyroid tissue	Metastatic thyroid carcinoma Struma ovarii, teratoma containing functional thyroid tissue, results in mild features of thyrotoxicosis (mildly elevated serum free T_4 and T_3; suppressed TSH)

Manifestations of hyperthyroidism

Investigation of thyrotoxicosis

- Thyroid function tests reveal elevated FT_4 and suppressed TSH (elevated free T_3 [FT_3] in T_3 toxicosis).
- Thyroid antibodies—📖 see Table 2.4 (p. 10)
- Radionucleotide thyroid scan if necessary to confirm Graves ' hyperthyroidism and exclude other causes (i.e., painless thyroiditis) (📖 see p. 169)

Manifestations of Graves' disease (in addition to those in Box 3.1)

- Diffuse goiter
- Ophthalmopathy (📖 see Graves' ophthalmopathy, p. 39)
  - A feeling of grittiness and discomfort in the eye
  - Retrobulbar pressure or pain, eyelid lag or retraction
  - Periorbital edema, chemosis,* scleral injection*
  - Exophthalmos (proptosis)*
  - Extraocular muscle dysfunction*
  - Exposure keratitis*
  - Optic neuropathy*

Box 3.1 Manifestations of hyperthyroidism (all forms)

Symptoms
- Hyperactivity, irritability, altered mood, insomnia
- Heat intolerance, sweating
- Palpitations
- Fatigue, weakness
- Dyspnea
- Weight loss with increased appetite (weight gain in 10% of patients)
- Pruritus
- Increased stool frequency
- Thirst and polyuria
- Oligomenorrhea or amenorrhea; loss of libido

Signs
- Sinus tachycardia, atrial fibrillation
- Fine tremor, hyperkinesia, hyperreflexia
- Warm, moist skin
- Palmar erythema, onycholysis
- Hair loss
- Muscle weakness and wasting
- Congestive (high-output) heart failure, chorea, periodic paralysis (primarily in Asian males), psychosis (rare)

---

* A combination of these suggests congestive ophthalmopathy. Urgent action is necessary if there is corneal ulceration, congestive ophthalmopathy, or optic neuropathy (📖 see Graves' ophthalmopathy, p. 39).

- Localized dermopathy (pretibial myxedema, 📖 see Graves' dermopathy, p. 43)
- Lymphoid hyperplasia
- Thyroid acropachy (📖 see Thyroid acropachy, p. 43)

Conditions associated with Graves' disease
- Type 1 diabetes mellitus
- Addison's disease
- Vitiligo
- Pernicious anemia
- Alopecia areata
- Myasthenia gravis
- Celiac disease (4.5%)
- Other autoimmune disorders associated with the HLA-DR3 haplotype

Treatment

Medical treatment

In general, the standard policy in Europe is to offer a course of antithyroid drugs (ATD) first. In the United States, radioiodine is more likely to be offered as first-line treatment. See the American Thyroid Association (ATA) Treatment Guidelines for Patients with Hyperthyroidism and Hypothyroidism (1995) for further details.

Aims and principles of medical treatment

- To induce remission in Graves' disease
- Monitor for relapse off treatment initially every 6–8 weeks for 6 months, then every 6 months for 2 years, and then annually thereafter or sooner if symptoms return.
- For patients who relapse, consider definitive treatment such as radioiodine or surgery. A second course of ATD rarely results in remission.

Choice of drugs—thionamides

Methimazole has a longer duration of action and can be given as a single dose. Carbimazole, the drug of choice in the UK, is converted to methimazole by cleavage of a carboxyl side chain on first liver passage. Methimazole and propylthiouracil are used widely in the United States and elsewhere in the world. Propylthiouracil is limited by tid dosing.

During pregnancy and lactation *propylthiouracil* (PTU) is the drug of choice given the association between PTU and fatal hepatotoxicity, PTU may be the drug of choice during the first trimester, however this remains an area of controversy. Methimazole is often recommended for second and third trimester although does have associated risks, such as aplasia cutis.

Action of thionamides

Thyroid hormone synthesis is inhibited by blockade of the action of thyroid peroxidase. Thionomides are especially actively accumulated in thyrotoxic tissue.

Propylthiouracil also inhibits extrathyroidal conversion of T_4 to T_3 by type 1 deiodinase, and thus may have advantages when given at high doses in severe thyrotoxicosis.

Dose and effectiveness

A does of 5 mg of carbimazole is roughly equivalent to 50 mg of propylthiouracil. Carbimazole dosing is ~40% higher than methimazole. Propylthiouracil has a theoretical advantage of inhibiting the conversion of T_4 to T_3, and T_3 levels decline more rapidly after starting the drug.

According to the ATA, initial daily doses of methimazole range from 10–40 mg daily and for PTU 100–600 mg daily.

Most ATDs as primary therapy are given for 6 months to 2 years, as there is no established standard for duration of therapy with ATDs.

From 30 to 40% of patients treated with an ATD remain euthyroid 10 years after discontinuation of therapy. If hyperthyroidism recurs after treatment with an ATD, there is little chance that a second course of treatment will result in permanent remission. Young patients, smokers, and those with large goiters, ophthalmopathy, or high serum concentrations of thyrotropin receptor antibody at the time of diagnosis are unlikely to have a permanent remission.

β-Adrenergic antagonists

Propranolol 10–40 mg up to four times daily or longer-acting β-blockers can be used to control symptoms such as anxiety, tremor, and palpitations. Relief may be appreciated in the initial 4–8 weeks of treatment.

Atrial fibrillation (AF)

AF should convert to sinus rhythm—otherwise, cardiovert after 4 months euthyroid.

Side effects

ATDs are generally well tolerated. Uncommonly, patients may complain of gastrointestinal (GI) symptoms or changes in sense of taste and smell.

Agranulocytosis represents a potentially fatal but rare side effect of ATD occurring in 0.1–0.5% of patients. Because cross-reactivity between ATDs has been reported, and may be idiosyncratic and dose dependent, it is not recommended to switch from one ATD if agranulocytosis has developed to another. It is controversial whether agranulocytosis is more frequent with methimazole or propylthiouracil.

Agranulocytosis usually occurs within the first 3 months after initiation of therapy (97% within the first 6 months, especially on higher doses). Although rare, it is important to be aware of the documented cases, which have occurred a long time after starting treatment.

As agranulocytosis occurs very suddenly and is potentially fatal, routine monitoring of complete blood count (CBC) is thought to be of little use. Patients typically present with fever and evidence of infection, usually in the oropharynx, and each patient should therefore receive *written instructions to discontinue antithyroid drug therapy and contact their doctor for a CBC should a severe sore throat and fever arise.*

Neutrophil dyscrasias occur more frequently in males; however these are more often fatal in the elderly.

Allergic-type reactions are more common in the form of rash, urticaria, and arthralgia, which occur in 1–5% of patients taking these drugs. These side effects are often mild and do not usually necessitate drug withdrawal, although one ATD may be substituted for another in the expectation that the second agent may be taken without side effects.

Thionamides may cause cholestatic jaundice; elevated serum aminotransferases and fulminant hepatic failure have also been reported. However, hepatic necrosis due to PTU and cholestatic jaundice due to methimazole is rare enough that routine liver function tests monitoring is unnecessary, according to the American Thyroid Association.[1]

All patients should be given written and verbal warnings about the potential side effects of thionamides.

Rarely, antineutrophil cytoplasmic antibody (ANCA)-positive vasculitis develops with propylthiouracil therapy, manifesting as arthralgias,

---

1 Singer PA, Cooper DS, Levy EG, et al. (1995). Treatment guidelines for patients with hyperthyroidism and hypothyroidism. *JAMA* 273:808–812.

skin lesions, glomerulonephritis, fever, and/or alveolar hemorrhage. Skin lesions include ulcers. Biopsy reveals vasculitis. Treatment is discontinuation of propylthiouracil and initiation of steroids if needed.

Treatment regimen

Two alternative regimens are practiced for Graves' disease: dose titration and block and replace.

Dose titration regime

The primary aim is to achieve a euthyroid state with relatively high drug doses and then to maintain euthyroidism with a low stable dose.

The dose of methimazole or propylthiouracil is titrated according to the thyroid function tests performed every 4–8 weeks, aiming for a serum free T_4 in the normal range and a detectable TSH. High serum TSH indicates the need for a dose reduction. TSH may remain suppressed for weeks or months.

The typical starting dose of methimazole is 10–20 mg/day. Higher initial doses (40 mg) may be indicated in severe hyperthyroidism.

When the plasma FT_4 level returns to normal, the dose should be adjusted to maintain normal FT_4 levels. No consensus exists on the optimal duration of therapy, although 12 months to 24 months is most common.

Relapses are most likely to occur within the first year and may be more likely in the presence of a large goiter and high T_4 level at the time of diagnosis, or the presence of TSH-receptor antibodies at the end of treatment (see p. 33.)

Patients with multinodular goiters and thyrotoxicosis frequently relapse on cessation of antithyroid medication, and definitive treatment with radioiodine or surgery is usually advised. Long-term low-dose thionamide therapy is also an option.

Block and replace regimen

After achieving an euthyroid state on methimazole or PTU alone, T_4 at a dose of 100 mcg can be prescribed. The patient can be continued on the combination of antithyroid drug and T_4 for an additional 12–24 months. If the size of the gland returns to normal or the former time period is reached, the drugs are discontinued. The main advantages of this regimen are fewer hospital visits for checks of thyroid function and shorter duration of treatment.

Most patients achieve an euthyroid state within 4–6 weeks of carbimazole therapy.

During treatment, FT_4 values are measured 4 weeks after starting thyroxine and the dose of thyroxine is altered, if necessary, in 25 mcg increments to maintain FT_4 in the normal range. Most patients do not require any dose adjustment.

The originally reported higher remission rate was not confirmed in a large, prospective, multicenter European trial when combination treatment was compared to carbimazole alone, but side effects were more common.[2]

Relapses are most likely to occur within the first year.

2 Reinwein D, Benker G, Lazarus JH, et al. (1993). A prospective randomized trial of antithyroid drug dose in Graves' disease therapy. European Multicenter Study Group on Antithyroid Drug Treatment. *J Clin Endocrinol Metab* 76:1516–1521.

Table 3.2 Recommended activity of radioiodine

Etiology	Comments	Guide dose (MBq)
Graves' disease	• First presentation; no significant eye disease • Moderate goiter (40–50 g)	8–16 mCi (400–600 MBq)
Toxic multinodular goiter in older person	Mild heart failure; atrial fibrillation or other concomitant disease, e.g., cancer	13.5–21.6 mCi (500–800 MBq)
Toxic adenoma	Usually mild hyperthyroidism	13.5 mCi (500 MBq)
Severe Graves' disease with thyroid eye disease	• Postpone radioiodine until eye disease is stable. • Prednisone 40 mg daily to be administered at same time as radioiodine and for further 4–6 weeks (see below)	13.5–21.6 mCi (500–800 MBq)
Ablation therapy	• Severe accompanying medical condition such as heart failure, atrial fibrillation, or other concurrent medical disorders (e.g., psy-chosis)	13.5–21.6 mCi (500–800 MBq)

Reprinted with permission from Weetman AP (2007), Radioiodine treatment for benign thyroid diseases. *Clin Endocrinol* 66(6):757–764.

Radioiodine treatment—radioiodine therapy
📖 See Table 3.2.

Indications
• Definitive treatment of multinodular goiter or adenoma
• Relapsed Graves' disease

Contraindications
• Young children, because of the potential risk of thyroid carcinogenesis
• Pregnant and lactating women
• Situations where it is clear that the safety of other people cannot be guaranteed

Graves' ophthalmopathy
There is some evidence that Graves' ophthalmopathy may worsen after the administration of radioactive iodine, especially in smokers. In cases of moderate to severe ophthalmopathy, radioiodine may be avoided.

Alternatively, steroid cover in a dose of 40 mg prednisone daily should be given on the day of administering radioiodine, with taper over the next 1–2 months following radioiodine treatment. It is essential that euthyroidism be closely maintained following radioiodine to avoid worsening of ophthalmopathy.

Caveats

- The control of disease may not occur for a period of weeks or a few months.
- More than one treatment may be needed in some patients, depending on the dose given; 15% require a second dose and a few patients require a third dose. The second dose should only be considered at least 6 months after the first dose.
- Compounds that contain iodine, such as amiodarone, block iodine uptake for a period of several months following cessation of therapy. Iodine uptake measurements may be helpful in this instance in determining the activity required and the timing of radioiodine therapy.
- Women of childbearing age should avoid pregnancy for a minimum of 6 months following radioactive iodine ablation.
- The prevalence of hypothyroidism is about 50% at 10 years and continues to increase thereafter.

Side effects are rare

- Anterior neck pain caused by radiation-induced thyroiditis
- Transient rise (72 hours) in plasma T_4 may occur within the first 2 weeks after therapy, which may exacerbate heart failure if present.

Hypothyroidism after radioiodine

After radioiodine administration, ATDs may be restarted. The ATDs should be withdrawn gradually, guided by TFTs every 6–8 weeks. Early post-radioiodine hypothyroidism may be transient. TSH should be monitored initially, then annually after radioiodine therapy to determine late-onset hypothyroidism.

In patients treated for autonomous toxic nodules, the incidence of hypothyroidism is lower since the toxic nodule takes up the radioactive iodine; the surrounding tissue will recover normal function once the hyperthyroidism is controlled, though this is disputed by some experts.

Cancer risk after radioiodine therapy

In a recent large series, no overall excess risk of cancer was found. It is unclear whether the risk of death from thyroid cancer is slightly higher.

Clinical guidelines

The goal is to administer enough radioiodine to achieve euthyroidism with the acceptance of a moderate rate of hypothyroidism, e.g., 15–20% at 2 years.

Instructions to patients before treatment

Discontinue ATDs 2–7 days before radioiodine administration, since their effects last for 24 hours or more, though PTU has a prolonged radioprotective effect. ATDs may be restarted 3–7 days after radioiodine administration without significantly affecting the delivered radiation dose.

Administration of radioiodine (Table 3.2)

- Radioactive iodine-131 is administered orally as a capsule or a drink.
- No universal agreement exists regarding optimal dose. Dosing according to size alone is not successful in 90% of cases.

- A dose of 10–21.6 mCi (400–800 MBq) should be sufficient to cure hyperthyroidism in 90%.
- Most patients are treated with 10–16 mCi (400–600 MBq) as the first dose.
- It is contraindicated in women who are pregnant and/or breast-feeding.
- For precaution, 📖 see Table 3.3.

Outcomes of radioiodine treatment
In general, 50–70% of patients have restored normal thyroid function within 6–8 weeks of receiving radioiodine. Shrinkage of goiter occurs but is slower.

Surgery

Thyroidectomy is rarely recommended for patients with Graves' disease. Indications for subtotal or total thyroidectomy include patients with very large, multinodular goiters causing obstruction of the airway, or those who cannot tolerate or are noncompliant with antithyroid drugs. Pregnant women with severe Graves' disease allergic to antithyroid therapy may be advised to undergo surgery.

There is disagreement regarding which operation to perform. Often patients require LT4 following thyroidectomy. See Box 3.2.

Indications
- Documented suspicious or malignant thyroid nodule by FNAC
- Pregnant mothers who are not adequately controlled by ATDs or in whom serious allergic reactions develop while being treated medically. Thyroidectomy is usually performed in the second trimester.

Thyroidectomy is also indicated in the following patients:
- Those who reject or fear exposure to radiation
- Those with poor compliance to medical treatment
- Those in whom a rapid control of symptoms is desired

Box 3.2 **Complications of thyroidectomy**

Immediate
- Recurrent laryngeal nerve damage
- Hypoparathyroidism
- Thyroid crisis
- Local hemorrhage, causing laryngeal edema
- Wound infection

Late
- Hypothyroidism
- Keloid formation

---

1 Royal College of Physicians of London Working Group (2007). Radioiodine in the management of benign thyroid disease. London: Royal College of Physicians of London[JH2].

- Those with severe manifestations of Graves' ophthalmopathy, since total and subtotal thyroidectomy does not worsen eye manifestations
- Those with relapsed Graves' disease
- Those with local compressive symptoms that may not improve rapidly with radioiodine. Operation removes these symptoms in most patients.
- Those with large thyroid glands and relatively low radioiodine uptake

Preparation of patients for surgery

ATDs should be used preoperatively to achieve euthyroidism (approximately 6 weeks).

β-blockers can be added as preparation for surgery, especially in those patients where surgery must be performed sooner than achieving euthyroid state.

Potassium iodide, 5 drops twice daily, can be used during the preoperative period (for 7–10 days) to reduce the vascularity of the gland. Operating later than this can be associated with exacerbation of thyrotoxicosis as the thyroid escapes from the inhibitory effect of the iodide. In practice, it is rarely needed, as good control of thyrotoxicosis can be achieved with ATDs in the majority of patients.

In patients who are noncompliant with ATDs and thyrotoxic prior to surgery, hospital inpatient admission may be necessary for supervised administration of high-dose ATDs, together with β-blockade, and measurement of FT_4 and FT_3 twice weekly. There is a risk of thyroid crisis, or storm, if a patient undergoes operation when thyrotoxic.

Most patients can be rendered euthyroid within 2–4 weeks and potassium iodide can be administered as above to coincide with the timing of surgery.

Additional measures are as for thyroid storm.

Thyroid crisis (storm)

Thyroid crisis represents a rare but life-threatening exacerbation of the manifestations of thyrotoxicosis. It should be promptly recognized since the condition is associated with a significant mortality; see Box 3.3. Thyroid crisis develops in uncontrolled hyperthyroid patients who

- Have a complicating acute infection.
- Undergo thyroidal or non-thyroidal surgery or (rarely) radioiodine treatment.

Thyroid crisis should be considered in a very sick patient if there is

- Recent history suggestive of thyrotoxicosis.
- Acute stressful precipitating factor such as surgery.
- History of previous thyroid treatment.

Laboratory investigations

- Routine hematology may indicate a leukocytosis, which is well recognized in thyrotoxicosis even in the absence of infection.
- The biochemical screen may reveal a raised alkaline phosphatase and mild hypercalcaemia.
- Thyroid function tests and thyroid antibodies should be requested, although treatment should not be delayed while awaiting the results.
- Thyroid hormone levels will be raised but may not be grossly elevated and are usually within the range of uncomplicated thyrotoxicosis.

Treatment

General supportive therapy

The patient is best managed in an intensive care unit where close attention can be paid to cardiorespiratory status, fluid balance, and cooling.

Standard antiarrhythmic drugs may need to be used, including digoxin (usually in higher than normal dose) after correction for hypokalemia.

Broad-spectrum antibiotics should be given if infection is suspected.

Specific treatment

The aim is to inhibit thyroid hormone synthesis completely.

- Antithyroid drugs in large doses (propylthiouracil or methimazole) i.e., PTU 200–300 mg every 6 hours via nasogastric (NG) tube if necessary. Propylthiouracil is preferred because of its ability to block T_4-to-T_3 conversion in peripheral tissues. Alternatively, methimaole 60 mg every 24 hours can be given. ATDs should be started first and quickly.

Box 3.3 Clinical signs suggestive of a thyroid storm

- Alteration in mental status
- High fever
- Tachycardia or tachyarrhythmias
- Severe clinical signs of hyperthyroidism
- Vomiting, jaundice, and diarrhea
- Multisystem decompensation: cardiac failure, respiratory distress, congestive hepatomegaly, dehydration, and renal failure

- Potassium iodide 10 drops, twice daily, *after* starting antithyroid drugs, will inhibit thyroid hormone release.
- β-Adrenergic blocking agents are essential in management to control tachycardia, tremor, and other adrenergic manifestations.
  - Propranolol 160–480 mg/day in divided doses or as an infusion at a rate of 2–5 mg/h.
- Calcium channel blockers can be tried in patients with known bronchospastic disease or severe heart failure when β-blockade is contraindicated.
- High doses of glucocorticoids are capable of blocking T_4-to-T_3 conversion: prednisone 60 mg daily or hydrocortisone 50 mg IV every 6 hours.
- Plasmapheresis and peritoneal dialysis may be effective in cases resistant to the usual pharmacological measures in order to remove high levels of circulating thyroid hormones.
- Colestyramine (3 g tid) reduces the enterohepatic circulation of thyroid hormones and may help improve thyrotoxicosis.

Subclinical hyperthyroidism

Values of thyroid hormones should be repeated to exclude nonthyroidal illness.

Subclinical hyperthyroidism is defined as undetectable thyrotropin (TSH) concentration in patients with normal levels of T_4 and T_3. Subtle symptoms and signs of thyrotoxicosis may be present.

It may be classified as endogenous in patients with thyroid hormone production associated with nodular thyroid disease or underlying Graves' disease, and as exogenous in those with undetectable serum thyrotropin concentrations as a result of treatment with levothyroxine.

Subclinical hyperthyroidism is a risk factor for development of atrial fibrillation or osteoporosis.[1]

The increased risk of fracture reported in older women taking thyroid hormone disappears when those with a history of hyperthyroidism are excluded.

In many patients with endogeneous subclinical hyperthyroidism who do not have nodular thyroid disease or complications of excess thyroid hormone, treatment is unnecessary, but TFTs should be performed every 6 months.

In older patients with atrial fibrillation or osteoporosis that could have been caused or exacerbated by mild excess of thyroid hormone, ablative therapy with ^{131}I is the best initial option.

In patients with exogenous subclinical hyperthyroidism, the dose of levothyroxine should be reduced, excluding those with prior thyroid cancer in whom thyrotropin suppression may be required. The dose of levothyroxine used for treating hypothyroidism may also be reduced if the patient develops the following:

---

1 Parle JV, Maisonneuve P, Sheppard MC, et al. (2001). Prediction of all-cause and cardiovascular mortality in elderly people from one low serum thyrotropin result: a 10-year cohort study. *Lancet* 358(9285):861–865.

- New-onset atrial fibrillation, angina, or cardiac failure
- Accelerated bone loss
- Borderline high serum T_3 concentration

Thyrotoxic periodic paralysis (TPP)

TTP is more common in Asians (5–10% of all with thyrotoxicosis due to Graves' disease or multinodular goiter) (0.1–0.2% of non-Asian Europeans/ North Americans). The etiology is probably disordered function of ion channels in muscle cell membranes.

TPP is the most common form of acquired periodic paralysis. The usual age of onset is 20–40 years and it occurs mostly in men.

There are recurrent episodes of painless muscle weakness lasting minutes to days. Flaccid paralysis occurs, usually spreading from the legs proximally, with depressed or absent deep tendon reflexes.

Clinical manifestations of thyrotoxicosis may be few, thus TSH should be checked in anyone presenting with periodic paralysis The condition improves as thyrotoxicosis is treated.

Serum potassium is low during attacks. Creatine phosphokinase (CPK) is ↑ during the recovery phase.

TPP is precipitated by carbohydrate intake, insulin, cold, and vigorous exercise.

Treatment is with potassium replacement, usually by oral route. However, in treatment of thyrotoxicosis, one needs to avoid overtreatment of hypokalemia resulting in hyperkalemia.

Symptoms usually improve within 2–4 hours; full resolution in 24–48 hours.

Nonselective β-blockers, such as propranolol (3 mg/kg), help reverse attacks as well as prevent attacks until a euthyroid state is achieved.

Thyrotoxicosis in pregnancy

📖 Also see p. 53.

Thyrotoxicosis occurs in about 0.2% of pregnancies. Graves' disease accounts for 90% of cases.

Less common causes include toxic adenoma and multinodular goiter. Other causes are gestational hyperthyroidism (hyperemesis gravidarum) and trophoblastic neoplasia.

Diagnosis of thyrotoxicosis during pregnancy may be difficult or delayed due to the normal physiological changes of pregnancy, which are similar to those of hyperthyroidism

Total T_4 and T_3 are elevated in pregnancy secondary to an elevated level of TBG. Free hormone assays can be used to better assess thyroid function.

Physiological features of normal pregnancy include an increase in basal metabolic rate, cardiac stroke volume, palpitations, and heat intolerance.

Serum free T_3 concentrations remain within the normal range in most pregnant women; serum TSH concentration decreases during the first trimester.

Symptoms

Hyperemesis gravidarum may cause mild hyperthyroidism, also known as "gestational thyrotoxicosis." Tiredness, palpitations, insomnia, heat intolerance, proximal muscle weakness, shortness of breath, and irritability may be presenting symptoms.

Thyrotoxicosis may occasionally be diagnosed when the patient presents with pregnancy-induced hypertension or congestive heart failure.

Signs

- Failure to gain weight despite a good appetite
- Persistent tachycardia with a pulse rate >90 beats/min at rest
- Other signs of thyrotoxicosis as described previously

Natural history of Graves' disease in pregnancy

There is aggravation of symptoms in the first half of the pregnancy, amelioration of symptoms in the second half of the pregnancy, and often recurrence of symptoms in the postpartum period.

Transient hyperthyroidism of gestational hyperthyroidism (hyperemesis gravidarum)

The mechanism is likely due to raised β-hCG level, which activates the TSH receptor.

β-hCG, luteinizing hormone (LH), follicle-stimulating hormone (FSH), and TSH are glycoprotein hormones that contain a common α-subunit and a hormone-specific β-subunit. There is an inverse relationship between the serum levels of TSH and hCG, best seen in early pregnancy. Structural homology exists between the TSH and hCG receptors.

Serum free T_4 concentration may be ↑ and the TSH levels suppressed in women with hyperemesis gravidarum.

Thyroid function tests recover after the resolution of hyperemesis.

Pregnant women with gestational hyperthyroidism (hyperemesis gravidarum), accounting for 2/3 of hyperemesis, are not usually given ATD treatment but managed supportively with fluids, antiemetics, and nutritional support.

There is no ↑ risk of thyrotoxicosis in subsequent pregnancies.

This condition can be differentiated from Graves' disease by the absence of a goiter, antithyroid antibodies, family history of Graves' disease, history of other autoimmune phenomena, or a previous history of ophthalmic Graves' disease.

Management of Graves' disease in the mother

The aim of treatment is alleviation of thyroid symptoms and normalization of thyroid function tests in the shortest time. Patients should be seen every 4–8 weeks and TFTs performed. Serum free T_4 is the best test to follow the response to ATDs. Block and replace regimen should not be used, as this will result in fetal hypothyroidism.

Both propylthiouracil (250 mg daily in divided doses or less) and methimazole control the disease in pregnancy; however, given the recent data regarding the risk of fatal hepatotoxicity with PTU, in an alert issued on 6/4/2009, the FDA recommended that given the risk of fetal hepatotoxicity, "PTU may be more appropriate for patients with Graves' disease who are in their first trimester of pregnancy." The choice of antithyroid agent during pregnancy remains controversial. PTU is more bound to plasma proteins and theoretically less of the drug would be transferred to the fetus than would methimazole. In addition, methimazole has been associated with aplasia cutis. A β-blocker (propranolol 20–40 mg q6–8h) is effective in controlling the hypermetabolic symptoms but should be used only for a few weeks until symptoms abate.

The dosage of ATDs is frequently adjusted during the course of the pregnancy; therefore, thyroid tests should be done at 2- to 4-week intervals, with the goal of keeping free thyroid hormone levels in the upper 1/3 of the reference range.

Thyroid tests may normalize spontaneously with the progression of a normal pregnancy as a result of immunological changes.

The use of iodides and radioiodine is contraindicated in pregnancy because it crosses the placenta and may cause toxicity to the fetal thyroid gland.

Surgery is rarely performed in pregnancy. It is reserved for patients not responding to ATDs. It is preferable to perform surgery in the second trimester.

Breast-feeding mothers should be treated with the lowest possible dose of propylthiouracil or methimazole. The low levels of ATD in breast milk do not affect the fetal thyroid gland.

Pre-pregnancy counseling

Hyperthyroid women who want to conceive should attain euthyroidism before conception, since uncontrolled hyperthyroidism is associated with an ↑ risk of congenital abnormalities (most seriously, stillbirth and cranial synostosis). 📖 See Table 3.3.

There is no evidence that radioactive iodine treatment given to the mother 6 months or more before pregnancy has an adverse effect on the fetus or on offspring in later life.

Antithyroid medication requirements decrease during gestation; in about 50–60% of patients, the dose may be discontinued in the last few weeks of gestation.

The risk of recurrent hyperthyroidism should be discussed with the patient. The rare occurrence of fetal and neonatal hyperthyroidism should be included during counseling sessions and the diagnosis of Graves' hyperthyroidism conveyed to the obstetrician and neonatologist.

Management of the fetus

The hypothalamic–pituitary–thyroid axis is well developed at 12 weeks gestation but remains inactive until 18–20 weeks. Circulating TSH receptor antibodies (TSH-RAb) in the mother can cross the placenta. The risk of hyperthyroidism to the neonate can be assessed by measuring TSH-RAb in the maternal circulation at the beginning of the third trimester. Antithyroglobulin antibodies and thyroid peroxidase antibodies have no effect on the fetus.

Long-term follow-up studies of children whose mothers received either methimazole or propylthiouracil have not shown an ↑ incidence of any physical or psychological defects.

Monitoring of the fetal heart rate and growth rate is the standard means by which fetal thyrotoxicosis may be detected. A rate >160 beats/min is suspicious of fetal thyrotoxicosis in the third trimester. Fetal thyrotoxicosis may complicate the latter part of the pregnancy of women with Graves' disease even if they have previously been treated with radioiodine or surgery, since TSH receptor antibodies may persist.

If there is evidence of fetal thyrotoxicosis, the dose of ATD should be increased. If this causes maternal hypothyroidism a small dose of T_4 can be added since, unlike methimazole, T_4 crosses the placenta less. A pediatrician should be involved to monitor neonatal thyroid function and detect thyrotoxicosis.

Hypothyroidism in the mother should be avoided because of the potential adverse effect on subsequent cognitive function of the neonate; 📖 see Table 3.3.

If the mother has been treated with methimazole, the post-delivery levels of T_4 may be low and neonatal levels of T_4 may only rise to the

Table 3.3 Potential maternal and fetal complications in uncontrolled hyperthyroidism in pregnancy

Maternal	Fetal
• Pregnancy induced hypertension	• Hyperthyroidism
• Preterm delivery	• Neonatal hyperthyroidism
• Congestive heart failure	• Intrauterine growth retardation
• Thyroid storm	• Small-for-gestational age
• Miscarriage	• Prematurity
• Abruptio placentae	• Stillbirth
• Accidental hemorrhage	• Cranial synostosis

thyrotoxic range after a few days. In addition, TSH is usually absent in neonates who subsequently develop thyrotoxicosis.

Clinical indicators of neonatal thyrotoxicosis include low birth weight, poor weight gain, tachycardia, and irritability. Methimazole can be given and withdrawn after a few weeks after the level of TSH-RAb declines.

Postpartum thyroiditis

This is defined as a syndrome of postpartum thyrotoxicosis or hypothyroidism in women who were euthyroid during pregnancy.

Postpartum thyroid dysfunction, which occurs in women with autoimmune thyroid disease, is characterized in 1/3 by a thyrotoxic phase in the first 3 months postpartum, followed by a hypothyroid phase occurring 3–6 months after delivery, followed by spontaneous recovery. In the remaining 2/3, a single-phase pattern or the reverse occurs.

Approximately 5 to 7% of women develop biochemical evidence of thyroid dysfunction after delivery. An ↑ incidence is seen in patients with type I diabetes mellitus (25%) and other autoimmune diseases, in the presence of anti-TPO antibodies, and in the presence of a family history of thyroid disease.

Hyperthyroidism due to Graves' disease accounts for 10–15% of all cases of postpartum thyrotoxicosis. In most cases, hyperthyroidism occurs later in the postpartum period (>3–6 months) and persists.

Providing the patient is not breast-feeding, a radioiodine uptake and scan can differentiate the two principal causes of autoimmune thyrotoxicosis by demonstrating ↑ uptake in Graves' disease and low uptake in postpartum thyroiditis.

Graves' hyperthyroidism should be treated with ATDs. Propylthiouracil is preferable if the patient is breast-feeding. Thyrotoxic symptoms due to postpartum thyrotoxicosis are managed symptomatically using propranolol.

One-third of affected women with postpartum thyroiditis develop symptoms of hypothyroidism and may require LT$_4$ for 2–3 months followed by a trial of 4–6 weeks off of LT4 and measurement of plasma TSH. There is a suggestion of an ↑ risk of postpartum depression in those with hypothyroidism.

Histology of the thyroid in the case of postpartum thyroiditis shows lymphocytic infiltration with destructive thyroiditis, predominantly occurring at 16 weeks in women with positive antimicrosomal antibodies.

Subsequent permanent hypothyroidism occurs in 25–30% of patients with postpartum thyroiditis. Given the increased risk, these patients should be followed up with annual TSH measurements.

Hyperthyroidism in children

Epidemiology

Thyrotoxicosis is rare before the age of 5 years. Although there is a progressive increase in incidence throughout childhood, it is still rare and accounts for <5% of all cases of Graves' disease.

Clinical features

Behavioral abnormalities, hyperactivity, and declining school performance may bring the child to medical attention. Features of hyperthyroidism are as described under Manifestations of hyperthyroidism (p. 19).

Accelerated growth rate is common in patients and presents as increasing height percentiles on growth charts. The disease may be part of McCune–Albright syndrome, myasthenia gravis, Down syndrome, diabetes mellitus, or other associated diseases.

Clinical exam should include examination for café-au-lait pigmentation, precocious puberty, and bony abnormalities.

Investigations

The primary cause of thyrotoxicosis in children is Graves' disease (positive antibodies to thyroid-stimulating antibodies, thyroglobulin, and/or thyroid peroxidase). Thyroiditis and toxic nodules have been described and a radioiodine scan may be useful if the diagnosis is not clear.

Hereditary syndromes of thyroid hormone resistance, often misdiagnosed as Graves' disease, are now increasingly recognized in children.

Treatment

ATDs represent the treatment of choice for thyrotoxic children. Therapy is generally started with propylthiouracil 6–8 mg/kg in three divided doses or methimazole (0.6–0.8 mg/kg per day).

Since relapse after withdrawal of ATDs is common, these drugs may be continued long term, until education is complete and definitive treatment with surgery or radioiodine can be offered (if ATDs result in serious side effects or if there is a recurrence after thyroidectomy).

Secondary hyperthyroidism

An elevated serum free T_4 and non-suppressed serum TSH are characteristic of TSH-secreting adenomas or resistance to thyroid hormone These conditions must be differentiated (Table 3.4).

TSH-secreting pituitary tumors

These tumors account for <1% of all pituitary tumors. Characteristically, there are *elevated* serum free T_4 and T_3 concentrations and *non-suppressed* (inappropriately normal or frankly elevated) serum TSH levels.

Among the 280 TSHomas reported in the literature (until 1998), 72% secreted TSH alone; the remainder co-secreted growth hormone (GH) (16%), prolactin (11%), or, rarely, gonadotropins. Approximately 90% were macroadenomas (>1 cm in diameter) and 71% exhibited suprasellar extension, invasion, or both into adjacent tissues (📖 see p. 131).

Patients with pure TSHomas may present with typical symptoms and signs of thyrotoxicosis and the presence of a diffuse goiter.

Patients may exhibit features of oversecretion of the other pituitary hormones, e.g., most commonly, prolactin or growth hormone. Headaches, visual field defects, menstrual irregularities, amenorrhea, delayed puberty, and hypogonadotropic hypogonadism have also been reported.

Careful establishment of the diagnosis is key to treatment. Inappropriate treatment of such patients with subtotal thyroidectomy or radioiodine administration not only fails to cure the underlying disorder but may also be associated with subsequent pituitary tumor enlargement and an ↑ risk of invasiveness into adjacent tissues.

Table 3.4 Tests useful in the differential diagnosis of TSHomas, PRTH, and GRTH

Test	TSHomas	PRTH	GRTH
Clinical thyrotoxicosis	Present	Present	Absent
Family history	Absent	Present	Present
TSH response to TRH	No change	Increase	In-crease
TSH response to T_3 (100 mcg/day + β-blockers)	No change	Decrease	Decrease
SHBG	Elevated–92%*	Normal†	Normal
α-Subunit	Elevated–65%	2% elevated	
Pituitary MRI	Tumor–30% micorade-noma†	Normal	Normal
Fall in TSH on octreotide LAR 20 mg/month for 2 months	95%	No change	No change

*Not usually raised in mixed GH/TSH tumor.
†Peripheral markers of toxicosis sometimes affected (8% SHBG elevated).
†The best biochemical test is an elevated A-subunit.

Treatment options are as follows:

- Transphenoidal surgery
- Pituitary radiotherapy if surgical results are unsatisfactory or surgery is contraindicated or not desired
- Medical therapy with somatostatin analogs such as octreotide or lanreotide may be useful preoperatively and suppresses TSH secretion in 80% of the cases.

Resistance to thyroid hormones

Patients with generalized resistance to thyroid hormone (GRTH) may present with mild hyperthyroidism, deaf mutism, delayed bone maturation, raised circulating thyroid hormone concentrations, non-suppressed TSH, and failure of TSH to decrease normally upon administration of supraphysiological doses of thyroid hormones.

Most patients present with goiter or incidentally found abnormal TFTs. Treatment is determined by thyroid status.

In selective pituitary resistance to thyroid hormones (PRTH), the thyroid hormone resistance is more pronounced in the pituitary. Thus the patient exhibits definite clinical manifestations of thyrotoxicosis.

About 90% of thyroid hormone resistance syndromes result from mutations in the gene encoding TRβ. Mutant receptors have a reduced affinity for T_3 and are functionally deficient. It is usually inherited in an autosomal dominant pattern with the affected individuals being heterozygous for the mutation.

A subset of RTH receptors has been identified that are capable of inhibiting wild-type receptor action. When coexpressed, the mutant proteins are able to inhibit the function of their wild-type counterparts in a dominant negative manner.

Common features of patients with thyroid hormone resistance syndromes include goiter (most commonly) and, less frequently, tachycardia, hyperkinetic behavior, emotional disturbances, ear, nose, and throat infections, language disabilities, auditory disorders, low body weight, cardiac abnormalities, and subnormal intelligence quotients.

Treatment options in RTH are not usually necessary.

In PTRH, treatment may be needed, but this is uncommon. Treatment is with chronic suppression of TSH secretion with LT_4, triiodothyroacetic acid, octreotide, or bromocriptine. If this is ineffective, thyroid ablation with radioiodine or surgery can be tried, with subsequent close monitoring of thyroid hormone status and pituitary gland size.

Further reading

Allahabadia A, Heward JM, Nithiyananthan R, et al. (2001). MHC class II region, CTLA4 gene, and ophthalmopathy in patients with Graves' disease. *Lancet* 358(9286):984–985.

Brent GP (2008). Grave's disease. *N Engl J Med* 358:2594–2605.

Brix TH, Kyvik KO, Hegedus L (1998). What is the evidence of genetic factors in the etiology of Graves' disease? A brief review. *Thyroid* 8:727–734.

Franklyn JA, Maisonneuve P, Sheppard MC, et al. (1998). Mortality after the treatment of hyperthyroidism with radioactive iodine. *N Engl J Med* 338:712–718.

Franklyn JA, Maisonneuve P, Sheppard MC, et al. (1999). Cancer incidence and mortality after radioiodine treatment for hyperthyroidism: a population-based cohort study. *Lancet* 353:2111–2115.Gunji K, Kubota S, Swanson J, et al. (1998). Role of the eye muscles in thyroid eye disease: identification of the principal autoantigens. *Thyroid* 8:553–556 [erratum *Thyroid* 1998; 8:1079].

Helfgott S, Smith RN (2002). Case records of the Massachusetts General Hospital. Weekly clinico-pathological exercises: Case 21-2002: a 21-year-old man with arthritis during treatment for hyper-thyroidism. *N Engl J Med* 347(2):122–130.

Parle JV, Maisonneuve P, Sheppard MC, et al. (2001). Prediction of all-cause and cardiovascular mortality in elderly people from one low serum thyrotropin result: a 10-year cohort study. *Lancet* 358(9285):861–865.

Panzer C, Beazley R, Braverman L (2004). Rapid preoperative preparation for severe hyperthyroid Graves' disease. *J Clin Endocrinol Metab* 89(5):2142–2144.

Pearce SH (2004). Spontaneous reporting of adverse reactions to carbimazole and propylthiouracil in the UK. *Clin Endocrinol* 61(5):589–594.

Rivkees SA, Sklar C, Freemark M (1998). The management of Graves's disease in children, with special emphasis on radioiodine treatment. *J Clin Endocrinol Metab* 83:3767–3776.

Ron E, Doody MM, Becker DV, et al. (1998). Cancer mortality following treatment for adult hyper-thyroidism. Cooperative Thyrotoxicosis Therapy Follow-up Study Group. *JAMA* 280:347–355.

Toft AD (2001). Clinical practice. Subclinical hyperthyroidism *N Engl J Med* 345(7):512–516.

Weetman AP (2000). Graves's disease. *N Engl J Med* 343(17):1236–1248.

Weetman AP, Pickerill AP, Watson P, et al. (1994). Treatment of Graves' disease with the block-replace regimen of antithyroid drugs: the effect of treatment duration and immunogenetic suscep-tibility on relapse. *QJM* 87:337–341.

Graves' ophthalmopathy, dermopathy, and acropachy

Graves' ophthalmopathy

See European Working Group on Graves' Ophthalmopathy at www. EUGOGO.org.

This organ-specific autoimmune disorder is characterized by swelling of the extraocular muscles, lymphocytic infiltration, late fibrosis, muscle tethering, and proliferation of orbital fat and connective tissue. The lesions are due to localized accumulation of glycosaminoglycans.

The disorder is clinically evident in 30% of patients. Most have mild disease, but 5% have severe disease that threatens sight.

Incidence is higher in women (except for severe disease, for which there is equal sex-incidence). There is a bimodal age distribution in women, with peak onsets between 40–44 years and 60–64 years. In men, a single peak incidence occurs at 65–69 years.

There are two stages in the development of the disease: an active inflammatory (dynamic) stage and a relatively quiescent static stage. 5% of patients with Graves' ophthalmopathy have hypothyroidism and 5% are euthyroid. 75% of patients develop Graves' disease within a year of developing Graves' ophthalmopathy.

The temporal relationship between the onset of thyroid dysfunction and ophthalmopathy is variable. In a minority of patients, there is a lag period between the presentation of hyperthyroidism and the appearance of eye findings.

Smoking and hypothyroidism moderately worsen Graves' ophthalmopathy, and current smokers (>20 cigarettes/day) are more likely to develop ophthalmopathy.

The endocrinologist should be prepared to identify ocular emergencies, such as corneal ulceration, congestive ophthalmopathy, and optic neuropathy.

Clinical features

Retraction of eyelids is extremely common in thyroid eye disease. The margin of the upper eyelid normally rests about 2 mm below the limbus. Retraction can be suspected if the upper eyelid margin is either level with or above the superior limbus, thus allowing the sclera to be visible below the lid. Additionally, the lower lid normally rests at the inferior limbus, and retraction can be suspected when the sclera is visible above the lower eyelid.

Proptosis or exopthalmos can result in failure of lid closure, thereby increasing the likelihood of exposure keratitis and a gritty eye sensation.

Damage to the eye can be confirmed with a fluorescein or rose Bengal stain.

Fundoscopy should be performed to rule out papilledema. Proptosis may result in periorbital edema and chemosis because the displaced orbit results in less efficient orbital drainage.

Persistent visual blurring may indicate an optic neuropathy requiring urgent treatment. Severe conjunctival pain may indicate corneal ulceration requiring urgent referral.

Features are unilateral in approximately 15% of cases.

Investigation of proptosis

The NOSPECS classification is not universally accepted; for detailed classification see ⫛ www.EUGOGO.org and The European Group on Graves' Orbitopathy.[1]

Documentation using a Hertel exophthalmometer

The feet of the apparatus are placed against the lateral orbital margin as defined by the zygomatic bones. The distance between the lateral angle of the bony orbit and an imaginary line tangent to the most anterior aspect of the cornea is recorded.

A normal result is considered <20 mm (<18 mm in Asians, <22 in Afro-Carribeans). A reading of 21 mm or more is abnormal, and a difference of 2 mm between the eyes is suspicious.

Soft tissue involvement

Soft-tissue signs and symptoms include conjunctival hyperemia, chemosis, and foreign-body sensation.

CT or MRI scan of the orbit

This demonstrates enlargement of the extraocular muscles, which can be useful in cases of diagnostic difficulty. This is also more accurate for demonstration of proptosis.

Examining for possible ophthalmoplegia

Patients may complain of diplopia due to ocular muscle dysfunction caused by either edema during the early active phase or fibrosis during the later phase. Assessment using a Hess chart may be helpful.

Intraoptic pressure may increase on upgaze and result in compression of the globe by a fibrotic inferior rectus muscle. Ocular mobility may be restricted by edema during the active inflammatory phase or by fibrosis during the fibrotic stage.

The two most common findings are defective eye elevation caused by fibrotic contraction of the inferior rectus muscle, and a convergence defect caused by fibrotic contraction of the medial rectus. Disorders of the medial rectus, superior rectus, and lateral rectus muscle produce typical signs of defective adduction, depression, and abduction, respectively.

---

1 The European Group on Graves' Orbitopathy (2006). Clinical assessment of patients with Graves' orbitopathy: recommendations to generalists, specialists and clinical researchers. *Eur Endocrinol* 155(3):387–389.

Examining for possible optic neuropathy

History of poor vision, a recent or rapid change in vision, and poor color vision are reasons for prompt referral. A visual acuity of <6/18 warrants referral to an ophthalmologist.

For color vision, each eye should be evaluated using a simple 15-plate Ishihara color vision test. Color vision is a subtle indicator of optic nerve function. Failure to identify >2 of the plates with either eye is an indication for referral. This is unhelpful in the 8% of men who may be color blind.

Marcus Gunn pupil: The "swinging flashlight" test detects the presence of an afferent pupillary defect.

Medical treatment

See Box 4.1.

Lid retraction

Most patients do not require any treatment, as clinical signs usually improve with treatment of hyperthyroidism or spontaneously with time (40%).

- Sunglasses help with photophobia and excess tears.
- In patients with significant lid retraction and exposure keratopathy, topical lubricants improve symptoms (surgery to reduce the vertical lid fissures can be considered).
- Botulinum toxin injection may reduce upper lid retraction.
- Head elevation during sleep and diuretics may help congestion.
- Tape eyelids at night to avoid corneal damage

Active ophthalmopathy threatening sight

- Glucocorticoids at high doses (e.g., prednisone 60–80 mg/day) improve ophthalmopathy in 60–75% of cases.
- Effectiveness of glucocorticoids is more likely in those with diplopia at neutral gaze and an inflammatory component to ophthalmoplegia.
- Treatment should be given for 2 weeks and then tapered gradually.
- Urgent referral to an ophthalmologist is indicated for any suspicion of optic neuropathy or corneal ulceration.

Orbital radiotherapy

- Indications for lens-sparing orbital radiotherapy are similar to those for high-dose glucocorticoids.
- Radiotherapy probably works by reducing the activity and number of activated T lymphocytes in the retrobulbar tissues.
- 20 Gray administered in 10 doses of 2 Gray over 2 weeks
- Treatment with both radiotherapy and glucocorticoids is more effective than either alone.
- Effectiveness in 60% of patients <40 years of age

Other medical therapies

- Other immunosuppressive regimens have no proven place in the general management of Graves' ophthalmopathy.
- Use of depot octreotide has been shown to be of no benefit in management.

Box 4.1 Treatment of Graves' ophthalmopathy

General measures
- Smoking cessation
- Dark glasses, with eye protection
- Control of thyroid function

Specific measures

Problem	Treatment
Grittiness	Artificial tears and simple eye ointment
Eyelid retraction	Tape eyelids at night to avoid corneal damage. Surgery if risk of exposure keratopathy
Proptosis	Head elevation during sleep Diuretics Systemic steroids Radiotherapy Orbital decompression
Optic neuropathy	Systemic steroids Radiotherapy Orbital decompression
Ophthalmoplegia	Prisms in lenses in the acute phase Orbital decompression Orbital muscle surgery

Surgical treatment
See Box 4.1.

Surgery for decompression
- Orbital decompression may be indicated for urgent treatment of optic neuropathy.
- Posteromedial wall of orbit is usually removed.
- Complications include dysmotility of the eye, blindness, orbital cellulitis, cerebrospinal fluid (CSF) leak, cerebral hematoma, obstruction to nasolacrimal flow, and anosmia.

Surgery for strabismus
- Should be performed after any necessary orbital decompression
- Aims are to allow correct binocular vision
- Performed when eyes are in a quiescent phase for at least 6 months after active disease
- Involves alteration, loosening or tightening of eye muscles, often over several operations, to improve binocular vision.

Eyelid surgery
This is the final stage of any surgical approach. The aims are to adjust the upper and lower eyelid position to improve comfort and appearance.

Graves' dermopathy

This is a rare complication of Graves' thyrotoxicosis (0.5%). It is usually pretibial in location (99%) and hence called *pretibial myxedema*. It is associated with ophthalmopathy (97%) and acropachy (18%).

Typically, raised, discolored, and indurated lesions are on the front or back of the legs or on the dorsum of the feet. Occasionally, these have been described in other areas, including the hands and face.

Lesions are due to localized accumulation of glycosaminoglycans. It is now recognized that there is a lymphocytic infiltrate. Lesions are characteristically asymptomatic, but they can also be pruritic, tender, and disfiguring.

Treatment

This condition is usually not treated. Potent topical fluorinated steroids such as fluocinolone acetonide may be effective (4–8 weeks) for treatment of localized pain and tenderness and occasionally may result in resolution of the visible skin signs. Surgery may worsen the condition.

One-quarter of cases remit completely; 50% are chronic on no therapy. The effect of topical steroids on remission rates is unclear.

Thyroid acropachy

This is the rarest manifestation of Graves' disease. It presents as painless clubbing of the digits and subperiosteal new bone formation. The soft-tissue swelling is similar to that seen in localized myxedema and consists of glycosaminoglycan accumulation.

Patients almost inevitably have Graves' ophthalmopathy or pretibial myxedema. If not, an alternative cause of clubbing should be looked for.

There is no effective treatment.

Further reading

European Group on Graves' Orbitopathy (2006). Clinical assessment of patients with Graves' orbitopathy: recommendations to generalists, specialists and clinical researchers. *Eur J Endocrinol* 155(3):387–389.

Schwartz KM, Fatourechi V, Ahmed DD, et al. (1992). Dermopathy of Graves' disease (pretibial myxedema): long-term outcome. *J Clin Endocrinol Metab* 87(2):438–446.

Tellez M, Cooper J, Edmonds C (1992). Graves' ophthalmopathy in relation to cigarette smoking and ethnic origin. *Clin Endocrinol* 36:291–294.

Multinodular goiter and solitary adenomas

Background

Nodular thyroid disease denotes the presence of single or multiple palpable or nonpalpable nodules within the thyroid gland.

Prevalence rates range from 5 to 50% depending on the population studied and sensitivity of detection methods. Prevalence increases linearly with age and exposure to ionizing radiation and iodine deficiency.

Clinically apparent thyroid nodules are evident in 4–7% of the U.S. population. Incidence of thyroid nodules is about 4× more common in women.

Thyroid nodules always raise the concern of cancer, although <5% are cancerous.

Nodules are more likely to be malignant in patients <20 or >60 years of age. Thyroid nodules are more common in women but approximately 4× more likely to be malignant in men.

Clinical evaluation

An asymptomatic thyroid mass may be discovered either by a clinician on routine neck palpation or by the patient during self-examination.

History should concentrate on the following:

- An enlarging thyroid mass
- A previous history of radiation, especially childhood head and neck irradiation
- A family history of thyroid cancer
- Development of hoarseness or dysphagia

Physical findings suggestive of malignancy include a firm or hard non-tender nodule, a recent history of enlargement, fixation to adjacent tissue, and the presence of regional lymphadenopathy.

Pemberton's sign is facial erythema and jugular venous distension upon raising the arms. It is a sign of superior venacaval obstruction caused by a substernal mass.

A hot nodule on a radioisotope scan makes malignancy less likely.

See Table 5.1 for the etiology of thyroid nodules.

Clinical features raising suspicion of thyroid malignancy

- Age (<20 or >60 years)
- Rapidly enlarging nodule
- Local symptoms including dysphagia, stridor, or hoarseness
- Previous exposure to radiation
- Positive family history of thyroid cancer or multiple endocrone neoplasia (MEN) syndrome

Table 5.1 Etiology of thyroid nodules

Common causes	Uncommon causes
• Colloid nodule	• Granulomatous thyroiditis
• Cyst	• Infections
• Lymphocytic thyroiditis	• Malignancy
	• Medullary
	• Anaplastic
	• Metastatic
	• Lymphoma
• Benign neoplasms	
• Hurthle cell	
• Follicular	
• Malignancy	
• Papillary	
• Follicular	

- Gardner's syndrome (familial large intestinal polyposis)
- Familial polyposis coli
- Cowden syndrome (autosomal dominantly inherited hamartoma syndrome)
- Lymphadenopathy
- History of Hashimoto's disease (Increased incidence of lymphoma)

Studies

- FNA (see p. 14)
- Serum TSH concentration. If TSH is suppressed, a radioisotope thyroid scan should be performed.
- Serum calcitonin if there is a family history of medullary carcinoma or MEN 2A or 2B
- Respiratory flow loop, especially for a large goiter possibly causing tracheal obstruction
- CT scan or MRI if there are concerns about retrosternal goiter or tracheal compression

Treatment

Toxic multinodular goiter or nodule

ATDs

ATDs are effective in controlling the hyperthyroidism but are not curative. As the hot nodules are autonomous, the condition will recur after stopping the drugs.

Methimazole and propylthiouracil are useful treatments to gain control of the disease in preparation for surgery or radioiodine treatment or as long-term treatment in those patients unwilling to accept radioiodine or surgery.

Radioiodine

This form of treatment is often considered the first choice for definitive treatment. ^{131}I is preferentially accumulated in hot nodules but not in normal thyroid tissue, which, because of the thyrotoxic state, is nonfunctioning.

Radioiodine treatment commonly induces a euthyroid state as the hot nodules are destroyed and the previously nonfunctioning follicles gradually resume normal function. A dose of 14–16 mCi for small to medium goiters and 16–22 mCi for medium to large goiters is recommended.

Surgery

The aim of surgery is to remove as much of the nodular tissue as possible and, if the goiter is large, to relieve local symptoms. Postoperative follow-up should involve checks of thyroid function.

Goiter recurrence, although rare, does occasionally occur.

Nontoxic multinodular goiter or nodule

Surgery

This is the preferred treatment for patients with the following:
- Local compression symptoms
- Cosmetic disfigurement
- Solitary nodule with FNA suspicious for malignancy

Radioiodine

This may be indicated in elderly patients for whom surgery is not appropriate. It may require admission. Up to 50% shrinkage of goiter mass has been reported in recent studies.

Hypothyroidism following radioiodine is relatively low but is still recognized.

Box 5.1 Etiology of goiter

- Autoimmune thyroid disease
- Sporadic
- Endemic (iodine deficiency, dietary origins)
- Pregnancy
- Drug induced (ATDs, lithium, amiodarone)
- Thyroiditis syndromes

Medical treatment
Use of T_4 to suppress TSH is associated with a risk of cardiac arrhythmias and bone loss. T_4 is useful only if TSH is detectable but is not generally indicated.

Pathology

Thyroid nodules may be described as *adenomas* if the follicular cell differentiation is enclosed within a capsule, and as *adenomatous* when the lesions are circumscribed but not encapsulated.

Thyroid nodules in pregnant mothers

- Increase in size during gestation
- Increase in number
- Need FNA as higher risk of malignancy
- Can be operated on in second trimester or postpartum

Thyroiditis

Background

The term *thyroiditis* refers to a varied group of disorders all characterized by some form of thyroid inflammation (Table 6.1). It includes conditions characterized by thyroid pain and tenderness (i.e., subacute granulomatous, infectious, traumatic, and radiation-induced thyroiditis) and those characterized primarily by thyroid dysfunction or goiter without pain (i.e., painless, postpartum, drug-induced and fibrous thyroiditis, chronic lymphocytic thyroiditis [Hashimoto's]).

Inflammation of the thyroid gland often leads to a transient thyrotoxicosis followed by hypothyroidism (Table 6.2).

Table 6.1 Causes and characteristics of thyroiditis

Cause	Characteristic features
Chronic lymphocytic thyroiditis (Hashimoto's)	Grossly lymphocytic and fibrotic thyrotoxicosis or hypothyroidism
Postpartum thyroiditis	Lymphocytic thyroiditis, transient thyrotoxicosis or hypothyroidism
Drug induced	Particularly with amiodarone
Subacute granulomatous (de Quervain)	Thought to be viral in origin, multinuclear giant cells
Riedel thyroiditis	Extensive fibrosis of the thyroid
Radiation thyroiditis	Radiation injury, transient thyrotoxicosis
Pyogenic	*Staph. aureus*, streptococci, *E. coli*, tuberculosis, fungal

Table 6.2 Clinical presentation of thyroiditis

Form of thyroiditis	Clinical presentation	Thyroid function
Suppurative (acute)	Painful, tender thyroid, fever	Usually normal
Subacute granulomatous (de Quervain)	Painful anterior neck, arthralgia, antecedent upper respiratory tract infection; generalized malaise.	Early thyrotoxicosis, occasionally late hypothyroidism
Chronic autoimmune	Hashimoto's: goiter Atrophic: no goiter	Usually hypothyroid Sometimes euthyroid Rarely early thyrotoxicosis
Riedel	Hard woody consistency of thyroid	Usually normal

Chronic autoimmune thyroiditis

See Tables 6.1 and 6.2.

Hashimoto's thyroiditis

This is characterized by a painless, variably sized goiter with rubbery consistency and an irregular surface. The normal follicular structure of the gland is extensively replaced by lymphocytic and plasma cell infiltrates with formation of lymphoid germinal centers.

The patient may have normal thyroid function, or subclinical, or overt hypothyroidism. Occasional patients present with thyrotoxicosis in association with a thyroid gland that is unusually firm and with high titers of circulating antithyroid antibodies.

Atrophic thyroiditis

This probably indicates end-stage thyroid disease. These patients do not have goiter and are antibody positive. Biochemically, the picture is that of frank hypothyroidism.

Studies

- Thyroid function tests
- Thyroid antibodies (antithyroglobulin antibodies positive in 20–25%, and antithyroperoxidase antibodies in >90%).
- FNA to exclude malignancy in patients who present with a goiter and dominant nodule

Prognosis

The long-term prognosis of patients with chronic thyroiditis is good, because hypothyroidism can easily be corrected with T_4 and the goiter is not usually of sufficient size to cause local symptoms.

In the atypical situation where Hashimoto's thyroiditis presents with rapidly enlarging goiter and pain, a short course of prednisone at a dose of 40 mg daily may prove helpful.

Other types of thyroiditis

Silent thyroiditis

This is associated with transient thyrotoxicosis or hypothyroidism. A significant percentage of patients have a personal or family history of autoimmune thyroid disease. It may progress to permanent hypothyroidism.

Postpartum thyroiditis

Also see p. 34. Thyroid dysfunction occurs within the first 6 months postpartum. Prevalence ranges from 5 to 7%. Postpartum thyroiditis develops in 30–52% of women who have positive thyroid peroxidase (TPO) antibodies.

Most patients have a complete remission but some may progress to permanent hypothyroidism. It is three times as common in patients with type I diabetes mellitus.

Chronic fibrosing (Riedel's) thyroiditis

This rare disorder is characterized by intense fibrosis of the thyroid gland and surrounding structures, leading to induration of the tissues of the neck. It may be associated with mediastinal and retroperitoneal fibrosis, salivary gland fibrosis, sclerosing cholangitis, lachrymal gland fibrosis, and parathyroid gland fibrosis leading to hypoparathyroidism.

Patients are usually euthyroid. The main differential diagnosis is thyroid neoplasia.

Management

Corticosteroids are usually ineffective. Surgery may be needed to relieve obstruction and to exclude malignancy. Tamoxifen may be of benefit.

Pyogenic thyroiditis

This disorder is rare; it is usually preceded by a pyogenic infection elsewhere. It is characterized by tenderness and swelling of the thyroid gland, redness and warmth of the overlying skin, and constitutional signs of infection.

Piriform sinus should be excluded. Excision of the tract is preferable to incision and drainage.

Treatment consists of antibiotic therapy and incision and drainage if a fluctuant area within the thyroid should occur.

Subacute thyroiditis (granulomatous or de Quervain thyroiditis)

This condition is most likely viral in origin. Symptoms include pronounced asthenia, malaise, pain over the thyroid, or pain referred to the lower jaw, ear, or occiput. Less commonly, the onset is acute with fever, pain over the thyroid, and symptoms of thyrotoxicosis.

Characteristic signs include exquisite tenderness and nodularity of the thyroid gland. There is often an elevated erythrocyte sedimentation rate (ESR) and depressed radionuclide uptake. Biochemically, the patient may be initially thyrotoxic, though later the patient may become hypothyroid (15%).

In mild cases, nonsteroidal anti-inflammatory agents offer symptomatic relief. In severe cases, glucocorticoids (prednisone 20–40 mg/day) are effective. Propranolol can be used to control associated thyrotoxicosis. Treatment can be withdrawn when T_4 returns to normal.

T_4 replacement is required if the patient becomes hypothyroid. Treatment with methimazole or propylthiouracil is not indicated.

Drug-induced thyroiditis

Causes

- Amiodarone
- Lithium
- Interferon-α (15% develop thyroid peroxidase antibodies and or thyroid dysfunction)
- Interleukin 2

Further reading

Lazarus JH, Hall R, Othman S, et al. (1996). The clinical spectrum of postpartum thyroid disease. *QJM* 89:429–435.

Muller AF, Drexhage HA, Berghout A (2001). Postpartum thyroiditis and autoimmune thyroiditis in women of child-bearing age: recent insights and consequences for antenatal and postnatal care. *Endocr Rev* 22:605–630.

Pearce EN, Farwell AP, Braverman LE (2003). Thyroiditis. *N Engl J Med* 348(26):2646–2655.

Weetman AP (2000). Autoimmune thyroid disease. In DeGroot LJ, Jameson JL (eds.), *Endocrinology*, Vol. 2. Philadelphia: WB Saunders.

Hypothyroidism

Background

Hypothyroidism results from a variety of abnormalities that cause insufficient secretion of thyroid hormones (Table 7.1). The most common cause is autoimmune thyroid disease.

Myxedema is severe hypothyroidism in which there is accumulation of hydrophilic mucopolysaccharides in the ground substance of the dermis and other tissues leading to thickening of the facial features and doughy induration of the skin.

Subclinical hypothyroidism refers to elevated TSH levels in the presence of normal concentrations of free thyroid hormones.

Epidemiology

In community surveys, approximately 0.1–2% of adults have overt hypothyroidism.

In the United States Nation Health and Nutrition Examination Survey (NHANES III), 4.3% of people without known thyroid disease had subclinical hypothyroidism, and 0.3% had overt hypothyroidism.

Incidence is higher in whites than in Hispanics or African-American populations. Incidence is higher in areas of high iodine intake.

An elevated TSH is associated with higher serum lipid concentrations, which may be an additional reason to initiate therapy,

Table 7.1 Classification of the causes of hypothyroidism

	TSH	Free T$_4$
Nongoitrous	↑	↓
Postablative (radioiodine, surgery)		
Congenital development defect		
Atrophic thyroiditis		
Postradiation (e.g., for lymphoma)		
Goitrous	↑	↓
Chronic thyroiditis (Hashimoto's thyroiditis)		
Iodine deficiency		
Drug elicited (amiodarone, aminosalicylic acid, iodides, lithium aminoglutethimide, interferon-α, thalidomide, bexarotene, stavudine—antiretroviral)		
Heritable biosynthetic de-fects		
Maternally transmitted (antithyroid agents, iodides)		
Pituitary	↓	↓
Panhypopituitarism		
Isolated TSH deficiency		
Hypothalamic	↓	↓
Neoplasm		
Infiltrative (sarcoidosis)		
Congenital defects		
Infection (encephalitis)		
Self-limiting	↑	↓
Following withdrawal of suppressive thyroid therapy		
Subacute thyroiditis and chronic thyroiditis with transient hypothyroidism		
Postpartum thyroiditis		

Clinical picture

Adult

- Insidious nonspecific onset
- Fatigue, lethargy
- Constipation
- Cold intolerance
- Muscle stiffness, cramps, carpal tunnel syndrome
- Menorrhagia, later oligo- or amenorrhea
- Slowing of intellectual and motor activities
- ↓ Appetite and weight gain
- Dry skin, hair loss
- Deep hoarse voice
- ↓ Visual acuity
- Obstructive sleep apnea
- Depression

Myxoedema

- Dull, expressionless face, sparse hair, periorbital puffiness, macroglossia
- Pale, cool skin that feels rough and doughy
- Enlarged heart (dilation and pericardial effusion)
- Megacolon/intestinal obstruction
- Cerebellar ataxia
- Prolonged relaxation phase of deep tendon reflexes
- Peripheral neuropathy.
- Encephalopathy
- Hyperlipidemia
- Hypercarotenemia (also caused by hyperlipidemia, diabetes mellitus, and porphyria)
- Psychiatric symptoms, e.g., depression, psychosis

Myxedema coma

- Predisposed to by cold exposure, trauma, infection, administration of central nervous system (CNS) depressants
- Marked respiratory depression with increased arterial P_{CO_2}
- Hyponatremia from impaired water excretion and disordered regulation of vasopressin secretion

Treatment of hypothyroidism

Normal metabolic state should be restored gradually as a rapid increase in metabolic rate may precipitate cardiac arrhythmias. The average replacement dose is 1.6 mcg/kg per day.

In younger patients, start levothyroxine at 50–100 mcg. In the elderly, with a history of ischemic heart disease, an initial dose of levothyroxine 25–50 mcg can be increased by 25-mcg increments at 4-week intervals until normal metabolic state is attained.

The optimum dosage is determined by clinical criteria, the objective of treatment being to restore serum TSH to the normal range.

TSH should be checked only 2 months after any dose change. Once stabilized, TSH should be checked on an annual basis.

In patients with secondary hypothyroidism, free T_4 is the most useful parameter to follow.

Dose requirements can increase by 25–50% in pregnancy because of the increase in thyroid-binding globulin (TBG). Recent data have shown that mild maternal hypothyroidism in the first trimester is associated with slightly impaired cognitive function in offspring. Thus, some now recommend a routinely increased levothyroxine dose by 25 mcg in any women on replacement therapy when she learns she is pregnant.

Combined T_4 and T_3 replacement

Some studies have suggested that the additional replacement with T_3 and T_4 in combination improves well-being and cognitive function in patients compared to treatment with T_4 alone.

A recent meta-analysis of double-blind crossover studies showed no benefit of this therapy; thus it is not recommended.

Treatment of subclinical hypothyroidism

Treatment is indicated if the biochemistry is sustained in patients with a past history of radioiodine treatment for thyrotoxicosis or positive thyroid antibodies. In these situations, progression to overt hypothyroidism is almost inevitable (at least 5% per year of those with positive antithyroid peroxidase antibodies).

Two samples should be taken 2–3 months apart to distinguish from nonthyroidal illness.

There is controversy over the advantages of T_4 treatment in patients with negative thyroid antibodies and no previous radioiodine treatment. If treatment is not given, follow-up with annual thyroid function tests is important.

There is no generally accepted consensus of when patients should receive treatment. Some authorities suggest treatment when the serum TSH is >10 U/L, because of an increased rate of progression to overt hypothyroidism.

Increased incidence of cardiac risk is probably greater if >65 years old.

Management

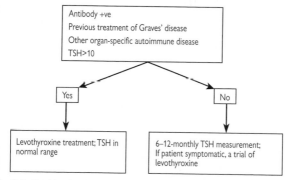

Fig. 7.1 Algorithm for management of subclinical hypothyroidism. Reprinted from *The Lancet*, Vol. 349, Lindsay RS and Toft AD, Hypothyroidism, pp. 413–417, Copyright 1997, with permission from Elsevier.

Management of myxedema coma

- Identify and treat concurrent precipitating illness.
- Give antibiotic therapy after blood cultures.
- Manage hypothermia with passive external rewarming.
- Manage patient in an intensive treatment unit if they are comatose.
- Give warm humidified oxygen by facemask. Mechanical ventilation is needed if the patient is hypoventilating.
- Aim for a slow rise in core temperature (0.5°C/h).
- Use a cardiac monitor for supraventricular arrhythmias.
- Correct hyponatremia (mild fluid restriction), hypotension (cautious volume expansion with crystalloid or whole blood), and hypoglycemia (glucose administration).
- Monitor rectal temperature, oxygen saturation, blood pressure (BP), central venous pressure (CVP), and urine output hourly.
- Take blood samples for thyroid hormones, TSH, and cortisol before starting treatment. If hypocortisolemic, administer glucocorticoids.

On thyroid hormone replacement no consensus has been reached. The following is an accepted regimen:
- T_4 300–500 mcg IV or by NG tube as a starting dose followed by 50–100 mcg daily until oral medication can be taken
- If no improvement within 24–48 hours, T_3 10 mcg IV q8h or 25 mcg IV q8h can be given in addition to above.

Give hydrocortisone 50–100 mg q6–8h in case of cortisol deficiency.

Management of persistently elevated TSH despite thyroxine replacement

See Fig. 7.2.
- Elevated TSH despite thyroxine replacement is common, most usually due to lack of compliance.

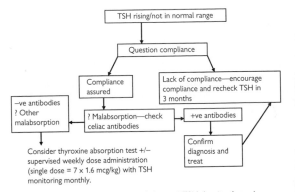

Fig. 7.2 Suggestions for investigations of elevated TSH despite thyroxine replacement therapy to >1.6 mcg/kg/day[N3].

- If TSH is still elevated when the levothyroxine dose is at 1.6 mcg/kg/day or higher, careful questioning of compliance is needed.
- Consider malabsorption.
- Consider other drugs that may interfere with levothyroxine absorption (Box 7.1).

Box 7.1 Interference with absorption of thyroxine

- Celiac disease
- Drugs—colestyramine, aluminum hydroxide, sucralfate, omeprazole, rifampicin, phenytoin, iron, and calcium carbonate
- Atrophic gastritis in *H. pylori* infection ($\downarrow$ T_4 by 30%)

Congenital hypothyroidism

Incidence is about 1 in 5000 neonates. All neonates should be screened.

Thyroid agenesis

This occurs in 1 in 1800 births.

Thyroid hormone dysgenesis

This is caused by inborn errors of thyroid metabolism. The disorders may be autosomal recessive, indicating single protein defects.

The disorder can be caused by inactivation of the TSH receptor, abnormalities of the thyroid transcription factors TTF1, TTF2, and PAX8, or defects in iodide transport, organification (peroxidase), coupling, deiodinase, or thyroglobulin synthesis.

In a large proportion of patients with congenital hypothyroidism, the molecular background is unknown.

Pendred's syndrome

This is characterized by overt or subclinical hypothyroidism, goiter, and moderate to severe sensorineural hearing impairment. The prevalence varies between 1 in 15,000 and 1 in 100,000. There is a partial iodide organification defect detected by increased perchlorate discharge.

Thyroid hormone synthesis is only mildly impaired and so may not be detected by neonatal thyroid screening.

Box 7.2 Clinical features and congenital hypothyroidism

The following features are late sequelae of congenital hypothyroidism. With routine screening now available, they should not be seen.
- Physiological jaundice
- Goiter
- Hoarse cry, feeding problems, constipation, somnolence
- Delay in reaching normal milestones of development; short stature
- Coarse features with protruding tongue, broad flat nose, wide-set eyes
- Sparse hair and dry skin, protuberant abdomen with umbilical hernia
- Impaired mental development, retarded bone age
- Epiphyseal dysgenesis, delayed dentition

Laboratory tests

- Neonatal screening by measurement of serum TSH
- Imaging procedure: ultrasonography or ^{123}I scintigraphy
- Measurement of serum thyroglobulin and low molecular weight iodopeptides in urine to discriminate between various types of defects
- Measurement of neonatal and maternal autoantibodies as an indication of possible transient hypothyroidism

Treatment

Irrespective of the cause of congenital hypothyroidism, early treatment is essential to prevent cerebral damage. Sufficient T_4 should be given to maintain TSH in the normal range.

Further reading

Clyde PW, Harari AE, Getka EJ, et al. (2003). Combined levothyroxine plus liothyronine compared with levothyroxine alone in primary hypothyroidism: a randomized controlled trial. *JAMA* 290(22):2952–2958.

de Vijlder JJM, Vulsma T (2000). In DeGroot LJ, Jameson JL (ed.), *Endocrinology*, Vol. 2. Philadelphia: WB Saunders.

Escobar-Morreale HF, Botella-Carretero JI, Escobar del Rey F, et al. (2005). Treatment of hypothyroidism with combinations of levothyroxine plus liothyronine. *J Clin Endocrinol Metab* 90(8):4949–4954.

Escobar-Morreale HF, Botella-Carretero JI, Gomez-Bueno M, et al. (2005). Thyroid hormone replacement therapy in primary hypothyroidism: a randomized trial comparing L-thyroxine plus liothyronine with L-thyroxine alone. *Ann Intern Med* 142(6):412–424.

Roberts CG, Ladenson PW (2004). Thyroxine adherence in primary hypothyroidism. *Lancet* 363(9411):793–803.

Amiodarone and thyroid function

Background

Amiodarone is a potent antiarrythmic drug used to treat various tachyarrhythmias. It is a benzofuranic derivative with a high concentration of iodine, and it bears structural resemblance to thyroxine. Each 200 mg tablet contains approximately 75 mg of organic iodine.

Amiodarone is distributed in several tissues from where it is slowly released. In one study, terminal elimination half-life of amiodarone averaged 52.6 days with a standard deviation of 23.7 days.

Abnormalities of thyroid function occur in up to 14–18% of patients[1] (Table 8.1). In the UK and United States, 2% of patients on amiodarone develop thyrotoxicosis and about 13% develop hypothyroidism.

Patients residing in areas with high iodine intake develop amiodarone-induced hypothyroidism (AIH) more often than amiodarone-induced thyrotoxicosis (AIT), but AIT occurs more frequently in regions with low iodine intake. AIT can present several months after discontinuing the drug because of its long half-life.

Hypothyroidism is more common in women and in patients with thyroid autoantibodies.

Thyroid function tests should be monitored initially and then every 6 months in patients taking amiodarone.

Table 8.1 Thyroid function tests in clinically euthyroid patients after administration of amiodarone

Tests	1–3 months	>3 months
Free T_3	Decreased	Remains slightly decreased, but within normal range
TSH	Transient increase	Normal
Free T_4	Modest increase	Slightly increased compared to pretreatment values, may be in normal range or slightly increased.
Reverse T_3	Increased	Increased

1 Gopalan M, Burks J (2009). Thyroid dysfunction induced by amiodarone therapy: differential diagnoses and workup, *eMedicine* July 2, 2009.

Pathogenesis

The high iodine content of amiodarone may either inhibit thyroid hormone synthesis and release, thus causing AIH (failure to escape the Wolff-Chaikoff effect), or may result in iodine-induced thyrotoxicosis (Jod–Basedow phenomenon).

Thyrotoxicosis resulting from iodine excess and therefore increased hormone synthesis is referred to as *AIT type I*. Thyrotoxicosis due to a direct toxic effect of amiodarone is referred to as *AIT type II* (Table 8.2).

Drug-induced destructive thyroiditis results in leakage of thyroid hormones from damaged follicles into the circulation and, like subacute thyroiditis, can be followed by a transient hypothyroid state before euthyroidism is restored.

Table 8.2 Characteristics of AIT*

	AIT type I (10%)	AIT type II (90%)
Etiology	Iodine toxicity	Thyroiditis
Signs of clinical thyroid disease	Yes	No
Goiter	Frequent	Infrequent
Thyroid antibodies	Positive	Negative
Radioiodine uptake	Normal	Decreased
Thyroglobulin	Normal or slightly elevated	Very elevated
Serum IL6 (research test)	Normal	Very elevated
Late hypothyroidism	No	Possible
Vascularity (Doppler)	Increased/normal	Reduced

*Some patients have a mixed form and classification is not always possible.

Diagnosis and treatment

See Table 8.3. After chronic administration of amiodarone, a steady state is achieved, typically reflected in mild elevation of free T_4 and reduction in free T_3. Thus in clinically euthyroid patients on amiodarone, a slightly elevated T_4 is not indicative of hyperthyroidism, nor is a low T_3 indicative of hypothyroidism.

Hyperthyroidism is indicated by significantly ↑ free T_4, together with elevated free T_3 and suppressed serum TSH.

Hypothyroidism is indicated by elevation of TSH with low serum free T_4. See Box 8.1 for treatment.

Discontinuation of amiodarone does not always control the thyrotoxic state because of its long half-life (particularly in the obese) due to its very high volume of distribution and fat solubility.

Numerous complex published algorithms exist for management, but since classification into type I and type II is often difficult (see Table 8.2), in practice most patients are treated with ATDs ± glucocorticoids (see Table 8.4).

Table 8.3 Side effects and complications of amiodarone therapy

Side effect	Incidence (%)
Corneal microdeposits	100
Anorexia and nausea	80
Photosensitivity; blue/gray skin discoloration	55–75
Ataxia, tremors, peripheral neuropathy	48
Deranged liver function tests	25
Abnormal thyroid function tests	14–18
Interstitial pneumonitis	10–13
Cardiac arrhythmias	2–3

Box 8.1 Treatment of amiodarone-induced hypothyroidism

Underlying thyroid abnormality (usually Hashimoto's thyroiditis)
- Amiodarone therapy can be continued.
- Add thyroxine replacement therapy.

Apparently normal thyroid
- Discontinue amiodarone if possible and follow up for restoration of euthyroidism.
  - If amiodarone cannot be withdrawn, start thyroxine replacement therapy.

Table 8.4 Treatment of amiodarone-induced thyrotoxico-sis

	Type 1 AIT	Type 2 AIT
Step 1 Aim: restore euthyroidism	Methimazole up to 40 mg/day or propylthiouracil 400 mg/day. If possible, discontinue amiodarone*	Discontinue amiodarone if possible* Prednisone 40 mg/day In mixed forms, add methimazole or pro-pylthiouracil as in type 1 AIT
Step 2: Definitive treatment	Radioiodine treatment or thyroidectomy	Follow up for possible spontaneous progression to hypothyroidism

*If amiodarone cannot be withdrawn and medical therapy is unsuccessful, consider total thyroidectomy.

The first line of treatment is ATDs (methimazole or propylthiouracil). A combination of corticosteroids and ATDs may be effective in AIT type II. A high dose of prednisone, 40–60 mg daily, may be required for 8–12 weeks; studies where steroids have been discontinued after 2–3 weeks have been associated with a high relapse rate.

Potassium perchlorate may be of additional benefit, but it is currently not available in the United States

Radioiodine is not usually effective because of reduced uptake by the thyroid gland, reflecting the iodine load associated with the drug.

Surgery remains a very successful form of treatment, with euthyroidism being restored within a matter of days. Achieving preoperative euthy-roidism may be difficult, however.

Cardiac function may be compromised by propranolol used in combination with amiodarone, since this may produce bradycardia and sinus arrest.

Further reading

Bartalena L, Brogioni S, Grasso L, et al. (1996). Treatment of amiodarone-induced thyrotoxicosis, a difficult challenge: results of a prospective study. *J Clin Endocrinol Metab* 81:2930–2933.

Martino E, Bartalena L, Bogazzi F, et al. (2001). The effects of amiodarone on the thyroid. *Endocr Rev* 22(2):240–254.

Newman CM, Price A, Davies DW, et al. (1998). Amiodarone and the thyroid. *Heart* 79:121–127.

Wiersinga WM (1997) Amiodarone and the thyroid. In Weetman AP, Grossman A (eds.), *Pharmacotherapeutics of Thyroid Gland.* Berlin: Springer-Verlag, pp. 225–287.

Thyroid cancer

Epidemiology

Clinically detectable thyroid cancer is rare. It accounts for <1% of all cancer and <0.5% of cancer deaths. Thyroid microcarcinoma (diameter <1 cm) may be found in multinodular goiters.

Thyroid cancers are most common in adults aged 40–50 and are rare in children and adolescents. Women are affected more frequently than men.

See Table 9.1 for classification of thyroid cancer and Table 9.2 for a comparison of the various types of carcinoma.

Table 9.1 Classification of thyroid cancer

Cell of origin	Tumor type	Frequency (%)
Papillary	Differentiated	
	Papillary	>80
	Follicular	10
	Undifferentiated (anaplastic)	1–5
C cells	Medullary	5–10
Lymphocytes	Lymphoma	1–5

Table 9.2 Comparison of papillary, follicular and anaplastic carcinomas of the thyroid

Characteristic	Papillary Ca	Follicular Ca	Anaplastic Ca
Age at presentation	30–50 (mean 44)	40–50	60–80
Spread	Lymphatic	Hematogenous	Hematogenous
Prognosis	Good	Good	Poor
Treatment	Initially: near total thyroidectomy Postoperative TSH suppression High-risk patient: ^{131}I remnant ablation Postoperative total body radioiodine scan	Initially: near total thyroidectomy Postoperative TSH suppression ^{131}I remnant ablation Postoperative total body radioiodine scan	Total thyroidectomy with lymph node clearance Chemotherapy with doxorubicin and cisplatin External beam irradiation

Etiology

Irradiation

There does not appear to be a threshold dose of external irradiation for thyroid carcinogenesis; doses of 200–500 rad seem to produce thyroid cancer at a rate of about 0.5%/year.

There is no evidence that therapeutic or diagnostic ^{131}I administration can induce thyroid cancer, although there is a small increase in death rates from thyroid cancer after ^{131}I. At present it is unclear whether this is due to an effect of ^{131}I or part of the natural history of the underlying thyroid disease.

External irradiation at an age <20 years is associated with an increased risk of thyroid nodule development and thyroid cancer (most commonly papillary). The radioactive fallout from the Chernobyl nuclear explosion in 1986 resulted in a 4.7-fold increase in thyroid cancer in the regions of Belarus from 1985 to 1993, including a 34-fold increase in children. Most of these were papillary carcinomas.

The risk is greater for women and when irradiation occurs at a younger age.

There is a latency of at least 5 years with maximum risk at 20 years following exposure, though this was not seen following the Chernobyl disaster.

Other environmental factors

Most investigators agree that iodine supplementation has resulted in a decrease in the incidence of follicular carcinoma.

Genetic syndromes and oncogenes

RET/PTC1 proto-oncogene abnormalities in the long arm of chromosome 10 are associated with some papillary tumors (5–30%), especially after irradiation (60–80%). It is similar to the abnormality associated with medullary thyroid carcinoma in MEN2A.

Two new proto-oncogenes have been have been identified: *RET/PTC2* and *RET/PTC3* TRK (less common).

The tumor suppressor gene *p53* has been found to be mutated in some de-differentiated cancers.

Overexpression of the *ras* and *PTTG* oncogenes is found in papillary thyroid cancers. These were found to be markers for adverse prognosis.

c-myc mRNA expression has been correlated with histological markers of papillary cancer aggression.

Papillary microcarcinoma of the thyroid (PMC)

PMC is defined by the World Health Organization (WHO) as a tumor focus of 1.0 cm or less in diameter. It is detected coincidentally on histopathological examination of resected thyroid

Autopsy studies show the following:
- Prevalence ranges from 1 to 35.6%.
- No significant difference in the prevalence rates of PMC has been demonstrated between the sexes.
- PMC rarely progresses to clinically apparent thyroid cancer with advancing age.

- PMC can be multifocal.
- Cervical lymph node metastasis from PMC ranges from 4.3 to 18.2%.
- Lymph node metastasis was most often associated with multifocal tumors.

Although exposure to irradiation increases the likelihood of developing papillary thyroid cancer, the tumors will usually be >1.0 cm in diameter and thus not PMC.

Follow-up studies suggest that PMC is a slow-growing lesion that rarely spreads to distant sites and carries a good prognosis. The recommendations for treatment of PMC vary widely:

- The low morbidity and long survival mean that collection of randomized, prospective data has never been performed and comparisons of therapies are based on retrospective studies.
- The treatment of PMC should not cause more morbidity than the disease process itself.
- Surgical treatment recommendations range from simple excision to ipsilateral lobectomy.
- With adjuvant therapy, the consensus is routine use of T_4 but not the use of radioiodine, as there is no difference in the recurrence rate. There is some evidence to keep TSH below the reference range, but robust supporting data are not available.

Papillary thyroid carcinoma

Papillary carcinoma constitutes approximately 80% of all thyroid cancers. It is more common in women (3:1).

It is rare in childhood Peaks occur in the second and third decades and again in later life (bimodal frequency).

Incidence is 3–5 per 100,000 population.

Pathology

The carcinoma is slow growing and usually non-encapsulated and may spread through the thyroid capsule to structures in the surrounding neck, especially regional lymph nodes.

Recognized variants are follicular, papillary, dorsal, columnar cell, tall cell, and diffuse sclerosing.

It is confined to the neck in over 95% of cases, although 15–20% have local extra thyroidal invasion.

Metastases (1–2% of patients) occur via lymphatics to local lymph nodes and more distantly to lungs.

Histology

The tumor contains complex branching papilla that have a fibrovascular core covered by a single layer of tumor cells.

Nuclear features include the following:

- Large size with pale staining, "ground-glass" appearance (*Orphan Annie–eye nucleus*)
- Deep nuclear grooves

The characteristic and pathognomonic cytoplasmic feature is the *psammoma body*, which is a calcified, laminated, basophilic, stromal structure.

Staging of DTC

TNM

See Table 9.3.

Table 9.3 Tumor, node, metastasis (TNM) staging

	Patient age <45 years	Patient age >45 years
Stage I	Any T, any N, M0	T1, N0, M0
Stage II	Any T, any N, M1	T2, N0, M0
Stage III		T3, N0, M0
		T1, N1a, M0
		T2, N1a, M0
		T3, N1a, M0
Stage IVA		T4a, N0, M0
		T4a, N1a, M0
		T1, N1b, M0
		T2, N1b, M0
		T3, N1b, M0
		T4a, N1b, M0
Stage IVB		T4b, Any N, M0
Stage IVC		Any T, Any N, M1

Surgery

Indeterminate nodules
- Lobectomy as initial approach
- Total thyroidectomy if >4 cm, marked atypia on biopsy, "suspicious for papillary cancer," family history of thyroid cancer, history of radiation exposure, bilateral nodular disease

Malignancy
- Lobectomy if <1 cm, low-risk, unifocal, intrathyroidal papillary thyroid carcinomas (PTC) in the absence of prior head and neck irradiation or radiological or clinically involved cervical nodal metastases
- Total thyroidectomy if >1 cm unless contraindications

Completion thyroidectomy
- Offer completion thyroidectomy to all patients for whom a total thyroidectomy would have been recommended had the diagnosis been available before initial surgery (all patients with thyroid cancer except those with unifocal subcentimeter disease that was completely intrathyroidal and node negative)

Neck dissection
- Central (level VI) dissection for patients with clinically involved central or lateral neck lymph nodes
- Prophylactic central dissection in patients with T3, T4 PTC
- No central dissection for T1, T2 PTC when noninvasive, clinically node-negative PTCs/most follicular cancer
- Lateral neck dissection for biopsy-proven metastatic lateral cervical lymphadenopathy

Postoperative thyroid hormone therapy

For stage TNM I and II disease, the serum TSH concentration should be at or slightly below the lower half of the reference range (0.1–2.0 mU/L).

For stage III and IV disease, the serum TSH should be <0.1 mU/L.

The presence of heart disease or low bone density may necessitate a lower level of TSH suppression with smaller doses of thyroxine.

The dose also may be decreased to allow the TSH to rise into the normal range in low-risk patients who remain disease-free for 5 to 10 years after primary therapy.

Radioactive iodine therapy

Postoperative radioactive iodine (RAI) ablation is generally performed 1–3 months after total thyroidectomies without remnant thyroid tissue.

RAI is indicated for almost all nonpapillary histologies (i.e., follicular, Hurthle) as well as various papillary histologies (Table 9.4).

* High-risk features (think about when "selective use")

- Worrisome histological subtypes (tall cell, columnar, insular, solid, poorly differentiated)
- Intrathyroidal vascular invasion
- Gross or microscopic multifocal disease
- Recombinant TSH is used for routine RAI remnant ablation
- Levothyroxine (LT$_4$) withdrawal is used if patient has known gross residual disease or distant metastases
  - Discontinue LT$_4$ ~4 weeks before rechecking the TSH (must be >30 mU/L) and proceeding with RAI ablation or scanning.
  - Supplement with T$_3$ 25 mcg bid for 2 weeks after stopping T$_4$, followed by a 2-week T$_3$ withdrawal prior to RAI ablation.
  - LT$_4$ may be resumed on second or third day after RAI administration.
- The patient is placed on a low iodine diet for 1–2 weeks to facilitate the uptake of the radioisotope

Pretreatment scan

- Either 2–5 mCi 131-I with whole body scan (WBS) 48–72 hours later or 1.3–5 mCi 123-I with WBS 6–24 hours later (may be skipped if very low risk of metastases and the goal is to ablate remnants)

If using rTSH: obtain a 24-hour 123-I scan on day 3 prior to that day's administration of RAI ablation. For example:

- Day 1: rhTSI I 0.9 mg IM
- Day 2: rhTSH 0.9 mg IM + 1.5 mCi 123-I
- Day 3: pretreatment WBS then 150 mCi 131-I
- Day 10: post-treatment WBS

Dosing (maximum lifetime dose: 600–800 mCi)

- Low risk: 30–75 mCi (primarily patients under age 45 with tumors confined to the thyroid gland)
- Intermediate risk: 100 mCi
- High risk of recurrence or death: 100–150 mCi
- Pulmonary metastases: 150 to 200 mCi
- Skeletal metastases: 200 mCi

Post-treatment scan

A post-treatment scan is used to confirm tumor uptake of the treatment dose 2–8 days later.

Directions after treatment:

- <30 mCi: 5 feet distance for 7 days

Table 9.4 Major factors impacting decision making in remnant ablation

Factors	Description	Expected benefit			RAI ablation usually recommended	Strength of evidence
		Decreased risk of death	Decreased risk of recurrence	May facilitate initial staging and follow-up		
T1	1 cm or less, intrathyroidal or microscopic multifocal	No	No	Yes	No	E
	1–2 cm, intrathyroidal	No	Conflicting data[a]	Yes	Selective use[a]	I
T2	>2–4 cm, intrathyroidal	No	Conflicting data[a]	Yes	Selective use[a]	C
T3	>4 cm					
	<45 years old	No	Conflicting data[a]	Yes	Yes	B
	≥45 years old	Yes	Yes	Yes	Yes	B
	Any size, any age, minimal extrathyroidal extension	No	Inadequate data[a]	Yes	Selective use[a]	I

Factors	Description	Expected benefit				Strength of evidence
		Decreased risk of death	Decreased risk of recurrence	May faciliate initial staging and follow-up	RAI ablation usually recommended	
T4	Any size with gross extrathyroidal extension	Yes	Yes	Yes	Yes	B
Nx, N0	No metastatic nodes documented	No	No	Yes	No	I
N1	<45 years old	No	Conflicting data[a]	Yes	Selective use[a]	C
	>45 years old	Conflicting data	Conflicting data[a]	Yes	Selective use[a]	C
M1	Distant metastasis present	Yes	Yes	Yes	Yes	A

[a]Because of either conflicting or inadequate data, we cannot recommend either for or against RAI ablation for this entire subgroup. However, selected patients within this subgroup with higher risk features may benefit from RAI ablation (see modifying factors in the text).

Reprinted with permission from Cooper DS, Doherty GM, Haugen BR, et al. Revised American Thyroid Association Management Guidelines for Patients with Thyroid Nodules. Thyroid 2009; 19(11):1167–1214. The publisher for this copyrighted material is Mary Ann Liebert, Inc. publishers.

- >30–100 mCi: 10 feet distance for 7 days, sleep alone for 2 days, drink fluids
- Avoid IV contrast for 6–8 weeks, pregnancy for 6–12 months

Side effects
- *Short term:* nausea, local neck pain, dry mouth (salivary gland toxicity), bone marrow toxicity, pulmonary toxicity, gastritis, thyroiditis, salty saliva
- *Long term:* salivary and bone toxicity, secondary malignancies, fertility, teratogenicity, dry eyes/conjunctivitis. If xerostomia occurs, see dentist to avoid dental caries

Management of recurrent disease

Locoregional metastases
- Persistent or recurrent disease confined to the neck: therapeutic comprehensive lateral and/or central neck dissection
- Patients with recurrent disease who have already undergone prior comprehensive dissection or external beam radiation therapy (EBRT): limited lateral and/or central neck dissection

Aerodigestive invasion
- Surgery and RAI and/or EBRT

Pulmonary metastases
- RAI therapy 100–200 mCi repeated every 6–12 months as long as disease continues to concentrate RAI and respond clinically

Bone metastases
- Surgical resection (especially if age <45), RAI, glucocorticoids.
- If not amenable to surgery, RAI, EBRT, intra-arterial embolization, radiofrequency ablation (RFA), frequent pamidronate or zolendronate infusions

Brain metastases
- Surgical resection regardless of RAI avidity
- If not amenable to surgery, EBRT
- If RAI avid, RAI (with prior EBRT and concomitant glucocorticoid therapy)

Follicular thyroid carcinoma (FTC)

FTC constitutes 15% of all thyroid cancers. The mean patient age in most studies is 50 years. FTC is more common in women (2:1).

It is relatively more common in endemic goiter areas.

Pathology

Follicular carcinoma is a neoplasm of the thyroid epithelium that exhibits follicular differentiation and shows capsular or vascular invasion.

Differentiation of benign follicular adenoma from encapsulated low-grade or minimally invasive tumors is difficult, particularly for the cytopathologist, and therefore surgery is often necessary for a follicular adenoma. FTC may be minimally invasive or widely invasive.

Metastases (15–20% cases) are more likely to be spread by hematogenesis to the lung and bones and less likely to local lymph nodes.

Hurthle cell carcinoma is an aggressive type of follicular tumor with a poor prognosis because it fails to concentrate [131]I.

Treatment

Treatment is as for papillary thyroid carcinoma.

Follow-up of papillary and follicular thyroid carcinoma

For patients with differentiated thyroid cancer (DTC) who undergo subtotal thyroidectomy or total thyroidectomy without RAI:
- Follow periodic thyroglobulin (Tg) and perform ultrasound.
- Rising Tg over time is suspicious.

For DTC patients after undergoing total thyroidectomy and remnant ablation, the following schedule is recommended.

6–12 months
- Clinical examination, serum TSH, free thyroxine, neck ultrasound, thyroglobulin (Tg), and thyroglobulin antibodies while on T4
  - If the neck ultrasound is suspicious for lymph nodes or nodules >5–8mm, send for biopsy for cytology and Tg wash
    - If biopsy positive, send for compartment dissection
    - If biopsy negative, monitor size of lymph nodes or nodules
  - If the ultrasound is negative and TgAb are negative, send for rhTSH or THW Tg stimulation and diagnostic RAI WBS
    - If negative WBS but stimulated Tg>5–10, send for neck/check CT or PET/CT
      - If imaging negative, consider repeat 1–131 therapy
      - If imaging positive, consider surgery, 1–131 therapy, EBRT, clinical trial or tyrosine kinase inhibitor therapy
    - If negative WBS and stimulated Tg<5–10, monitor Tg and neck ultrasound. If Tg rising, consider repeat 1–131 therapy
    - If positive WBS, consider repeat 1–131 therapy
  - If the ultrasound is negative but Tg Ab are positive, follow TgAb and neck ultrasound

Years 2–10
- Clinical examination, measurements of serum free thyroxine, TSH, and thyroglobulin annually
- Neck ultrasonography every 1–2 years or less frequently in low-risk patients with no evidence of disease
- Thyrogen-stimulated Tg and WBS if serum Tg increases or there is other evidence of recurrence

Years 11–20
- Clinical examination and measurements of serum free thyroxine, TSH, and thyroglobulin annually
- Neck ultrasonography every 1–3 years or less frequently in low-risk patients with no evidence of disease
- Thyrogen-stimulated Tg and WBS if serum Tg increases or there is other evidence of recurrence

Years 21+

- Clinical examination and measurements of serum free thyroxine, TSH, and thyroglobulin annually
- Neck ultrasonography every 3–5 years or less frequently in low-risk patients with no evidence of disease
- Thyrogen-stimulated Tg and radioiodine imaging if serum Tg increases or there is other evidence of recurrence

---

Box 9.1 Thyroid cancer in children

- Uncommon, with an incidence of 0.2–5 per million per year
- >85% are papillary, but with more aggressive behavior than in adults (local invasion and distant metastases are more common)
- An ↑ incidence reported in children in Belarus and Ukraine following the Chernobyl nuclear accident in 1986. RET oncogene rearrangements are common in these tumors.
- Management is similar to that for adults, with a similar controversy as to the extent of initial surgery.
- Various studies report an overall recurrence rate of 0–39%; disease-free survival of 80–93%; and disease-specific mortality of 0–10%.
- Evidence is lacking on the independent risks or benefits of radioactive iodine or extensive surgery.
- Many investigators recommend lifelong follow-up with a combination of thyroglobulin and radionuclide scanning.

Thyroid cancer and pregnancy

The natural course of thyroid cancer developing during pregnancy may be different from that in nonpregnant women. Any woman presenting with a thyroid nodule during pregnancy appears to have an ↑ risk for thyroid cancer.

Evaluation should be undertaken with FNAC. Radioiodine scan is contraindicated.

Lesions <2 cm diameter or any lesion appearing after 24 weeks' gestation should be treated with TSH suppression and further evaluations carried out postpartum.

If FNAC is suspicious or diagnostic, operation should be performed at the earliest safe opportunity—generally the second trimester or immediately postpartum.

^{131}I ablation should be scheduled for the postpartum period and the mother advised to stop breast-feeding. She should avoid pregnancy for 6 months after any ^{131}I ablation.

Medullary thyroid carcinoma (MTC)

Also see Chapter 92, MEN type 2 (p. 503).

Accounts for 5–10% of all thyroid cancers. Should be managed by a dedicated regional service.

Presentation
- Lump in neck
- Systemic effects of calcitonin including flushing and diarrhea

Diagnosis
- FNAC
- Unsuspected at surgery
- Comprehensive family history and screening in search for features of MEN-2 is needed.
- Pathology specimens show immunostaining for calcitonin and staining for amyloid.

Management
- Baseline plasma calcitonin
- Baseline biochemical investigations for pheochromocytoma and hyperparathyroidism
- Genetic screening
- Staging with thoracoabdominal CT/MRI
- MIBG and pentavalent ^{99m}Tc DMSA scintography may also be used.

Treatment
- Total thyroidectomy and central node dissection is the preferred treatment modality.
- Germline RET mutation carriers should ideally undergo thyroidectomy before 5 years of age.

Adjuvant therapy
- Radioiodine and TSH suppression do not play a role.
- External radiotherapy and systemic chemotherapy have not been shown to be of benefit.
- Therapeutic MIBG may help in some cases.

Follow-up
All patients should have lifelong follow-up at the dedicated regional service.

Anaplastic (undifferentiated) thyroid cancer

- Rare
- Peak incidence: seventh decade. $\female:\male$ = 1:1.5
- Characterized by rapid growth of a firm/hard fixed tumor
- Often infiltrates local tissue such as larynx and great vessels and so does not move on swallowing. Stridor and obstructive respiratory symptoms are common.
- Aggressive, with poor long-term prognosis—7% 5-year survival rate and a mean survival of 6 months from diagnosis
- Optimal results occur following total thyroidectomy. This is usually not possible and external irradiation is used, sometimes in association with chemotherapy.

Lymphoma

- Uncommon
- Almost always associated with autoimmune thyroid disease (Hashimoto's thyroiditis). Occurs more commonly in women and in patients aged >40 years.
- Characterized by rapid enlargement of the thyroid gland
- May be limited to thyroid gland or part of a more extensive systemic lymphoma (usually non-Hodgkin's lymphoma). Trucut-needle biopsy may be required.
- Treatment with radiotherapy alone or chemotherapy if more extensive often produces good results.

Further reading

British Thyroid Association (2007). *Guidelines for the Management of Thyroid Cancer*, 2nd ed. London: Royal College of Physicians.

British Thyroid Association (nd). Guidelines/statement. Available at: www.british-thyroid-association.org/Guidelines/

Cooper DS, Doherty GM, Haugen BR, et al., for American Thyroid Association (2009). Revised American Thyroid Association management guidelines for patients with thyroid nodules. *Thyroid* 19(11):1167–1214.

Hay I, Wass JAH (2008). *Clinical Endocrine Oncology*, 2nd ed. Blackwell-Wiley. pp. 109–171.

Mazzaferri EL, Robbins RJ, Spencer CA, et al. (2003). A consensus report of the role of serum thryoglobulin as a monitoring method for low-risk patients with papillary thyroid carcinoma. *J Clin Endocrinol Metab* 88(4):1433–1441.

Sherman SI (2003). Thyroid carcinoma. *Lancet* 361(9356):501–511.

Wartofsky L, Sherman SI, Gopal J, et al. (1998). The use of radioactive iodine in patients with papillary and follicular thyroid cancer. *J Clin Endocrinol Metab* 83:4195–4203.Table 9.4 (*Contd.*)

Part 2

Pituitary

Janice M. Kerr

Pituitary gland anatomy and physiology

Embryology and anatomy

The anterior gland comprises ~2/3 of the pituitary gland and is derived from the oral ectoderm (Rathke's pouch). The posterior pituitary gland is derived from the diencephalon.

The pituitary gland resides in a portion of the sphenoid bone called the *sella turcica* and is covered by dura (diaphragma sella).

The pituitary gland is contiguous with the hypothalamus via the pituitary stalk. Anatomically, the pituitary gland is adjacent to several critical structures, including the optic chiasm (superiorly), the cavernous sinuses (laterally, and which contain the internal carotid arteries and cranial nerves [oculomotor(III), trochlear (IV), abducens (VI) and the trigeminal branches(V1 and V2]) and the sphenoid sinus (inferiorly).

The anterior pituitary gland is vascularized by superior hypophyseal arteries that form a capillary bed (hypophyseal-portal circulation) into which hypothalamic releasing and inhibitory factors are delivered.

The pituitary stalk and posterior pituitary gland receive direct arterial blood supply via the middle and inferior hypophyseal arteries.

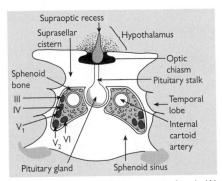

Fig. 10.1 The sellar region. Reproduced with permission from by Weatherall DJ, Ledingham JGG, and Warrell DA (Eds.) (1996). *Oxford Textbook of Medicine*, 3rd ed. Oxford: Oxford University Press.

Anterior gland physiology

See Table 10.1. The pituitary gland consists of five differentiated cell types that secrete six hormones important for growth, metabolism, stress responses and reproductive function.

Prolactin (PRL)

PRL is a single-chain polypeptide that belongs to the somatotropin/prolactin family. PRL has a diurnal pattern of secretion, with a sleep-associated augmentation of PRL levels.

Growth hormone (GH)

GH is a single-chain polypeptide of which the 22 KDa variant is the major isoform. Pulsatile GH secretions are usually undetectable in the serum apart from 5–6 noctural bursts, which occur during early sleep stages.

Luteinizing hormone and follicle stimulating hormone (LH/ FSH)

These are glycoprotein hormones with an α chain common to LH, FSH, TSH and hCG, but a β chain that is specific for each hormone. LH and FSH have complex pulsatile secretion patterns, particularly during puberty and across the menstrual cycle.

Thyroid stimulating hormone (TSH)

TSH is secreted in a circadian pattern and has increased pulse amplitudes at night.

Adrenocorticotropic hormone (ACTH)

ACTH is derived from a larger precursor polypeptide, proopiomelanocortin (POMC), which also encodes for β endorphins and melanocyte stimulating hormone. ACTH has a circadian pattern of secretion, with a peak level at 6–0 A.M. and a nadir level between 11 and 12 P.M. (with normal sleep-wake cycles).

Table 10.1 Anterior pituitary gland physiology

Cell Type (Hormone)	% Pit	+ Regulation	– Regulation	Targets	Effects
Somatotropes (growth hormone) GH	45–50	Growth hormone–releasing hormone (GHRH)	Insulin-like growth factor (IGF-1) and somatostatin	Liver, Cartilage, Muscle, Fat, Skin	Linear and somatic growth. Metabolism (lipids and proteins carbohydrates)
Lactotropes (prolactin) PRL	15–25 (↑ in pregnancy)	Thyrotropin-releasing hormone (TRH) and estrogen	Dopamine	Breast	Lactation
Gonadotropes (luteinizing hormone and follicle-stimulating hormone) FSH/LH	10–15	Gonadotropin-releasing hormone (GnRH) Estrogen-late follicular phase of menstrual cycle	Estrogen Progesterone Testosterone (on FSH) Inhibin	Gonads	Sex steroids production. Folliculogenesis and ovulation (♀) Spermatogenesis (♂)
Thyrotropes (thyroid-stimulating hormone) TSH	5–10	TRH	T_4, T_3, Somatostatin	Thyroid	Thyroid hormone production
Corticotropes (adrenocorticotropin) ACTH	15–20	Corticotropin-releasing hormone (CRH)	Cortisol	Adrenal gland	Glucocorticoid and DHEA production

Posterior gland physiology

The posterior pituitary gland secretes antidiuretic hormone and oxytocin, which are synthesized in the hypothalamic neurons of the supraoptic and paraventricular nuclei.

Antidiuretic hormone (ADH)

ADH is a nonapeptide that is released in response to hyperosmotic and hypovolemic stimuli. ADH acts on V2 renal collecting tubule receptors to mediate free water retention, and acts on V1 blood vessel receptors, at higher concentrations, to cause vasoconstriction. ADH also acts synergistically with corticotropin-releasing hormone (CRH) to augment ACTH release.

Oxytocin

In women, oxytocin facilitates uterine contraction, during parturition, and milk let-down in the post-partum period. In men, oxytocin has no known function but may aid in seminal vesicle contractions.

Further reading

Aron DC, Findling JW, Tyrrell JB (2007). Hypothalamus and pituitary gland. In Gardner DG, Shoback D (Eds.), *Greenspan's Basic and Clinical Endocrinology*, 8th ed, New York: McGraw Hill, pp. 101–140.

Imaging

Background

High-resolution, contrast-enhanced, thin-cut (3mm) magnetic resonance imaging (MRI) provides the optimal evaluation of the sellar and parasellar regions.

Coronal and sagittal T_1-weighted images, before and after gadolinium administration, are recommended. T_2-weighted imaging is usually unnecessary, but may assist in the diagnosis of cystic lesions. In addition, axial imaging may be helpful to define lateral extension with large tumors.

Computed tomography (CT) scans are most useful for patient with contra-indications to MRIs. In addition, they may demonstrate boney destruction and calcification with some tumors (e.g., meningiomas and craniopharyngiomas).

MRI appearances

See Figure 11.1.

The size, shape and signal characteristics of the pituitary gland vary with age, gender and physiological status. Non-contrasted T_1 images of the anterior pituitary gland are isointense with cerebral white matter, whereas the posterior pituitary gland appears hyperintense (as a bright spot), in most normal subjects.

Following contrast administration, the pituitary gland and stalk enhance, because they are below the blood–brain barrier.

▶ There is significant overlap in the imaging characteristics of adenomas, and other pituitary diseases such as craniopharyngiomas, inflammatory/infiltrative lesions and cysts.

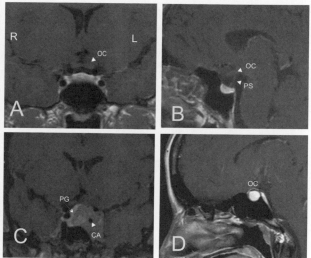

Fig. 11.1 Normal and abnormal pituitary MRI images. A. Normal coronal, post-contrast T_1 image showing optic chiasm (OC). B. Normal saggital image showing pituitary stalk (PS) and OC. C. Pituitary macroadenoma with evidence of pituitary gland (PG) compression, left cavernous sinus invasion, and encroachment of carotid artery (CA). D. Rathke's cleft cyst—bright T_1 image consistent with mucinous, proteinaceous or blood products.

Pituitary adenomas

See Figure 11.1.

Microadenomas are best appreciated on contrast-enhanced, T_1 weighted, coronal MRI images. They appear as hypointense signals, and often with associated pituitary gland asymmetry and stalk deviation (contralateral to the tumor).

Macroadenomas are characterized radiographically by their size and extrasellar extension. Important considerations include the proximity of the adenoma to the optic chiasm and any radiological evidence for cavernous sinus invasion. Macroadenomas are frequently heterogenous appearing and may undergo spontaneous necrotic and/or hemorrhagic changes. On T_1-weighted images:

- Low-intensity areas indicate necrotic or cystic changes.
- High-intensity signals indicate hemorrhage (particularly after the acute phase, days 1-2).
- The normal pituitary gland enhances more avidly with contrast than tumors, so is commonly seen as an enhanced signal that is peripherally located.

Craniopharyngioma/Rathke's cleft cyst

Craniopharyngiomas are typically suprasellar in location. They vary in content from cystic to mixed solid/cystic (most commonly) to predominantly solid. Imaging characteristics vary with the tumor composition. Calcifications are a distinguishing feature of adamantinomatous craniopharyngiomas, and are best detected by CT scans.

Rathke's cleft cysts (RCC) are typically intrasellar, but may extend into the suprasellar space. MRI images vary by cyst content from hypointense (with serous fluid), to hyperintense (with mucinous, proteinaceous or blood products) on T_1-weighted images.

Further reading

Naidich MJ, Russell EJ (1999). Current approaches to imaging of the sellar region and pituitary. *Endocrinol Metab Clin North Am* 28:45–79.

Pituitary function testing

Background

- Pituitary function is best assessed with basal concentrations of the pituitary hormones and their corresponding target gland hormones.
  - Pituitary hormone deficiency is established by a low target hormone level in the setting of a low, or an inappropriately normal pituitary hormone level. In equivocal cases, stimulation tests are used to assess the pituitary hormone reserve (e.g., Insulin tolerance test for GH deficiency).
  - Pituitary hormone excess (or less commonly, resistance to target organ hormone) is established by a high target hormone level in the setting of an inappropriately normal or a high pituitary hormone level. In equivocal cases, suppression tests are used to assess for a hyper-secretory state. (e.g., OGTT for acromegaly).

Lactotropes

Basal testing
Lactotrope function is best assessed by a fasting PRL level.

Dynamic testing
None is used.

Thyrotropes

Basal testing
Thyrotrope function is best assessed with concomitant TSH and circulating thyroid hormone levels (free T_4 and less commonly, T_3).

Dynamic testing
None is used; TRH is not commercially available in the United States.

Gonadotropes

Basal testing

Gonadotrope function is best assessed with concomitant gonadotropin (FSH and LH) and sex steroid levels: estradiol (in females) and testosterone (in males).

In premenopausal females, because the gonadotropin levels differ significantly across the menstrual cycle, hormone testing should be performed in the early follicular phase (days 1–5 after the onset of menses), when the LH and FSH levels are approximately equal.

In males, testosterone levels are best assessed in the early morning (7–9 A.M.), which corresponds to normal peak levels.

Dynamic testing

Gonadotropin-releasing hormone (GnHR) testing is most commonly used to assess pubertal disorders, particularly precocious puberty.

Corticotropes

Basal testing

Basal cortisol levels have a broad normal range: 3–18 mcg/dL. Random A.M. cortisol levels <3 mcg/dL indicate adrenal insufficiency, whereas levels >18 mcg/dL exclude adrenal insufficiency. A stimulation test is indicated for equivocal cortisol values to exclude adrenal insufficiency.

Midnight salivary or serum cortisol levels, which correspond to the normal nadir level, are used as screening tests for cortisol excess (Cushing's syndrome).

Stimulation testing

Insulin tolerance test (ITT) and metyrapone tests are the gold standards for assessing corticotrope deficiency.

The ITT is based on the physiological stressor of insulin-induced hypoglycemia on CRH–ACTH–cortisol activation (and GH release) and assesses the complete hypothalamic–pituitary–adrenal (HPA) axis.
- Test protocol: Insulin bolus (0.1-0.15 units/kg IV). Goal glucose <40 mg/dL. Normal serum cortisol >18 mcg/dL
- ITT has the disadvantages of being labor intensive, requiring close monitoring and having a number of important contraindications.

Contraindications to ITT

- Abnormal ECG
- Ischemic heart disease
- Seizures
- Elderly

Metyrapone test protocol: Metyrapone (30 mg/kg) is given at 11–12 P.M., and 11-dexocycortisol (DOC), ACTH and cortisol are measured the next morning.
- Normal response: 11-DOC >7 mcg/dL, ACTH >50 pg/mL and cortisol < 5 mcg/dL.
▶ Metyrapone must be obtained by written request from Novartis in the U.S.

- Cosyntropin stimulation test: The Synacthen® test is performed with synthetic ACTH (amino acids 1–24) which stimulates the adrenal glands See Box 12.1.
▶ Importantly, the Cosyntropin test is unreliable for assessing adrenal dysfunction attributable to acute CRH/ACTH deficiencies (within several weeks).

CRH test for Cushing's disease

Administration of 100 mcg of CRH (IV) leads to an exaggerated rise in cortisol (20%, above basal at 30/45 minutes (mean)) and ACTH (35% above basal at 15/30 minutes (mean)) in patients with Cushing's disease.

The test sensitivity and specificity are 91% and 88%, respectively.

Box 12.1 Cosyntropin stimulation test

- The test can be done at any time of the day.
- Prednisone and hydrocortisone, but **not** dexamethasone, interfere with the cortisol assay.
- Synacthen® is administered 250 mcg IV, and cortisol is measured at 0, 30 and 60 minutes.
- A normal post-stimulation cortisol level should increase to >18 mcg/dL.
- Controversy still exists regarding the utility of the low-dose (1 mcg) ACTH test, although this test is limited by the lack of a commercially-available preparation. In addition, a number of studies showed comparable test performance characteristics between the high-dose (250 mcg) and the low-dose ACTH tests.

Suppression tests for Cushing's syndrome

- 1 mg dexamethasone suppression test: 1 mg dexamethasone is given between 11 and 12 P.M., and a serum cortisol is drawn the following morning (8 A.M.).
  - Interpretation: cortisol <1.8 mcg/dL (with a sensitive cortisol assay) excludes Cushing's syndrome
- 8 mg dexamethasone suppression test is used to distinguish ectopic Cushing's from Cushing's disease. 8 mg dexamethasone is given at 11–12 P.M., and a random cortisol is drawn the following morning.
  - Interpretation: A ≥ 50% decreases in basal cortisol level is suggestive of CD, although ~20% of ectopic ACTH tumors (particularly bronchia Carcinoids) may suppress to this degree.
- DEX-CRH test is used to distinguish pseudo-Cushing's disease from Cushing's disease: Dexamethasone (0.5 mg q6h x 8 doses) starting at 12 noon, followed by CRH administration (1 mcg/kg) at 8 A.M. (2 hours after the final dexamethasone dose).
  - Normal cortisol suppression will be observed in pseudo-Cushing's disease: cortisol <1.4 mcg/dL (5-15 minutes after CRH), but not in Cushing's disease. Test sensitivity and specificity are 98% and 70%, respectively.

Somatotropes

Basal testing

Insulin-like growth factor-1 (IGF-1) represents integrated GH secretion and varies significantly with age and gender.

▶ IGF-1 is generally not a good indicator for GH deficiency in adults >40 years of age.

Random growth hormone levels are generally not useful unless very low (excludes acromegaly) or very elevated [(suggestive of acromegaly) and excludes growth hormone deficiency (GHD)].

Patients with ≥3 pituitary hormone deficiencies, and a low IGF-1 level, have a >95% probability of GHD and can generally forego GH stimulation testing.

Suppression test for acromegaly

Oral glucose (75 g) is given after an overnight fast, followed by serial GH measurements every 30 minutes × 2 hours. Normal response is GH <1 mcg/dL (with RIA) and <0.30 mcg/dL (with ultrasensitive GH assays).

Stimulation tests for growth hormone deficiency

The insulin tolerance test is the gold standard for GHD testing, although it has limited use because of the disadvantages stated above. GHRH plus arginine (Semorelin) is the second-best provocative test for GH deficiency, but is no longer commercially available in the U.S.

- **Glucagon and arginine**, although suboptimal GH secretagogues, are now commonly used to assess GHD.
- Glucagon test protocol: Glucagon-1 mg IM is given, followed by serial GH measurements q 30 minutes for **3 hours**.
  - Normal response: GH level >3 mcg/dL (using an ultrasensitive assay). Test sensitivity and specificity are >95%.
- Arginine test protocol: Arginine 0.5g/kg (max 30 g) in 100 mL normal saline is infused IV over 30 minutes, followed by serial GH measurements q 30 minutes for 2 hours.
  - Normal response: GH level >0.4 mcg/dL. Test sensitivity is 87% and specificity is 91%.

Further reading

Gasco V, Corneli G, Rovere S, Croce C, et al. (2008). Diagnosis of adult GH deficiency. *Pituitary* 11:121–128.
Kola B, Grossman AB. (2008). Dynamic testing in Cushing's syndrome. *Pituitary* 11:155–162.

Hypopituitarism

Definition

Hypopituitarism is defined as the partial or complete deficiency of one or more pituitary hormones from hypothalamic or pituitary gland diseases.

Etiologies of hypopituitarism

▶ Pituitary tumors and/or their treatments account for ~75% of cases (in adults)
- Radiotherapy—hypothalamus, pituitary, skull base tumors
- Pituitary infarction/hemorrhage
- Infiltrative diseases—sarcoidosis, lymphocytic hypophysitis hemochromatosis, Langerhans' cell histiocytosis, metastases.
- Infection—tuberculosis, pituitary abscess, meningitis
- Traumatic brain injury
- Isolated hypothalamic releasing hormone deficiency—e.g., Kallmann's syndrome is congenital GnRH deficiency + anosmia
- Parasellar tumors—craniopharyngiomas, meningiomas, chordomas, gliomas, schwanomas
- Congenital pituitary transcription factor mutations: *POU1F1* gene mutations (GH, PRL, and TSH deficiencies). *PROP1* gene mutations (GH, PRL, TSH, FSH/LH ± ACTH deficiencies). Isolated ACTH deficiency (very rare)

Features

The clinical features of hypopituitarism depend on the severity of the hormone deficiency (from partial to complete) and the rate of development (from acute to chronic) (see Table 13.1).

▶The loss of anterior pituitary hormone function, from pituitary diseases and/or their treatments, generally follows a predictable order:

GH ≈ GnRH > ACTH ≈ TSH > PRL

- ADH deficiency is very rare with pituitary adenomas.
- The clinical features of hypopituitarism are generally similar to those of target gland insufficiency. A notable exception is the lack of pigmentation and hyperkalemia in secondary adrenal insufficiency vs. primary adrenal insufficiency.
- *Houssay phenomenon* is defined as the improvement of diabetes mellitus in patients with hypopituitarism due to a reduction in counterregulatory hormones (GH and cortisol).

Apoplexy

Apoplexy is the clinical syndrome of sudden headache, visual impairment, ophthalmoplegia, and/or altered mental status caused by hemorrhage or infarction of the pituitary gland. It occurs in ~10–15% of pituitary adenomas. Subclinical apoplexy is more common than clinically-apparent disease.

Treatment

Surgical decompression is indicated for patients with severe neuro-ophthalamologic signs, such as severely reduced visual acuity or a deteriorating level of consciousness. Secondary adrenal insufficiency complicates up to 70% of apoplectic patients, and is a major cause of morbidity and mortality in untreated cases.

Stress-dose glucocorticoids (50–100 mg IV hydrocortisone q 6–8 hours) are indicated for patients with proven or presumptive adrenal insufficiency (i.e., hemodynamic instability). Panhypopituitarism is common and should be evaluated and managed expectantly after an acute apoplectic event.

Empty sella syndrome (ESS)

ESS is defined as a sella that is partially or completely filled with CSF.
- Primary ESS is most often due to arachnoid herniation through a congenital diaphragmatic defect. Hyperprolactinemia occurs in ~10% of cases, but hypopituitarism is uncommon.
- Secondary ESS is due to a pituitary tumor and/or its treatment (e.g., apoplexy, surgery or radiotherapy). Hypopituitarism is common with this condition.

Traumatic brain injury (TBI)

TBIs associated with subarachnoid hemorrhage and skull-based fractures have a high incidence of hypopituitarism. In addition, patients with moderate-to-severe head traumas are also at increased risk for hypopituitarism. The most common deficiencies are GH and gonadotropins (10–15% of cases), and these are best assessed at 6–12 months, post-TBI.

Table 13.1 Clinical features of pituitary hormone deficiencies

Hormone deficiency	Clinical features
GH →↓ IGF-1	*In children:* short stature, decreased somatic maturation (e.g., bones and muscles)
	In adults: altered body composition (e.g., increased central adiposity/fat mass and reduced lean body mass), fatigue, reduced exercise capacity, impaired psychological well-being, reduced bone mineral density, pro-atherogenic lipid profile (↑ cardiovascular risk)
LH/FSH →↓ T and E	*In children:* delayed puberty
	In women: anovulatory cycles, oligo- or amenorrhea, vaginal dryness/atrophy, dyspareunia, hot flashes and breast atrophy
	In men: reduced libido, erectile dysfunction, testicular atrophy and decreased muscle mass and strength
	In both sexes: infertility, decreased bone mineral density and decreased body hair
ACTH →↓ cortisol ↓DHEA-S	Features as in Addison's disease, except lack of hyperpigmentation and hyperkalemia (📖 p. 196) *Acute:* fatigue, anorexia, weight loss, nausea, vomiting, abdominal pain, hypoglycemia and circulatory collapse *Chronic:* fatigue, weight loss, decreased axillary/pubic hair, decreased libido, myalgias and arthralgias
TSH →↓ T4/T3	Fatigue, dry skin, cold intolerance, constipation, weight gain, irregular menses (women), hair loss, brittle nails, bradycardia and normocytic anemia
PRL	Failure of lactation

Investigations

Basal levels

Basal concentrations of the anterior pituitary hormones and their target organ hormones should be measured. Pituitary hormone deficiencies are characterized by low levels of target hormones in the setting of low or inappropriately normal pituitary hormone levels.

- TSH and free T_4
- ACTH and A.M.Cortisol
- PRL
- LH, FSH, A.M. testosterone (♂), estradiol (♀)
- GH, IGF-1

Dynamic pituitary hormone testing

This testing is done to assess for GHD and adrenal insufficiency (📖 see p. 92).

Posterior pituitary function

- Serum sodium, serum osmolality, urine osmolality and 24-hour urinary volume
- A formal water deprivation test should be performed in cases of suspected diabetes insipidus.

Treatment

Hypopituitarism treatment involves management of the underlying etiology, and hormone replacement as indicated (📖 see p. 99)

Further reading

Marinis L, Bonadonna AB, Maira G, Giustina A (2005). Extensive clinical experience. Primary empty sella. *J Clin Endocrinol Metab* 90:5471–5477.

Popovic V, Aimaretti G, Casanueva FF, Ghigo E (2005). Hypopituitarism following traumatic brain injury. *Growth Hormone IGF Res* 15:177–184.

Toogood AA, Stewart PM (2008). Hypopituitarism: clinical features, diagnosis and management. *Endocrinol Metab Clin North Am* 37:235–261.

Rajasekaran S, Vanderpump M, Baldeweg WD, Narendra R, et al. (2011). UK guidelines for the management of pituitary apoplexy. *Clinic Endo* 74:9–20.

Anterior pituitary hormone replacement

Background
Anterior pituitary hormone deficiencies are usually repleted with the target hormones. Exceptions are GH replacement in adults, and gonadotropin replacement for fertility treatment.

Glucocorticoid replacement
See Table 14.1.
- Patients with ACTH deficiency need only glucocorticoid replacement, as mineralcorticoid secretion, via the renin–angiotension–aldosterone axis, is still intact.
- Prednisone and hydrocortisone are the most commonly used medications. Dexamethasone is generally avoided in secondary adrenal deficiency because of its long half-life (36 hours), and non-physiological profile.
- The goal for replacement is the lowest possible glucocorticoid dose that eliminates clinical features of glucocorticoid deficiency (see Table 13.1), and also avoids clinical signs and symptoms of glucocorticoid excess (e.g. Cushingoid features, weight gain, hypertension, dyslipidemia, impaired glucose tolerance and decreased bone mineral density).

⚠ Patients with concomitant thyroid hormone deficiency should initiate glucocorticoid replacement first, because T_4 accelerates cortisol metabolism and may precipitate an adrenal crisis.

Safety and stress-dose steroids
Patients with adrenal insufficiency should be encouraged to carry appropriate medical identification and should also be instructed in the indications for increased glucocorticoid dosing, as follows:
- Mild disease without fever: no change in glucocorticoid replacement
- Febrile illness: double or triple the replacement dose for the duration of fever. "3 × 3" day rule
- Vomiting or diarrhea: parenteral therapy and seek medical assistance
- Minor surgery (e.g., under local anesthetic, arthroscopy, dental procedure): 25 mg hydrocortisone at the time of the procedure, then usual replacement dose.
- Moderate surgical stress (e.g., cholecystectomy, joint replacement): 50–75 mg hydrocortisone QD × 2 days, then usual replacement dose
- Severe illness/major operation: parenteral therapy (IV) hydrocortisone 50–100 mg q6–8h × 2–3 days, with subsequent taper to maintenance glucocorticoid dose

Table 14.1 Pituitary hormone replacement regimens

Hormone or drug	Dosage
Hydrocortisone or	15–25 mg/day (in 2–3 divided doses)10–15 mg on waking, 5 mg at early afternoon
Prednisone	5–7.5 mg on waking
L-thyroxine (T$_4$)	1.6 mcg/kg/day replacement dose
GH	Age <30 years 400–500 mcg/day Age 30–59 years 300 mcg/dayAge >60 years 100–200 mcg/day
Estrogen/progesterone/testosterone	Formulation dependant
dDAVP	Intranasal spray (10 mcg BID) or oral tablets (100 mcg BID) are standard starting doses

Growth hormone replacement

✒ GH replacement has been approved for use in adult since 1996, but is still somewhat controversial regarding the cost–benefit ratio relative to other medical therapies for GHD-related comorbidities.

GH therapy is most likely to benefit those patients who have severe clinical and biochemical manifestations of GH deficiency.

Treatment and Monitoring

- Start with a low, age-appropriate GH dose, and titrate according to clinical response, IGF-1 levels and side effects.
- Goal: IGF-1 in the upper half of the normal range for age and gender
- Annual lipid level, fasting blood sugar, DEXA scans (every 1–2 years)
- Reversible, dose-dependent side effects: peripheral edema, headaches hypertension, arthralgias, carpal tunnel syndrome, impaired glucose tolerance or diabetes

► In general, premenopausal women and women taking oral estrogens require higher GH doses than do males, because estrogen antagonizes GH at the liver.

⚠ GH increases the conversion of T$_4$ to T$_3$, so GH replacement may decrease free T$_4$ levels. In addition, GH increases cortisol metabolism to cortisone, so GH replacement may unmask subclinical adrenal insufficiency.

Thyroid hormone replacement

This is as discussed in the section on primary hypothyroidism (📖 p. 58).

Monitoring

In central hypothyroidism, unlike in primary hypothyroidism, the TSH level cannot be used to assess the adequacy of thyroid hormone replacement, and instead the free T_4 level is used exclusively for monitoring.

• The free T_4 level should be maintained in the upper half or third of the normal range.

Sex hormone replacement

• 📖 See Hormone replacement therapy in females (p. 268).
• 📖 Androgen replacement therapy in males (p. 296).
• 📖 Fertility treatment in males and females (p. 324–325).

Further reading

Auernhammer CJ, Vlotides G (2007). Anterior pituitary hormone replacement therapy—a clinical review. *Pituitary* 10:1–15.

Crown A, Lightman S (2005). Why is the management of glucocorticoid deficiency still controversial: a review of the literature. *Clin Endocrinol* 63:483–492.

Molitch ME, Clemmons DR, Malozowski S, Merriam GR, et al. (2006). Evaluation and treatment of adult growth hormone deficiency: an Endocrine Society clinical practice guideline. *J Clin Endocrinol Metab* 91:1621–1634.

Pituitary tumor basics

Epidemiology

- Pituitary adenomas are the most common pituitary disease in adults (Box 15.1).
- Approximately 10% of the population harbors incidental adenomas, most commonly microadenomas (<5 mm).
- Clinically-apparent pituitary disease occurs in an estimated ~1:10,000 people/year.
- Pituitary carcinomas are very rare (<0.1% of tumors), and but most commonly involve ACTH and PRL-secreting tumors.

Classification

Size

- Microadenoma <1 cm
- Macroadenoma >1 cm

Box 15.1 Lesions of the sellar turcica and parasellar regions

Pituitary adenomas
(>90% of sellar lesions)
- Prolactinoma
- Gonadotropinoma
- Null cell adenoma
- GH-secreting adenoma
- ACTH-secreting adenoma
- TSHoma

Cell rest tumors
- Rathke's cleft cyst
- Craniopharyngioma
- Chordoma/chondrosarcoma
- Epidermoid cyst

Benign lesions
- Meningiomas
- Gangiocytoma
- Hypothalamic hamartoma
- Schwannoma

Granulomatous, infectious, inflammatory lesions
- Abscess
- Sarcoidosis
- Tuberculosis
- Histiocytosis X
- Granulomatous disease
- Lymphocytic hypophysitis

Metastatic tumors

Vascular aneurysms

Miscellaneous
- Empty sella syndrome
- Arachnoid cyst
- Gliomas, Germ cell tumor
- Lymphoma

Functional status

This is defined by clinical and biochemical evidence of hormone excess.

Tumor Types and Distribution

- Nonfunctioning adenomas (bonadotropinoma/null cell adenoma) 30–35%
- Prolactinoma: 35–40%
- Growth hormone adenoma (acromegaly): 10–15%
- ACTH adenoma (Cushing's disease): 10–15%
- TSH adenoma: <2%

Mass effects

Common with macroadenomas and include the following:

- Headache
- Visual field defects (uni- or bitemporal quadrantanopia or hemianopia)
- Hypopituitarism
- Ophthalmoplegia/cranial nerve palsies (CN III, IV and VI)
- Vision loss (optic nerve atrophy)
- CSF rhinorrhea (rarely from inferior tumor extension)

Pathophysiology

- Adenomas are monoclonally-derived tumors, and they are categorized by their hormone expression, as determined by clinical/biochemical features and immunohistochemical staining (on surgically-resected pathology specimens).
- The most important oncogene involved in sporadic pituitary adenomas tumorgenesis is *gsp*-which encodes a constitutively-active mutation in the α-subunit of the stimulatory G protein. This mutation occurs in ~40% of GH tumors.
- Various other mutations, including: growth factor receptors (FGFR4), tumor suppressor genes (ZAC, MEG3, menin, GADD45γ), oncogenes (PTTG), cell signaling pathways (BMP-4), and cell cycle regulators (p53, p27, p16, p18, cyclin D/E), have been detected in pituitary adenomas but do not account for most mutations. In addition, RAS mutations occur in rare pituitary carcinomas.
- Inheritable diseases associated with pituitary tumors are uncommon (<5%) and include MEN-1, McCune–Albright syndrome, Carney's complex and familial somatotropinoma syndromes. PRL- and GH-secreting tumors are the most common tumor types.

Investigations

- For microadenomas, evaluate clinically and biochemically for hormone excess. Check basal PRL TSH, free T4, FSH, LH, testosterone (in males), estradiol (in females) and IGF-1 levels. Screen for Cushing's disease if clinically indicated (see , 📖 p. 118).
- For macroadenomas, assess for hormone excess and deficiencies.
- Conduct formal visual field tests for patients with subjective vision loss and with tumors that abut the optic chiasm.

Management and natural history

Adenomas with excess hormone secretion (of any size) and non-functioning macroadenomas associated with mass effects require treatment.

- Medical therapy, with dopamine agonists, is first-line therapy for prolactinomas (micro- or macroadenomas).
- Transsphenoidal resection is indicated for all other functioning and non-functioning tumor types.
- For patients without specific indications for treatment, periodic MRI surveillance is recommended.
- Approximately 10% of incidentally-detected microadenomas and ~30–50% of macroadenomas will significantly enlarge, without treatment, over a 8 year period.

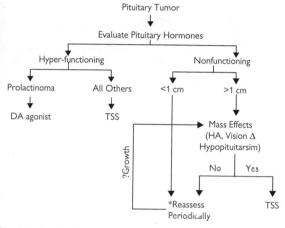

Fig. 15.1 Algorithm for pituitary tumor evaluation. * Reassessment period varies by tumor size and clinical status, but generally includes annual MRIs, particularly for macroadenomas. Transsphenoidal surgery (TSS) is recommended for continued macroadenoma growth, before the development of adverse mass effects.

Further reading

Asa SL, Ezzat S (2002). The pathogenesis of pituitary tumors. *Nat Rev Cancer* 2:836–849.

Karavitaki N, Collison K, Halliday J, Byrne JV, Price P, Cudlip S, Wass JA (2007). What is the natural history of nonoperated nonfunctioning pituitary adenomas? *Clin Endocrinol* 67:938–943.

Molitch ME (2009). Pituitary tumors: pituitary incidentaloma. *Best Pract Res Clin Endocrinol Metab* 23:667–675.

Dekkers OM, Pereira AM & Romijn JA (2008). Treatment and follow-up of clinically nonfunctioning pituitary macroadenomas. *J Clin Endocrinol Metab* 93:3717–3726.

Prolactinomas

Epidemiology

- Prolactinomas account for ~35–40% of pituitary tumors and are the most common functioning tumor
- Female-predominance 10:1, ♀:♂
- Microadenomas are more common in females, whereas macroadenomas are more common in males at the time of presentation.

Etiology/pathogenesis

See Box 16.1 for causes of hyperprolactinemia.

Prolactinomas are the most common pituitary tumor in MEN-1, occur in 20% of cases, and may be more aggressive than sporadic prolactinomas.

Clinical features

Hyperprolactinemia effects (microadenomas and macroadenomas)

- Galactorrhea (up to 90% of women, <10% of men)
- Hyperprolactinemia inhibits GnRH release, leading to hypogonadotropic hypogonadism.
- Women present with menstrual disturbance—amenorrhea, oligomenorrhea, reduced libido and infertility.
- Men present with loss of libido, erectile dysfunction and in fertility. Gynecomastia is uncommon.
- Hyperprolactinemia is associated with a long-term risk of ↓ bone mineral density.
- Hyperprolactinemia was an adverse effect on libido, independent from hypogonadism.

Mass effects (macroadenomas only).

- Headaches
- Visual field defects (uni- or bitemporal field defects)
- Hypopituitarism
- Cranial nerve palsies from cavernous sinus invasion
- Rarely, CSF leak or meningitis from tumor invasion of the sphenoid bone

Box 16.1 Causes of hyperprolactinemia

Physiological
- Pregnancy
- Sexual intercourse
- Nipple stimulation, suckling
- Physical and/or psychological stressors

Pituitary tumors
- Prolactinomas
- Mixed GH/PRL tumor
- Macroadenoma-related stalk compression

Parasellar causes
- Hypothalamic disease—stalk compression (craniopharyngioma, meningioma, germinoma, glioma)
- Infiltration—sarcoidosis, Langerhans' cell histiocytosis
- Pituitary Stalk section—traumatic head injury, neurosurgery
- Empty sella syndrome

Drug treatment
- Dopamine receptor antagonists (metoclopramide, domperidone)
- Neuroleptics (phenothiazines, butyrophenones, thioxanthenes, risperidone, molindone, olanzapine)
- Antidepressants (tricyclics, monoamine oxidase inhibitors, selective serotonin reuptake inhibitors)
- Antihypertensive drugs—verapamil, methyldopa, reserpine.
- Opiates and cocaine
- Estrogens

Metabolic
- Primary hypothyroidism—TRH increases PRL
- Chronic renal failure—reduced PRL clearance
- Severe liver disease—disordered hypothalamic regulation

Other
- Chest wall lesions—zoster, burns, trauma (stimulation of suckling reflex)
- Idiopathic hyperprolactinemia
- Macroprolactin (Ig6: PRL complex)

Investigations

Serum PRL
- Normative PRL levels differ by gender and are slightly higher in females (e.g., 20–25 ng/mL in females, and 15–20 ng/mL in males).
- A slightly elevated PRL may represent a stress response or a pulsed secretion and should be confirmed with additional PRL measurements.
- Serum PRL levels >100–150 ng/mL are suggestive of pituitary prolactinomas, whereas lower PRL levels are generally more consistent with non-tumoral etiologies (e.g., medications, renal insufficiency, stalk effect) or very small prolactinomas.
- PRL levels generally trend with adenoma size.
▶ Exclude GH co-secretion with a prolactinoma (20–25% of tumors) as clinically indicated.

Issue with PRL measurements

Hook effect
This is a lab artifact of a two-site immunoassay is which very high PRL levels (most commonly from giant [>4 cm] prolactinomas) saturate both the capture and the detection antibodies and prevent "sandwich" complex formation. The PRL levels are spuriously normal or only slightly elevated.
▶ PRL assays of large tumors, and suspected prolactinomas, should be performed as a 1:100–1000 diluted serum sample.

Hyperprolactinemia and drugs

Antipsychotics and antidepressants are among the most common medications that cause hyperprolactinemia (dopamine agonists are contraindicated with psychiatric diseases). For cases of medication-induced hyperprolactinemia that are complicated by hypogonadotropic hypogonadism, consideration could be given, under the guidance of a psychiatrist or a mental health professional, to a trial of an alternate psychiatric medication that is not associated with hyperprolactinemia. Alternatively, the hypogonadism could be treated with sex steroid replacement.

Idiopathic hyperprolactinemia

Hyperprolactinemia of unclear etiology is designated *idiopathic* but is likely due to an undetected microprolactinoma on imaging or to hypothalamic dysregulation. PRL normalizes in ~1/3 of idiopathic cases.

Treatment

Aims of therapy

Microprolactinomas
- Restoration of normal gonadal function and libido
- Relief from galactorrhea

Macroprolactinomas
- Reduction in tumor size and prevention of tumor growth
- Clinical improvement in signs and symptoms of tumor mass effects (e.g., headaches, vision impairment or hypopituitarism)
- Restoration of normal gonadal function and libido

Drug therapy—dopamine agonists

Dopamine agonist (DA) treatment (📖 see Dopamine agonists, p. 144) is first-line medical therapy for patients with prolactinomas and normalizes prolactin levels, and significantly decreases tumor size in >90% of cases. Dopamine agonist resistance is uncommon (see Box 16.2)

- *Cabergoline* (Dostinex) is the preferred therapy because of its greater efficacy at normalizing PRL levels and decreasing tumor size than bromocriptine. In addition, cabergoline is better tolerated and requires less frequent dosing (twice weekly).
- *Bromocriptine* (Parlodel) is recommended for women seeking fertility, because of the greater safety data in pregnancy.
- *Monitoring*: Adjust DA agonist every 1–2 months as needed to maintain PRL in the normative range. Repeat MRI at ~6–12 months, particularly with macroadenomas, to ensure that the tumor size decreases with the PRL levels. PRL normalization generally precedes a decreased tumor size by several weeks to months.

Sex steroids

Estrogen/progesterone replacement (in females) or testosterone therapy (in males), rather than dopamine agonist therapy, may be appropriate

---

Box 16.2 Dopamine agonist resistance

- *General definition:* failure to normalize prolactin and/or failure to decrease tumor size by <50%. More commonly, drug non-compliance or drug intolerance lead to an erroneous diagnosis of DA resistance.
- *Prevalence:* resistance is observed in ~11% and 5–10% of cabergoline-treated patients, respectively.
- *Etiology:* reduced tumor D_2 receptors concentration
- *Treatment options:* switch dopamine agonists, increase dose as tolerated, surgery, fertility treatment, sex steroid replacement or radiation therapy (for macroprolactinomas)

for patients with idiopathic hyperprolactinemia or microprolactinomas in whom fertility, galactorrhea and/or decreased libido are not of concerns.

Surgery

📖 See Transsphenoidal surgery (p. 140).

Transsphenoidal surgery is second-line therapy and is indicated for patients who are resistant to, or intolerant of, dopamine agonists. In addition, prolactinoma patients who have severe or vision-threatening apoplexy that is unresponsive to initial medical management are also potential surgical candidates.

- The surgical success rates vary by the tumor size, the neurosurgery expertise and previous treatment, but range between 73.3 ± 10.7% for microadenomas and 38.0 ± 21.3% for macroadenomas (in large surgical series).

Radiotherapy

📖 See Radiation therapy for pituitary tumors (p. 147).

Radiation therapy is generally indicated for patients with residual or recurrent prolactinomas after failed medical and surgical approaches.

Long-term management (see Box 16.3)

Pituitary Society Guidelines support attempted DA dose reduction or discontinuation if, after ~2 years of medical therapy, the PRL level remains normal and the MRI shows a marked tumor reduction.

- PRL should then be closely monitored for recurrence, which is usually observed in the first several months after drug withdrawal. The best predictor of reoccurrence is the presence of residual tumor on MRI.
- In cases of DA re-initiation or long-term use, patients should be maintained on the lowest possible DA dose that achieves the desired treatment goals.

Box 16.3 Cabergoline and cardiac valvulopathy

- Cabergoline, but not bromocriptine is a 5-hydroxytryptamine 2B receptor agonist.
- High doses of cabergoline (e.g., 3 mg/day for ≥6 months in Parkinson's patients) have been associated with valvular heart disease (aortic, mitral, and tricuspid regurgitations) via a 5-HT2B off-target effect.
- The risk of cardiac valvulopathy appears to be low in prolactinoma patients on standard doses of cabergoline (≤2 mg/week).
- For patients requiring higher cabergoline doses, annual clinical cardiac exams are warranted, and consideration should be given to periodic echocardiograms.

Management of prolactinomas in pregnancy

📖 See Prolactinoma in pregnancy (p. 354).

Further reading

Casanueva FF, Molitch ME, Schlechte JA, Abs R, et al. (2006). Guidelines of the Pituitary Society for the diagnosis and management of prolactinomas. *Clin Endocrinol* 65(2):265–273.

Cheung D, Heaney A (2009). Dopamine agonists and valvular heart disease. *Curr Opin Endocrinol Diabetes Obes* 16:316–320.

Colao A (2009). The prolactinoma. *Best Pract Res Clin Endocrinol Metab* 23:575–596.

Molitch ME (1992). Pathologic hyperprolactinemia. *Endocrinol Metabo Clin North Am* 21:877–910.

Molitch ME (2008). Drugs and prolactin. *Pituitary* 11:209–218.

Klibanski A (2010). Prolactinomas. *N Engl J Med* 362:1219–26.

Acromegaly

Definition

Acromegaly is the clinical condition resulting from prolonged exposure to excessive GH/IGF-1 levels in adults.

Epidemiology

Estimated annual incidence is 3–4 cases/million population. There is equal sex distribution. Acromegaly has an insidious onset which often results in a delayed diagnosis (~7–10 years).

Etiologies of acromegaly

- Pituitary adenoma (95% of cases)

Rare causes of GH excess
- GHRH secretion—hypothalamic tumor (gangliocytoma)
- Ectopic GHRH—carcinoid tumors (e.g., pancreas, lung), pheochromocytoma and medullary thyroid cancer
- Ectopic GH secretion—pancreatic islet cell tumor and lymphoma

Pathophysiology

- Constitutively-active mutations of the α-subunit of the stimulatory G protein are seen in ~30–40% of densely granulated GH tumors.
- Familial syndromes: MEN-1, Carney complex, and McCune–Albright syndrome can manifest with GH tumors in ~10% of cases.
- Isolated familial somatotropinomas are associated with aryl hydrocarbon receptor interacting protein (AIP gene) mutations in ~10–15% of cases.

Clinical features

The clinical features arise from the somatic and metabolic effects of prolonged excess GH/IGF-1 exposure.

Symptoms
- Hyperhidrosis (↑ Sweating)
- Headaches—independent of tumor effect

- Fatigue
- Arthralgias
- Increased ring or shoe size
- Carpal tunnel syndrome
- Muscle weakness and myopathy

Signs

- Facial appearance: coarse, acral features, frontal bossing, enlarged nose, deep nasolabial furrows, prognathism, jaw malocclusion and ↑ interdental spacing
- Deep voice: laryngeal thickening
- Macroglossia
- Musculoskeletal changes: enlargement of hands and feet, large joint and axial arthropathy, osteopenia/osteoporosis
- Goiter and other visceromegaly: liver, spleen, kidney, prostate
- Skin changes: oily skin, acanthosis nigricans, skin tags

Complications

- Hypertension
- Insulin resistance: impaired glucose tolerance and diabetes mellitus
- Sleep apnea: 1/3 central and 2/3 obstructive
- Kyphosis and vertebral fractures (attributable to hypogonadism)
- Hypertriglyceridemia
- Cardiovascular diseases: cardiomyopathy, arrhythmias, valvular heart disease and congestive heart failure
- Colonic polyps and colon cancer: slightly ↑ risk

Mass effects of tumor

- Visual field defects
- Hypopituitarism

Investigations

Insulin-like growth factor-1 (IGF-1)

IGF-1 is the single best screening test for acromegaly (Fig. 17.1). IGF-1 has a long half-life (18–20 hours), reflects integrated GH secretion, and correlates with clinical features of acromegaly. It is important to use age- and gender-based normative ranges for IGF-1.

▶ Etiologies for false negative (low) IGF-1 levels include: malnutrition, hypothyroidism, poorly controlled type I diabetes mellitus (DM), and chronic liver disease.

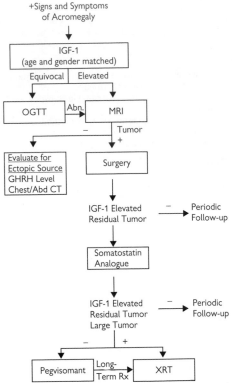

Fig. 17.1 Algorithm for the evaluation and management of acromegaly.

Oral glucose tolerance test (OGTT)

OGTT is a confirmatory test for acromegaly and is indicated for an equivocal IGF-1 level (on screening), or after transsphenoidal surgery to assess for disease control. An abnormal test is defined by a failure to suppress GH to <1 mcg/dL (in response to a 75 g oral glucose load), as assessed by GH measurements every 30 minutes over a 2-hour period. Lower cutoffs (<0.30 mcg/dL) are recommended for ultrasensitive GH assays.
► Etiologies for false positive results (failure to suppress GH) include: chronic renal and liver failure, malnutrition, anorexia, uncontrolled diabetes mellitus, heroin addiction, estrogen use, pregnancy and adolescence (due to high pubertal GH surges).

Random GH

This is generally not useful for the diagnosis of acromegaly, but a low random GH level (<0.40 mcg/dL with an ultrasensitive assay), in conjunction with a normal IGF-1 level, excludes the diagnosis.

MRI

MRI usually demonstrates a pituitary tumor (>95%), of which 80% are macroadenomas.

Pituitary function testing

Serum PRL may be elevated from stalk effect or GH/PRL tumors' co-secretion. In case of macroadenomas, assess other anterior pituitary hormones (e.g., free T4, cortisol, testosterone or estradiol) to exclude hypopituitarism.

GHRH

In cases where a pituitary tumor is not identified, a serum GHRH level and chest and abdomen imaging are recommend to identify a potential extrapituitary source of GH excess.

Comorbidities

Evaluate and treat potential comorbid conditions, including: impaired glucose intolerance/diabetes, dyslipidemia, sleep apnea, cardiac disease (baseline EKG and echocardiogram) and colonic polyps (colonoscopy).

Management

Transsphenoidal surgery

See Transsphenoidal surgery (p. 140). This is first-line therapy in most U.S. neurosurgery centers. Cure rates are generally 80–90% for microadenomas and 40–60% for macroadenomas.

Role of preoperative somatostatin analog treatment

There is limited evidence to recommend preoperative treatment to improve surgical outcomes or postoperative complications, although treatment can be considered for large, invasive tumors (if anticipated surgical delays), or for significant GH-related co-morbidities such as congestive heart failure or severe OSA.

Criteria for cure

Defined as

- Absence of clinical signs and symptoms of GH excess
- Normalization of IGF-1 levels
- GH nadir following OGTT to <1 mcg/dL (or <0.30 mcg/dL with an ultrasensitive GH assay)
  - Failed OGTT, with normal IGF-1, is a potential marker of recurrence risk.
  - ~30% discordance rates between the IGF-1 and the OGTT results have been observed in acromegalics:
    - High GH/normal IGF-1 is more common in young estrogen-sufficient females and somatostatin-treated patients.
    - Normal GH/high IGF-1 is more common in older patients and radiation-treated patients.

Medical therapies

Somatostatin analogs

📖 See Somatostatin analogs (p. 145).

- Somatostatin analogs are the first-line medical therapy after failed or incomplete surgical resection.
- They may be used as primary therapy in patients who are not surgical candidates.

Efficacy

- Normalizes IGF-1 levels in ~50–60% /of patients.
- **More efficacious with densely-granulated GH tumors than the sparsely-granulated GH sub-type.**
- Constrains tumor growth (>90%) and decreases tumor size (mild to moderately) in ~50% of patients.

GH receptor antagonists (pegvisomant)

📖 see Pegvisomant (p. 146).

- Indicated for somatostatin non-responders or intolerance
- Normalizes of IGF-1 levels in >90% of patients
- IGF-1 levels are used exausively to monitor therapy (not GH).

Dopamine agonists

📖 See Dopamine agonists (p. 144).
- Therapy is generally ineffective at normalizing IGF-1 levels, but may be useful for GH/PRL co-secretors.
- Only cabergoline is effective (not bromocriptine), but requires significantly higher doses than those used for prolactinomas (≥3 mg/week).

Radiotherapy

📖 Also see Technique (p. 147).

Generally this is third-line therapy after failed surgery and medical approaches, although radiation therapy can be used to decrease the need for lifelong medications.
- Normalization of GH hypersecretion may take several years (e.g., 5–10 years) with conventional radiotherapy, although it is likely faster with smaller tumors ± stereotactic radiosurgery.
- Adjunctive medical treatment (e.g., somatostatin analogs or pegvisomant) is usually required during the latency period after XRT.
- Prevention of tumor growth precedes control of GH hypersecretion by several months to years.

Mortality data

A recent meta-analysis found an overall ~72% increase in all-cause mortality in patients with acromegaly compared with the general population.
- Historically, major causes of mortality in acromegalic patients include cardiovascular diseases, respiratory diseases and malignancies.
- A greater awareness of acromegaly, newer medications and improved treatment strategies, over the past decade, have resulted in earlier diagnosis, better outcomes and decreased mortality rates.

Further reading

Alexopoulou O, Bex M, Abs R, Tsuen K, et al. (2008). Divergence between growth hormone and insulin-like growth factor-1 concentrations in the follow-up of acromegaly. *J Clin Endocrinol Metab* 93:1324–1330.

Dekkers OM, Biermasz AM, Pereira AM, Romijn JA, et al. (2008). Mortality in acromegaly: a meta-analysis. *J Clin Endocrinol Metab* 93:61–67.

Melmed S (2006). Medical progress: acromegaly. *N Engl J Med* 355:2558–2573.

Melmed S, Colao A, Barkan M, Molitch M, et al. (2009). Guidelines for acromegaly management: an update. *J Clin Endocrinol Metab* 94:1509–1517.

Verloes A, Stevenaert A, Teh BT, Petrossians P, et al. (1999). Familial acromegaly: case report and review of the literature. *Pituitary* 1:273–277.

Cushing's disease

Definition

Cushing's syndrome (CS) is a disease complex that results from chronic hypercortisolemia of any cause.

Cushing's disease (CD) is hypercortisolemia from an ACTH-secreting pituitary tumor chronic. Untreated hypercortisolemia leads to a ~3 to 5-fold increased mortality rate.

Epidemiology

- Annual incidence of CD is approximately 2–4/million population
- Female prevalence (3–15:1, ♀:♂)
- Age at diagnosis-20–40 years

☞ Subclinical CS may be more common than clinically-Apparent CS, although this is still a controversial area regarding definition, diagnosis and optimal management.

Differential diagnosis

- Iatrogenic etiologies (e.g., oral, inhaled or topical steroids) are the most common cause of CS
- *Pseudo-Cushing's disease*, defined as non-tumorous activation of the HPA axis from multiple potential stressors, including: psychiatric disorders (i.e., severe depression, anxiety disorder, obsessive-compulsive disorder), uncontrolled diabetes, alcoholism and severe obesity.
- Glucocorticoid resistance syndrome

Etiologies of CS

The majority of endogenous Cushing's syndrome is due to ACTH-secreting pituitary adenomas (Cushing's disease).

Box 18.1 Causes of endogenous Cushing's syndrome

ACTH-dependent
- Pituitary adenoma (Cushing's disease): 70–80%
- Ectopic ACTH syndrome: 10%
- Ectopic CRH secretion: <1%

ACTH-independent
- Adrenal adenoma: 10–20%
- Adrenal carcinoma: <5%
- Nodular (macro or micro) hyperplasia: 1%
  - Carney's complex
  - McCune–Albright syndrome
  - Aberrant adrenal receptor expression (e.g., GIP, LH, 5-HT4)

Clinical features of CS

Box 18.2 Clinical features of Cushing's syndrome

Features that best distinguish Cushing's syndrome
- Facial appearance: moon facie and plethoric complexion
- Spontaneous ecchymoses
- Violaceous striae: >1 cm on abdomen, thighs and axillae
- Proximal muscle weakness
- In children, weight gain with decreased growth velocity
- Early bone fractures, especially atraumatic rib or vertebral fractures

Clinical features less specific for Cushing's syndrome
- Fatigue
- Hypertension
- Impaired glucose tolerance, diabetes mellitus
- Osteopenia, osteoporosis
- Susceptibility to infections
- Mood disturbance —depression, irritability, insomnia, psychosis
- Menstrual disturbance
- Low libido and impotence
- Weight gain—truncal obesity, buffalo hump, supraclavicular fat pads
- Acne
- Hirsutism
- Polycystic ovarian syndrome

Investigations

Step 1. Conduct screening tests

Consider screening patients who have multiple and progressive 'high-discriminatory' features consistent with Cushing's syndrome, particularly with an early onset (Box 18.2). In addition, patients with an adrenal adenoma >1 cm should be screened.

▶ Note: All screening tests can give false-positive results with pseudo-Cushing's disease.

Outpatient screening tests (Fig. 18.1).

24-hour urinary free cortisol (UFC)

- At least two measurements
  - Upper limit of normal for cortisol is assay dependent (e.g., antibody-based
    > chromatography-based).

▶ Caveats: 1) Some medications can interfere with the cortisol assays (e.g., fenofibrate, carbamazepine and digoxin can give false-positive results on HPLC-based assays), and 2) reduced glomerular filtration rates (GFR) <60 mL/min may lead to false-negative results.

Overnight dexamethasone suppression test (DST)

- Administration of 1 mg dexamethasone (DEX) at 11–12 P.M., followed by a serum cortisol measurement the following morning (between 7 and 9 A.M.). A longer, low-dose dexamethasone suppression test (2 mg/day for 48 hours) is a comparable screening test.
  - Normal: Serum cortisol < 1.8 mcg/dL (with a sensitive cortisol assay)

▶ Caveats: The following interfering conditions should be excluded: ↓ dexamethasone absorption, hepatic enzyme inducers (e.g., phenytoin, carbamazepine, and rifampin), and ↑ (cortisol-binding globulin (CBG) (from oral contraceptive pills, which should be discontinued 6 weeks before testing or pregnancy). A morning dexamethasone level can be drawn to exclude rapid metabolism in specific cases.

Midnight salivary cortisol

- At least two measurements

▶ Caveats: Patients must have a normal sleep–wake cycle.

Step 2. Establish the cause

ACTH

A basal A.M. ACTH level should be measured to distinguish between ACTH-dependent vs. ACTH-independent Cushing's syndrome.
  - ACTH >10 pmol/mL indicate an ACTH-dependent etiology
  - ACTH levels are generally higher in ectopic patients, although 1/3 are within the normal range.
  - ACTH values <10 pmol/mL indicate an ACTH-independent tumor.
  - Equivocal ACTH values require additional testing.

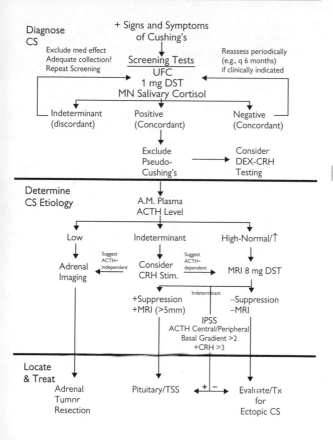

Fig 18.1 Algorithm for diagnosis of Cushing's syndrome. Adapted and Reprinted with permission from Liu H, Crapo L (2005). Update on the diagnosis of Cushing syndrome. *The Endocrinologist* 15(3):165–179.

Step 3. Localize the tumor

Pituitary imaging

80% of corticotrope adenomas are microadenomas, but MRI localizes these tumors in only ~ 50% of cases (with 1.5 Tesla MRI technology).

▶ Because ~ 10% of the normal population has a microadenoma (mostly <5 mm), patients with very small tumors or undetectable adenomas on

MRI should undergo an inferior petrosal sinus sampling (IPSS) for definitive diagnosis of Cushing's disease.

Inferior petrosal sinus sampling (Fig 18.2)

▶ IPSS is the single best test to distinguish Cushing's disease from ectopic CS, with a sensitivity and specificity of >95%. Comparatively, the 8 mg DST and CRH stimulation tests are inferior diagnostic tests.

- Bilateral IPSS involves the measurement of ACTH centrally and peripherally, in the basal state and following stimulation with CRH (100 mcg IV). A basal central-to-peripheral ACTH ratio of >2:1 (or >3:1 stimulated, 5-15 minutes after CRH injection) is diagnostic of CD.
- Ideally, IPSS should be performed only in experienced centers.

Abdominal CT

This is indicated for a suspected adrenal source.

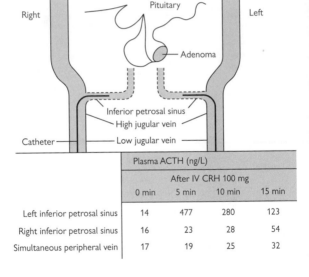

	Plasma ACTH (ng/L)			
	After IV CRH 100 mg			
	0 min	5 min	10 min	15 min
Left inferior petrosal sinus	14	477	280	123
Right inferior petrosal sinus	16	23	28	54
Simultaneous peripheral vein	17	19	25	32

Fig. 18.2 Inferior petrosal sinus sampling (IPSS). Simultaneous bilateral inferior petrosal sinus and peripheral vein sampling for ACTH. The ratio of >3 between the left central and peripheral vein confirms a diagnosis of Cushing's disease.
Right Basal Gradient ~1
ACTH stimulated (+CRH) gradient = 1.7
Left Basal Gradient ~1
ACTH stimulated (+CRH) gradient = 3.8
Reprinted with permission from Besser M, Thorner GM (1994). *Clinical Endocrinology*, 2nd ed. New York: Elsevier.

Abdominal and chest CT/MRI

These are indicated for suspected ectopic ACTH tumors and identify ~ 75% of tumors. Detection may be augmented by the complimentary use of functional studies, such as an octreotide scan or a positron emission tomography (PET) scan.

Additional tests

- *Serum potassium:* Hypokalemia is found in >95% of patients with ectopic, ACTH tumors but only 10% of patients with CD. Confounding issues for hypokalemia, such as diuretic use must be excluded.
- *High-dose dexamethasone suppression test* (🕮 see Pituitary function testing, p. 92).
- *Corticotropin-releasing hormone test* (🕮 see Pituitary function testing, p. 92).
- *Assess other pituitary hormones*: Hypercortisolism suppresses the thyroidal, gonadal and GH axes.
- *Assess and treat hypercortisolemia-associated co-morbidities:* impaired glucose tolerance, diabetes, hypertension, dyslipidemia and low bone mineral density

Treatment

Transsphenoidal surgery (TSS)
📖 Also see Transsphenoidal surgery (p. 140).

This is the first-line therapy in most Cushing's disease cases. Selective hypophysectomy is curative in up to 80–90% of microadenomas, and ~50% of macroadenomas.

A post-operative cortisol level of <2 mcg/dL is reassuring for short-term remission, although long-term studies indicate a recurrence rate for Cushing's disease of approximately 15-20% at 5 years.

Medical therapies (see Table 18.1)
To date, there are no effective tumor-directed therapies for Cushing's disease. Most of the adrenal-directed therapies are ineffective at normalizing hypercortisolemia and have poor side-effect profiles. As such, medical therapies are generally used as a temporizing measure (e.g., preoperatively or during the latency period after radiation therapy).

Pituitary radiotherapy (see p. 147)
Radiation therapy is usually third-line treatment following incomplete surgical resection and inadequate medical therapies.

Control of hypersecretion is frequently delayed (e.g., fractionated radiation therapy controls hypercortisolemia in ~50–60% of patients within 3–5 years).

Adrenalectomy
In ACTH-dependent Cushing's, bilateral adrenalectomy is the treatment of last resort, but may be indicated for patients with severe persistent hypercortisolism and/or an unlocalizable ectopic ACTH tumor.

Nelson's syndrome is caused by an enlargement of a pituitary adenoma (often aggressively), and may occur in up to 30% of Cushing's disease patients who have undergone a bilateral adrenalectomy. These tumors are associated with a marked increase in ACTH levels, hyperpigmentation and mass effects. Monitoring should be performed annually with a basal ACTH measurement and pituitary MRI (as indicated for signs and symptoms of mass effects or a markedly elevated ACTH level). Transsphenoidal surgery and radiation therapy are the main treatment options.

Table 18.1 Drug treatments for Cushing's syndrome

Drug	Dose	Action	Side effects
Metyrapone	1–4 g/day (usually given in 4 divided doses)	11β-hydroxylase inhibitor	Nausea, ↑ androgenic and mineralcorticoid precursors lead to hirsutism and hypertension Neutropenia.
Ketoconazole	200–400 mg tid first line in children. Avoid if taking H2 antagonists as acid is required to metabolize active compound	Direct inhibitor of P450 enzymes at several different sites	Abnormalities of liver function (usually reversible). Gynecomastia
Mitotane (o-p- DDD)	4–12 g/day (begin at 0.5–1 g/day and gradually increase dose)	Inhibits steroido-genesis at the side-chain cleavage, 11- and 18-hydroxylase and 3β-hydroxy-steroid dehydrogenase. Adrenolytic	Nausea & vomiting, Cerebellar disturbance, Somnolence, Hyper-cholesterolemia. May increase clearance of steroids. May be teratogenic. Avoid if fertility desired.
RU486 (mifepristone)	400–1000 mg/day	Glucocorticoid Antagonists	Amenorrhea Hypokalemia (antagonizes progesterone and androgen receptors)
Etomidate	0.03 mg/kg IV, followed by infusion of 0.1 mg/kg/h	Inhibits side-chain cleavage and 11β-hydroxylase	

Follow-up

- After a successful transsphenoidal tumor resection, periodic assessment of basal and stimulated cortisol levels are indicated to monitor for recovery from central adrenal insufficiency (which is typically prolonged [>1 year]).
- Monitor periodically for disease recurrence, particularly in patients at high risk for CD recurrence (i.e., non-suppressed post-op cortisol levels, rapid glucocorticoid taper, macroadenomas and/or failed intraoperative adenoma detection).
- ACTH-secreting macroadenoma are generally not cured with TSS and require subsequent radiation therapy ± medical therapies. In addition, "silent" ACTH adenomas are among the most aggressive tumors with ~30% recurrence rates.

Further reading

Biller BK, Grossman AB, Stewart PM, Melmed S, et al. (2008). Treatment of adrenocorticotropin-dependent Cushing's syndome: a concensus statement *J Clin Endocrinol Metab* 93:2454–2462.

Ilias I, Torpy DJ, Pacak K, Mullen N, et al. (2005). Cushing's syndrome due to ectopic corticotropin secretion: twenty years' experience at the National Institute of Health. *J Clin Endocrinol Metab* 91(2):371–377.

Nieman LK (2002). Medical therapy of Cushing's disease. *Pituitary* 5:77–82.

Nieman LK, Biller BM, Findling JW, Newell-Price J, et al. (2008). The diagnosis of Cushing's syndrome. An Endocrine Society clinical practice guideline. *J Clin Endocrinol Metab* 93:1526–1540.

Patil CG, Prevedello DM, Shivanand P, Vance ML et al. (2008). Late recurrences of Cushing's disease after initial successful transphenoidal surgery. 93:358–362.

Gonadotropinomas

Epidemiology

Gonadotropinomas are the most common non-functioning pituitary tumors and account for ~40–50% of all pituitary macroadenomas. They are most commonly diagnosed in middle-aged men.

Pathology

- Gonadotropinomas synthesize but generally do not efficiently secrete intact glycoprotein hormones (FSH, LH) or their free (α or β) subunits.
- Null cell tumors are defined by the absence of immunoreactive hormone expression and likely represent poorly differentiated gonadotrope cells.

Clinical features

Mass effects

- Headache
- Visual field defects (uni- or bitemporal quadrantanopia or hemianopia)
- Ophthalmoplegia (III, IV and VI cranial nerve palsies)
- Vision loss (optic nerve atrophy)
- Cerebrospinal fluid rhinorrhea (rarely)
- Hypopituitarism. At diagnosis, > 50% of patients are growth hormone and/or gonadotrope deficient. Adrenal and thyroid insufficiencies are less common (<30%).

Hormone effects

Rarely, gonadotropinomas can present with hormone hypersecretory syndromes, such as ovarian hyperstimulation syndrome, testicular enlargement or precocious puberty.

Investigations

- *Pituitary imaging:* Usually presents as a macroadenoma on MRI/CT
- *Visual fields assessment:* Vision field defects are observed in ~60–70% of patients.
- *PRL:* Mild hyperprolactinemia is common due to stalk compression.
- ❶ *Pituitary function:* Gonadotropinomas rarely present with elevated serum FSH, LH, and/or α-subunit levels, but may be confused with primary gonadal failure and or the postmenopausal state. Headaches, visual field disturbances and hypopituitarism are distinguishing features of a large gonadotropinoma.

Management

Surgery

Transsphenoidal resection is the preferred therapy in most cases.

Radiotherapy

Radiation therapy is indicated for invasive or recurrent tumors, after initial surgical resection, or for patients who are deemed poor surgical candidates.

- Conventional fractionated or stereotactic radiotherapies are effective at controlling tumor growth in (>80–90% of cases).
- XRT carries a long-term risk of hypopituitarism (~50% at 5–10 years with conventional XRT).

Medical treatment

Medical therapies, such as dopamine agonists, somatostatin analogs and GnRH agonist/antagonists are ineffective for gonadotropinomas.

- Hormone replacement therapy is required for any hypopituitarism (📖 see p. 98).

Follow-up and prognosis

- Surgical gross-total resection rates for gonadotropinomas are ~60–70%, with experienced neurosurgeons.
- Risk of tumor recurrence and growth are estimated at ~5–10% at 5 years following gross-total resection of gonadotropinomas, and 20–50% at 10 years with subtotal resection.
- Most patients with gonadotropinomas lack a detectable serum hormone marker (e.g., FSH/LH), so must be followed clinically and radiographically (with MRIs).
- For patients with asymptomatic/residual tumors or microadenomas, a watchful waiting approach with annual imaging is recommended Consideration should be given to repeat TSS, or XRT, for evidence of significant interval tumor growth.

Further reading

Chaidarun SS, Klibanski A (2002). Gonadotropinomas. *Semin Reprod Med* 20:339–348.

Dekkers OM, Pereira AM, Romijn JA (2008). Treatment and follow-up of clinically nonfunctioning pituitary macroadenoma. *J Clin Endocrinol Metab* 93:3717–3726.

Jaffe CA (2006). Clinically non-functioning pituitary adenomas. *Pituitary* 9:317–322.

Thyrotropinomas

Epidemiology

- Less than 2% of pituitary adenomas are thyrotropinomas (TSH-secreting).
- Female predominance-10:1,♀:♂.
- Thyrotropinomas are frequently misdiagnosed and treated as primary hyperthyroidism.

Clinical features

- Hyperthyroidism (☐ see p. 17)
- Most thyrotropinomas are macroadenomas at the time of diagnosis and present with mass effects, including headaches (20%), vision defects (25%) and hypopituitarism (50%).
- Goiter is common at presentation.

Differential diagnosis of elevated free T_4 /T_3 and non-suppressed TSH

- TSH-secreting tumor
- Thyroid hormone resistance
- Inherited abnormalities of thyroid-binding globulin proteins

Investigations

- Elevated Free T_4 and T_3 levels with an inappropriately normal or elevated TSH level
- Elevated glycoprotein hormone α-subunit/TSH molar ratio
- PRL and/or GH may be elevated in mixed tumors (~25%).
- Elevated sex hormone binding globulins (hyperthyroid effect)
- Failed suppression of TSH with T_3 (80–100 mcg × 8–10 days) with TSH-secreting tumor
- Pituitary imaging MRI

Management

Surgery

- First-line therapy, with >80% cure rates for microadenomas and ~50% cure rates for macroadenomas

Medical therapies

Somatostatin analogs

📖 See Medical therapies for pituitary tumors (p. 144).

- Somatostatin analogs, including octreotide LAR and lanreotide, are second-line therapy after failed or incomplete surgical resection.
- Normalizes TSH secretion in >80% of patients and decreases tumor size in ~40–50% of patients.

Antithyroid medications

- Short-term use only, for preoperative normalization of thyroid hormone levels. Long-standing use has potential adverse effects of tumor growth.
- β-blockers as needed for symptomatic hyperthyroidism.

Radiotherapy

Radiation therapy is used as adjuvant therapy following incomplete surgical resection or inadequate medical response.

Further reading

Beck-Peccoz P, Persani L (2008). Thyrotropinomas. *Endocrinol Metab Clin North Am* 37:123–134.

Craniopharyngiomas and Rathke's cleft cysts

Craniopharyngiomas

Epidemiology

Craniopharyngiomas comprise ~2–5% of all intracranial tumors and ~10% of all intracranial tumors in children. There is an equal gender prevalence, and a bimodal distribution, with peaks at ages 5–14 years and 50–74 years.

Pathology

Tumors arise from squamous epithelial remnants of Rathke's pouch. Histological classification includes two sub-types:
- Adamantinomatous—predominantly affects the young. Calcifications are common.
- Papillary—adult predominance. Calcifications are rare.

▶ Although craniopharyngiomas are benign tumors, they are biologically aggressive tumors which have a proclivity to invade and adhere to critical neurovascular structures (i.e., the hypothalamus and the third ventricle).

Clinical features

- Mass effects: headaches, vision loss or visual field deficits, cranial nerve palsies and obstructive hydrocephalus (in children)
- Pituitary disturbances:
  - Children commonly present with growth failure and delayed puberty.
  - Adults commonly present with hypopituitarism.
  - DI occurs in ~15–20% of cases.
- Hypothalamic syndrome: hyperphagia, severe obesity, cognitive impairment, thirst and water/electrolyte imbalances, temperature dysregulation and sleep disturbances.

Investigations

- MRI/CT (CT better depicts boney erosions and calcifications)
- Visual field testing
- Anterior and posterior pituitary assessment
- Neuropsychological testing (particularly in children)

Management

- Surgical resection is first-line therapy for most cases. The surgical approach (transfrontal vs. transsphenoidal) is dependent on the tumor size and suprasellar extension.
- Gross-total resection is feasible only for relatively small tumors with a predominantly intrasellar location.
- Subtotal resection, followed by adjuvant radiation therapy, is preferred over aggressive resection to minimize the potentially devastating effects of hypothalamic damage (see Hypothalamic syndrome, p. 130).
- Craniopharyngiomas are radiosensitive, and therefore radiation therapy is indicated for residual disease, recurrent tumor growth, or for patients who are deemed poor surgical candidates.
- Data regarding additional adjuvant therapies, including: intracavitary irradiation (brachytherapy), bleomycin and systemic chemotherapy are limited.
- Restoration of pituitary hormone deficiencies is unlikely following surgery, and the need for lifelong pituitary hormone replacement is common.

Follow-up

- Craniopharyngiomas have a high recurrence rate following surgery (~30% at 10 years), with most occurring in the first 3 years. Radiation therapy is very effective at constraining tumor growth.
- The recommended frequency of clinical evaluation, imaging and anterior pituitary hormone assessment depends on the disease status. In general, imaging is recommended initially at 6- to 12-month intervals.
- Patients who have received radiotherapy should undergone pituitary hormone testing biannually in anticipation of developing hypopituitarism. For patients on a stable pituitary hormone regimen, annual testing is usually sufficient.

Rathke's cleft cysts (RCC)

Epidemiology

Rathke's cleft cysts account for ~1% of primary intracranial tumors. There is a female predominance (2:1 ♀:♂), and the mean age at presentation is ~38 years.

Pathology

RCCs are derived from the remnants of Rathke's pouch and are lined by epithelial cells (ciliated cuboidal/columnar epithelium). Squamous metaplasia is associated with a higher risk of RCC recurrence.

Clinical features

- RCCs are usually asymptomatic
- Large cysts (>1 cm) can be associated with mass effects, including headaches (~65–85%) and vision problems (~20–40%).
- Rarely, RCCs are associated with apoplexy (see 📖 Apoplexy, p. 95).
- Pituitary dysfunction, with large cysts occurs in 30–60% of cases, with hyperprolactinemia and hypogonadism being the most common abnormalities. DI is uncommon.

Investigations

MRIs with variable signals characteristics are observed, depending on the cyst content (see 📖 Imaging, p. 88). RCCs may be indistinguishable from cystic adenomas or cystic craniopharyngiomas.

Management

- Transsphenoidal surgery is recommended for RCCs associated with mass effects (i.e., headaches or vision defects or pituitary hormone insufficiency).
  - Conservative decompression (cyst drainage and cyst wall biopsy) is preferred over aggressive cyst wall resection to minimize the risk of DI and hypopituitarism.
  - Transsphenoidal surgery results in >80% symptomatic improvements in headaches and vision defects and with low complication rates (see 📖 Transsphenoidal surgery, p. 140).
  - Hyperprolactinemia and hypogonadism commonly normalize after surgery whereas other pre-existing pituitary hormone abnormalities less commonly improve.

Follow-up

Recurrence rates for RCC vary by surgical procedure, definition of recurrence, and length of follow-up, but are generally low (<10% symptomatic recurrence rates at 5 years) at experienced neurosurgery centers.

Further reading

Kanter AS, Sansur CA, Jane JA, Laws ER Jr (2006). Rathke's cleft cysts. In Laws ER, Sheehan JP (eds.), *Pituitary Surgery—A Modern Approach. Frontiers of Hormone Research*, Vol 34. Basel: Karger Press, pp. 127–157.

Karivitaki N, Cudlip S, Adams CB, Wass JA (2006). Craniopharyngiomas. *Endocr Rev* 27:371–393.

Karavitaki N, Waas JA (2008). Craniopharyngiomas. *Endocrinol Metab Clin N Am* 37:173–193.

Oskouian RJ, Samii A, Laws ER Jr (2006). The craniopharyngioma. In Laws ER, Sheehan JP (Eds.), *Pituitary Surgery—A Modern Approach. Frontiers of Hormone Research*, Vol 34, Basel: Kager Press, pp. 105–126.

Lillehei KO, Widdel L, Arias-Astete C, Wierman ME, et al (2010). *J Neurosurg* Transphenoidal resection of 82 Rathke cleft cysts; limited value of alcohol cauterization in reducing recurrence rates. 27:1–8

Parasellar tumors

See ▢ Table 15.1, Lesions of the sellar turcica and parasellar region (p. 101).

Meningiomas

- Most common benign tumors of the sellar region, after adenomas
- Peak incidence between the ages of 40–70 years
- Strongly associated with previous radiation therapy
- Usually present with vision disturbances and occasionally with pituitary dysfunction
- Enhancing "dural tail" on contrasted T_1 MRI is highly characteristic of this tumor type.
- Management is surgical, when possible, and/or radiation therapy for persistent or recurrent tumors.
- Rarely transforms to malignant tumors (poor prognosis)

Germ cell tumor (GCT)

- Malignant tumors that most commonly present in the first two decades of life
- GCTs are classified as germinomas or nongerminomatous.
- Most develop around the third ventricle (80% in the region of the pineal gland), followed by suprasellar/hypothalamic locations.
- For pineal gland involvement and treatment, see ▢ Pineal gland (p. 161).
- Suprasellar GCT typically presents with DI, hypopituitarism and vision disturbances.
- Diagnosis is based on histological confirmation (gold standard) or elevated tumor markers (β-hCG, α-fetoprotein in germinomas) and imaging characteristics.
- A multimodal treatment approach, from among surgical resection, radiation therapy and chemotherapy, is used depending on tumor type and stage.

Gangliocytomas

- Neuroepithelial tumors comprised of ganglion cells either alone (gangliocytoma) or in combination with glial cells (ganglioglioma)
- Frequently found in association with hormonally active pituitary adenomas, particularly growth hormone tumors
- Surgical resection is usually first-line therapy.

Chordomas/condrosarcomas

- Cartilaginous tumors originating from the primitive notochord.
- Incidence: chordomas > chondrosarcomas
- Both tumors are locally aggressive and cause extensive boney destruction.
- Clinically, patients most commonly present with vision complaints (diplopia) and headaches.
- The preferred treatment is surgical resection followed by radiotherapy in most cases.

Hamartomas

- Hypothalamic hamartomas are congenital, neuronal-derived heterotopic tumors.
- They typically present in childhood with seizures—commonly gelastic (laughing).
- They may release GnRH, leading to precocious puberty, or very rarely secrete GHRH, leading to gigantism
- Treatment consists of surgical resection and medical therapies when indicated by harmonl hypersecretion (see 📖,p. 214).

Metastatic tumors to the pituitary

- Most commonly includes colon, lung and breast cancers (in 2/3 of the cases).
- Typically these tumors present in the sixth to seventh decades of life as part of widespread metastatic disease.
- DI is common (>70% of cases) and is a distinguishing characteristic.
- Mass effects and hypopituitarism are less commonly observed (<30%).
- Treatment is mainly palliative. Surgical debulking and radiation therapy are rarely indicated for pituitary mass effects.
- Pituitary hormone replacement, particularly dDAVP, glucocorticoids and thyroid hormone, as indicated for these deficiencies.

Further reading

Kaltsas GA, Evanson J, Chrisoulidou, Grossman AB (2008). The diagnosis and management of para-sellar tumors of the pituitary. *Endocr Relat Cancers* 15:885–903.

Komninos J, Vlassopoulou V, Protopapa D, Korfias S, et al. (2004). Clinical case seminar. Tumors metastatic to the pituitary gland: case report and literature review. *J Clin Endocrinol Metab* 89:574–580.

Inflammatory and infiltrative pituitary diseases

Background

Inflammatory, infiltrative and granulomatous diseases of the hypothalamus and pituitary gland are uncommon but should be considered in cases of systemic illnesses that are associated with pituitary enlargement, mass effects (e.g., headaches, vision disturbances) and neurogenic diabetes insipidus.

Box 23.1 Classification of hypophysitis

Lymphocytic hypophysitis
- Lymphocytic adenohypophysitis (LAH)
- Lymphocytic infundibuloneurophysitis (LINH)
- Lymphocytic panhypophysitis (LPH)

Xanthomatous—characterized by foamy histiocytes

Granulomatous
- Idiopathic—giant cell
- Infectious—tuberculosis (TB)
- Systemic granulomatous disease
  - Sarcoidosis
  - Wegner's granulomatosis
- Systemic histiocytosis
  - Langerhan's cell histiocytosis
  - Erdheim–Chester disease

Infectious disease (e.g., viral, fungal, syphilis)

Investigations

Inflammatory lesions typically appear as an enlarged pituitary gland and stalk and may mimic a pituitary mass. In contrast to adenomas, however, these lesions typically show marked enhancement on contrasted T_1-weighted MRI images. Biopsy of the pituitary lesion, by a transsphenoidal approach, may be indicated for a definitive diagnosis.

Lymphocytic hypophysitis

Lymphocytic hypophysitis is a disease characterized by lymphocytic infiltration of the hypothalamus and/or pituitary gland and is an autoimmune (T cell–mediated) process.

- It varies between focal (adenohypophysitis) and diffuse (panhypophysitis) processes.
- Lymphocytic hypophysitis is associated with other autoimmune conditions (e.g., Hashimoto's thyroiditis, Addison's disease, pernicious anemia) in >30% of cases.
- Anti-pituitary antibodies, although variably present, are not sensitive or specific markers.

Clinical presentation

LAH is associated with pregnancy (last trimester and within 1 year post-partum) in ~70–80% of cases. LINH has an equal gender distribution.

- Mass effects; headaches (60%) and visual disturbances (40%)
- ⚠ Hypopituitarism-ACTH and TSH deficiencies are slightly more common (60–65%), than gonadotropin and GH deficiencies (40–54%)
- PRL levels are variable: frequently elevated with mass effects (20–40%), or may be low with a destructive/infiltrative process.
- DI is common with neurohypophyseal involvement (e.g., LINH, LPH).

Treatment

An empiric trial of pharmacological glucocorticoids, early in the disease process (<6 months), has been advocated in the setting of mass effects and progressive pituitary dysfunction, although data are limited regarding its true benefit relative to the diseases' natural history.

- Transsphenoidal surgery is sometimes indicated for diagnostic confirmation and mass effects.
- Adjuvant therapies such as other immunosuppressive agents (e.g., azathioprine, methotrexate, cyclosporine A) and radiation therapy have been tried in selective cases and with variable success.

Pathology

Histopathology is the gold standard for the diagnosis and shows a lymphocytic infiltration of T cells, particularly CD4 cells.

Natural history

Outcomes vary between spontaneous resolution and normal pituitary gland function to progressive pituitary gland fibrosis and permanent hypopituitarism.

Sarcoidosis

Sarcoidosis is a chronic, multisystem disease of unknown etiology that is characterized by the presence of granulomas.

Clinical features
- Sarcoidosis affects young and middle-aged adults most commonly and has an equal gender prevalence.
- Most cases have multivisceral (e.g., lungs, cardiac, sinonasal, eye, skin) involvement at the time of diagnosis.
- Isolated CNS disease occurs in ~5% of cases and can involve the hypothalamus, pituitary gland, cranial nerves and leptomeninges.
- Hypopituitarism is common, including gonadotrope deficiencies, hyperprolactinemia and diabetes insipidus as early manifestations.
- Hypothalamic involvement may also manifest with disturbances in sleep, thirst (primary polydipsia/adipsia), appetite and temperature regulation.

Investigations
Serum and CSF angiotensin-converting enzyme (ACE) levels may be elevated, although these tests are not sensitive or specific for neurosarcoidosis. MRI findings are as described earlier under Investigations (see p. 137). In addition, MRI may demonstrate meningeal enhancement.

Management
Glucocorticoid therapy is the mainstay of treatment.
- Pharmacological doses of glucocorticoid (e.g., 1 mg/kg/day prednisone for 2–4 weeks) are recommended for initial treatment. Subsequent steroid dosage and duration are dependent on the disease response and severity.
- Adjuvant therapies, including azathioprine, methotrexate, infliximab, and radiation therapy, have been tried in selective cases and with variable success.

Natural history
The disease course varies from monophasic (66% of cases) to relapsing/remitting to progressive disease. Glucocorticoid therapy generally does not reverse the hormonal deficiencies.

Langerhans' cell histiocytosis

This rare, multisystemic disease is characterized by aberrant proliferation of dendritic cells (called *Langerhan's cells*).

Clinical features and treatment

- Incidence is 3–5 cases per million.
- Most cases occur in children; up to 50% manifest with pituitary disease, with DI and growth hormone deficiencies being the most common abnormalities.
- In adults, diffuse disease (e.g., skin, bone, lung) is usually present at the time of diagnosis and is associated with a 20% mortality rate.
- Standard Langerhan's-directed therapy of vinblastine and steroids does not reverse pituitary hormone deficiencies.

Hemochromatosis

This disorder is characterized by increased iron absorption and multi-organ deposition, including the heart, liver, pancreas and the pituitary gland.

Clinical features and treatment

- Hypogonadotropic hypogonadism is the most common pituitary manifestation of hemochromatosis and reflects a predilection for iron deposition in gonadotrope cells.
- MRI may show decreased T_1 and T_2 signaling from paramagnetic iron deposition.
- Phlebotomy is the mainstay of treatment and may reverse the pituitary dysfunction, although long-term sex steroid replacement is frequently required.

Further reading

Carpinteri R, Patelli I, Casanueva FF, Giustina A (2009). Inflammatory and granulomatous expansive lesions of the pituitary. *Best Pract Res Clin Endocrinol Metab* 23:639–650.

Molitch ME, Gillam MP (2007). Lymphocytic hypophysitis. *Hormone Res* 68:145–150.

Surgical treatment of pituitary tumors

Transsphenoidal surgery (TSS)

Minimally-invasive, endonasal TSS is the preferred approach, for pituitary tumors, and accounts for ~95% of pituitary surgeries. See Box 24.1 for indications. Compared to craniotomy, TSS has the following advantages:
- Reduced associated morbidity and mortality
- Better visualization of small tumors
- Reduced duration of hospital stay

Preoperative management
- Optimize medical comorbidities.
- In apoplexy, correct fluid, electrolyte and hormone deficiencies (as indicated), with an emphasis on glucocorticoid and thyroid hormone replacement.
- In macroadenomas, assess and treat hypopituitarism, particularly glucocorticoid and thyroid hormone deficiencies as indicated.

Box 24.1 Indications for transsphenoidal surgery (TSS)

- Nonfunctioning pituitary adenomas (usually macroadenomas)
  - Gonadotropinomas
  - Null cell adenomas
- Functioning pituitary adenomas
  - GH-secreting adenoma
  - ACTH-secreting tumor
  - Prolactinoma—if patient is dopamine agonist resistant or intolerant
  - TSH-secreting adenoma
  - Nelson's syndrome
- Pituitary apoplexy
- Recurrent pituitary tumors
- Parasellar tumors
  - Craniopharyngioma
  - Rathke's cleft cyst
  - Chordoma
  - Arachnoid cyst
- Pituitary biopsy for definitive diagnosis (e.g., hypophysitis, pituitary metastases)

- Discontinue antiplatelet therapies and substitute anticoagulants as needed.
- Consider preoperative medical treatment for severe Cushing's disease.
- Consider medical treatment of acromegalic patients with significant preoperative comorbidities (e.g., congestive heart failure [CHF], OSA).
- Establish euthyroid status for thyrotropinomas associated with hyperthyroidism.

Perioperative management

- Prophylactic antibiotics are given perioperatively to reduce the risk of meningitis.
- Immediate postoperative issues include monitoring for DI and neuro-ophthalmalogic complications.

▶ Patients with Cushing's disease require peri- and postoperative gluco-corticoid treatment because of persistent secondary adrenal insufficiency with successful tumor resection (see 🕮, Cushing's disease, p. 116).
- DVT prophylaxis is necessary for Cushing's patients because hypercortisolism induces a hypercoagulable state.

Complications of transsphenoidal surgery (see Table 24.1)

- The complication risks are highly dependent on the neurosurgeon and correlate inversely with TSS experience.
  - For experienced neurosurgeons (>200 transsphenoidal surgeries), mortality rates are low (<1%).
  - Morbidity related to fluid and electrolyte balances, such as DI, complicates an estimated 10–15% of transsphenoidal surgeries, but is usually transient.

Table 24.1 Potential complications of pituitary surgery

Complications of any surgical procedure	Anesthesia related Venous thrombosis and pulmonary embolism
Immediate	Hemorrhage/hematoma Hypothalamic damage Carotid injury Meningitis
Transient	DI CSF rhinorrhea Visual deterioration Epistaxis/septal perforation Sinusitis SIADH
Permanent	Visual deterioration or loss Cranial nerve damage Hypopituitarism DI

- Newer surgical techniques such as computerized navigation, endoscopy, and intraoperative imaging are used in selected cases and centers, although they are still not widely available.

Postoperative management

- Clinical evaluation on postoperative days 14, to assess for symptomatic improvement and to exclude complications (e.g., hyponatremia and sinusitis).
- Pituitary hormone function is preserved in most patients with preoperative normal function and may improve in ~30% of patients with pre-operative hypoprturtarism. This percentage is likely higher with an experienced neurosurgeon and for hypogonadism caused by hyperprolactinemia-related stalk effects.
- Vision improves in >80% of patients following optic nerve decompression but varies by disease duration and severity and may take several months to fully recover.
- A postoperative MRI and pituitary hormone testing (basal ± dynamic) are recommended at 3-month initially, and then annually for the first five years.

Box 24.2 Postoperative disorders of fluid balance

- Acute and transient DI
- Hyponatremia from excessive hypotonic fluid administration or SIADH
- Permanent DI "classic triphasic DI response:" initial DI due to axon shock (hours–days) followed by antidiuretic phase due to uncontrolled release of ADH from damaged posterior pituitary (2–14 days) followed by DI due to depletion of ADH. Permanent DI complicates <2% of TSS.
- Isolated SIADH phase, delayed hyponatremia at 7–10 days postoperative, usually mild and self-limiting. More common in the elderly population.

Transfrontal craniotomy

Indications

Craniotomy is often the preferred surgical approach for a giant pituitary tumor (>4 cm) or a purely suprasellar location (e.g., craniopharyngiomas, meningiomas).

Complications (see Table 24.1)

Craniotomy has higher complication rates than does TSS. The potential complications are as listed for TSS (Box 24.1), and include the following:
* Brain retraction may lead to cerebral edema or hemorrhage.
* Manipulation of the optic chiasm may lead to visual deterioration.
* Damage to the olfactory nerve.

Perioperative management

* Recovery is typically slower than after transsphenoidal surgery.
* Prophylactic anticonvulsants are commonly used.
* Patients are typically given dexamethasone over 1–2 weeks to minimize the risk of brain edema.

Further reading

Joshi SM, Cudlip S (2008). Transsphenoidal surgery. *Pituitary* 11:353–360.

Laws ER, Thapar K (1999). Pituitary surgery. *Endocrinol Metab Clin N Am* 28:119.

Vance ML (2003). Perioperative management of patients undergoing pituitary surgery. *Endocrinol Metab Clin N Am* 32:355–365.

Ciric I, Ragin A, Baumgartner A, Crain PA Pierce D (1997). Complications of transphenoidal surgery:results of a national survey, review of the literature and personal experience. *Neurosurgery* 40:225–237.

Medical treatment of pituitary tumors

Dopamine agonists (DA)

For indications for use see Prolactinomas (p. 107) and Acromegaly (p. 114).

DA formulations/doses

- Bromocriptine (Parlodel): short-acting, non-ergot derivative.
  Usually administered orally, twice daily. Therapeutic daily dose for
  prolactinomas ranges between 5.0 and 30 mg; usual dose is 10 mg
  a day. Bromocriptine is the preferred medication in women seeking
  fertility because of the greater safety data during pregnancy.
- Cabergoline (Dostinex): long-acting ergot derivative. Usually
  administered twice a week. The usual therapeutic dose is 1.0 mg a week.
  - Better side-effect profile and more efficacious than bromocriptine
- Pergolide (Permax): no longer available in the United States

Mechanism of action

DAs activate D_2 receptors, which are coupled to inhibitory G proteins,
and decrease cAMP production.

Side effects

Side effects, particularly with bromocriptine, may be minimized by starting
a low dose (e.g., 1.25 mg/day), and titrating up slowing. In females, vaginal
administration can be tried if GI intolerance is dose limiting.

Common side effects (>10%)

- Nausea
- Fatigue
- Headache

Less common side effects (<10%)

- Postural hypotension, dizziness, nasal stuffiness, constipation and a
  Raynaud-like phenomenon in the hands.
- Very rarely, patients develop hallucinations and psychosis (usually at
  higher doses).

Uncommon side effects

The problems of cardiac valvulopathy, as noted in Parkinson's patients on
high-dose cabergoline (>3 mg/day), is uncommon in prolactinoma patients
on standard cabergoline doses ($\leq$ 2 mg/week).

Somatostatin analogs

Box 25.1 Uses of somatostatin analogs

- Acromegaly
- Carcinoid tumors
- Pancreatic neuroendocrine tumors
- TSH-secreting pituitary tumors

Indications for use

See Acromegaly (p. 114).

Mechanism of action

- Analogs of the naturally-occurring GH inhibitor somatostatin, but with increased serum half-lives and higher somatostatin receptor affinities.
- The somatostatin analogs signal predominantly through somatostatin receptors subtypes 2 and 5.

Formulations/doses

- Octreotide LAR® (Sandostatin LAR) (10–30 mg intramuscular [IM]) administered every 4–6 weeks
- Lanreotide Autogel® (Somatuline) (60–120 mg deep subcutaneous [SC]) administered every 4–6 weeks
- SC octreotide (50–200 mcg) administered 3 × daily.
- Lanreotide SR (30 mg IM) administered every 7–14 days.

Side effects

- Gallstones or sludge develops in ~20–30% of patients, but only 1%/year develop symptomatic cholecystitis.
- Abdominal cramps, bloating and mild steatorrhea, due to inhibition of motor activity and pancreatic enzymes secretion, commonly occur early in treatment, although symptoms usually improve, or resolve, over the first few months.
- Transient worsening of diabetes (from inhibition of β-cell function).
- Injection site pain is minimized by allowing the medication to warm to room temperature before administration.
- Hair loss (<10%)

Issues

- The long-acting somatostatin analogs have similar efficacies and side-effect profiles.
- The need for dose titrations should be assessed at 3 month intervals, based on the IGF-1 levels.
- IGF-1 levels, but not GH-OGTT suppression tests, are recommended to monitor the therapeutic response to somatostatin analogs in acromegaly.

Growth hormone receptor antagonists

Indications for use include medical therapy for acromegalic patients who are incompletely responsive to, or intolerant of, somatostatin analogs.

Mechanism of action

- Mutated GH molecule that binds to peripheral GH receptors (predominantly on the liver) and blocks GH receptor signaling

Formulations and doses

- Pegvisomant (Somavert) 40 mg SC loading dose, followed by 10–40 mg SC administered daily

Side effects

- Abnormal liver function tests (transaminitis), in ~5%, but are usually transient
- Injection site reactions (i.e., atopic reactions or lipohypertrophy)

Issues

- High cost
- Successful weekly and biweekly administrations of pegvisomant have been reported, based on its long half-life (70 hours).

▶ Therapeutic response is assessed by IGF-1 levels only (GH levels are elevated on GH antagonist therapy).

- The need for dose titrations should be assessed at ~3-month intervals.
- Medication has no effect on tumor size. MRI of the pituitary is indicated 6 months after starting therapy and then annually thereafter. Long-term studies indicate a low risk for tumor growth (<5 % over 5 years).
- Pegvisomant can be given concomitantly with somatostatin analogs to control GH hypersecretion.

Further reading

Higham CE, Bidlingmaier M, Drake WM, Trainer PJ (2009). Successful use of weekly pegvisomant administration in patients with acromegaly. *Eur J Endocrinol* 161:21–25.

Melmed S, Colao A, Barkan M, Molitch M, et al. (2009) Guidelines for acromegaly management: an update. *J Clin Endocrinol Metab* 94:1509–1517.

Trainer PJ (2009). ACROSTUDY: the first 5 years. *Eur J Endocrinol* 161:S19–S24.

Trainer PJ, Drake WM, Katznelson L, Freda PU, et al. (2000). Treatment of acromegaly with the growth hormone receptor antagonist pegvisomant *N Engl J Med* 342:1171–1177.

Pituitary radiotherapy

Background

Pituitary radiotherapy is used to control pituitary tumor growth and excess hormone secretion for patients with residual or recurrent tumors that are not adequately treated by surgical and medical approaches.

Techniques

Conventional external beam radiation

A three-field crossfire technique is used to deliver ionizing irradiation. The standard 45–50 Gy dose is delivered in 25 fractions (~2 Gy/day) over ~5–6 weeks.

Stereotactic radiation therapy (see Box 26.1)

This therapy represents improved immobilization, radiation beam focusing and imaging techniques. Stereotactic irradiation can be given as a single-fraction radiosurgery (SRS) or delivered as fractionated doses. SRS is limited to relatively smaller tumors with tumor margins that are >5 mm from the optic apparatus.

Box 26.1 Stereotactic forms of radiotherapy

- *Gamma knife:* ionizing radiation from a cobalt 60 source delivered by convergent collimated beams
- *LINAC:* delivers photons via a linear accelerator and frequently incorporates a cyberknife.
- *Proton beam:* utilizes heavy-charge particle proton beams, produced by a cyccotron but has limited availability in the U.S.
- *Cyber knife:* a frameless, robotic radiosurgery delivery system

Efficacy

- Radiotherapy is effective and rapid in controlling pituitary adenoma growth, with progression-free survivals of 80–90% at 10 years.
- Effects of radiation therapy on normalizing hormone hypersecretion are delayed. For example, normalization of GH/IGF-1 levels is observed in ~30–50% of acromegalic patients at ~5–10 years after conventional radiation therapy.
- Stereotactic techniques have the theoretical advantage, over conventional radiation therapy, of decreased complication rates (i.e., hypopituitarism), and a more rapid normalization of hormone hypersecretion, although this is still a controversial area.
- To potentially optimize treatment efficacy, consideration should be given to the temporary discontinuation of pituitary-directed medications, such as somatostatin analogs (for at least 1 month) prior to radiation therapy.

Complications

Short-term

- Fatigue
- Nausea
- Headache
- Temporary hair loss at radiotherapy entry portals

Hypopituitarism

- Anterior pituitary hormone deficiency is the most common late complication of radiation therapy, and occurs in 30–60% of patients ~10 years after conventional radiation (Fig. 26.1).
- The loss of anterior pituitary hormones, after radiation therapy, generally develops in a predictable order: GH ~ FSH/LH >> ACTH ~ TSH
- Posterior pituitary deficiencies are rare after XRT.
- Expectant management is recommended for hypopituitarism with biannual pituitary hormone testing to include basal ACTH, cortisol, free T_4, IGF-1, testosterone (in males), and estradiol (in females). Cosyntropin stimulation test is indicted for an equivocal A.M. cortisol value.

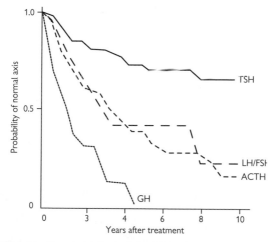

Fig 26.1 Life-table analysis indicating the probability of developing pituitary hormone deficiencies after conventional radiation therapy. Reproduced with permission from Littley MD, Shalet SM, Beardwell CG, Ahmed, SR, et al. (1989). *Q J Med* 70:145–160.

Visual impairment

The optic chiasm is radiosensitive, whereas cranial nerves are generally radioresistant. The risk of vision impairment is related to the total administered dose and the dose per fraction (highest with SRS). A standard total dose of 4500 cGy (and a daily dose of 180 cGy in conventional radiation) poses very little risk to the optic chiasm (<1% risk of blindness).

Long-term radiation complications

- Radiation is associated with the development of secondary brain tumors, particularly meningiomas and gliomas, with an estimated risk of 2.4% at 20 years.
- The effects of pituitary radiation on long-term neuro-cognitive and neuro-psychological function are not well defined.

● Increased cerebrovascular morbidity and mortality rates have been reported with conventional radiation treatment of pituitary adenomas, although the relative contribution of radiation to stroke risk remains to be determined.

Further reading

Darzy KH, Shalet SM (2009). Hypopituitarism following radiotherapy. *Pituitary* 12:40–50.

Gittoes N (2005). Pituitary radiotherapy: current controversies. *Trends Endocrinol Metab* 6:407–413.

Minniti G, Gilbert DC, Brada M (2009). Modern techniques for pituitary radiotherapy. *Rev Endocrinol Metab Disord* 10:135–144.

Minniti G, Traish AS, Gonsalves A, Brada M (2005). Risk of second brain tumor after conservative surgery and radiotherapy for pituitary adenomas: update after an additional 10 years. *J Clin Endocrinol Metab* 90:800–804.

Diabetes insipidus (DI)

Definition

DI is defined as the passage of large volumes (>40 ml/kg/day in adults) of dilute urine.

Classifications and etiologies (see Box 27.1)

Neurogenic
- Inadequate arginine vasopressin (AVP) secretion

Nephrogenic
- Inadequate renal response to AVP

Dipsogenic
- Compulsive polydipsia (psychogenic)
- Disorders of hypothalamic thirst center

Box 27.1 Etiologies of DI

Neurogenic
Congenital
- Autosomal dominant (AVP-neurophysin gene mutation)
- DIDMOAD syndrome (**d**iabetes **i**nsipidus, **d**iabetes **m**ellitus, **o**ptic **a**trophy, **d**eafness)

Acquired
- Trauma—head injury, neurosurgery
- Tumors—craniopharyngioma, metastatic, germinoma
- Inflammatory conditions—sarcoidosis, TB, Langerhans' cell histiocytosis, lymphocytic hypophysitis
- Infections—meningitis, encephalitis.
- Vascular—Sheehan's syndrome, cerebral hemorrhage or infarction
- Idiopathic

Nephrogenic
Congenital
- X-linked recessive—vasopressin receptor gene
- Autosomal recessive—aquaporin-2 gene

Acquired
- Drugs—lithium, demeclocycline, amphotericin B, cisplatin
- Metabolic—hypercalcemia, hypokalemia, hyperglycemia
- Infiltrating lesions—sarcoidosis, amylodosis
- Chronic renal disease
- Sickle cell anemia

Dipsogenic
- Psychogenic polydipsia
- Hypothalamic diseases—similar lesions as in neurogenic DI

Features

- Clinical presentation
  - Adults-polyuria, polydipsia and nocturia
  - Children-polyuria, polydipsia, enuresis and failure to thrive.
- Rapid dehydration and hypernatremia can occur if the patient does not have access to water or has impaired thirst mechanisms.
- Transient DI complicates an estimated 10–15% of pituitary surgeries, although permanent DI is uncommon (requires the destruction of >90% of AVP neurons).
- Pregnancy results in increased AVP metabolism from placental vasopressinase, but is generally not clinically relevant.

▶ Neurogenic DI may be masked by cortisol deficiency and uncovered by the administration of glucocorticoids.

Investigations

Diagnosis of DI

- Confirm large urine output (>40 mL/kg/day in adults) with a 24-hour urine collection.
- Exclude diabetes mellitus and renal failure (osmotic diuresis).
- Exclude hypokalemia and hypercalcemia (nephrogenic DI).
- Consider water deprivation test (see Box 27.2)
- Pituitary MRI is recommended for suspected neurogenic DI.

Box 27.2 Water deprivation test

1   The patient is water deprived in a monitored setting for ~8 hours.
2   Urine output and osmolality are monitored hourly, and plasma sodium and osmolality are measured every 2 hours.
3   The test is stopped when one of the following parameters is met:
    a. Urine osmolality is normal (>600 mOsm/kg), thereby excluding DI.
    b. The plasma osmolality or sodium values become clearly elevated.
    c. The urine osmolality is stable (<10% change) on three consecutive readings.
4   A plasma sample is sent for ADH measurement and dDAVP is administered (1–2 mcg SQ), followed by hourly measurements of urinary volume and urine osmolality × 2.

Treatment

Maintenance of adequate fluid input

In patients with partial DI, mild polyuria and an intact thirst mechanism, drug therapy may not be necessary.

Drug therapy

Neurogenic DI

- Arginine vasopressin (Pitressin): short half-life and vasopressor effect when administered intravenously limits its general utility.
- Desmopressin (1-deamino-8-D-arginine-vasopressin)
  - Vasopressin analog, acts predominantly on the V2 receptors in the kidney, and has the following advantages: longer half-life than the native hormone, increased antidiuretic efficacy, and no vasopressor (V1 receptor) activity.
  - In the hospital setting: 1–2 mcg parenteral (SQ, IM, or IV) administration is preferred.
  - Chronic administration: intranasal spray use is preferable (10–40 mcg/day in divided doses) or oral tablets (50–1200 mg/day).

Additional medications can be used to augment ADH release or actions (e.g., chlorpropamide, carbamazepine, clofibrate, NSAIDs), but these are less efficacious than dDAVP and may cause adverse side effects.

Nephrogenic DI

- Correct underlying causes and discontinue offending drug when possible.
- Low-sodium/protein diets
- Thiazide diuretic
- Amiloride (for lithium-induced DI)
- NSAIDs

Dipsogenic

Management is often difficult. Treat any underlying tumor or psychiatric disorder, when possible.

Caveats for water deprivation study

- Differentiating between partial neurogenic/nephrogenic DI and psychogenic polydipsia is best done by comparing the plasma AVP level with urinary and plasma osmolalities (using established nomograms) during a hyperosmotic state.
- Chronic psychogenic polydipsia may result in reduced urine-concentrating ability because of medullary solute washout.

Test interpretation

	After fluid deprivation Urine Osm ADH	After desmopressin Urine Osm
Complete neuro DI	-------No change-------	↑ (>100%) %
Complete nephro DI	No change ↑	No change (<10%)
Psychogenic polydipsia	↑	↑ No change (<10%)

Further reading

Loh JA, Verbalis JG (2008). Disorders of water and salt metabolism associated with pituitary disease. *Endocrinol Metab Clin North Am* 37:213–234.

Verbalis JG (2002). Managment of disorders of water metabolism in patients with pituitary tumors. *Pituitary* 5:119–132.

Hyponatremia

Incidence

Hyponatermia is the most common electrolyte abnormality in hospitalized patients. Mild to moderate hyponatremia (sodium 126–135 mmol/L) and severe hyponatremia (sodium <125 mmol/L) occur in 14% and 1% of hospitalized patients, respectively.

Etiologies

Box 28.1 Causes of hyponatremia

Excess water
- ↑ Water reabsorption: cirrhosis, congestive heart failure, nephrotic syndrome
- Reduced renal excretion of a water load: SIADH, glucocorticoid deficiency, hypothyroidism
- Excess water intake: primary polydipsia

Salt deficiency
- Renal loss: salt wasting nephropathy—tubulointerstitial nephritis, polycystic kidney disease, analgesic nephropathy, recovery phase of acute tubular necrosis, cerebral salt wasting, mineralcorticoid deficiencies
- Nonrenal loss: mucosal losses, burns, sweating, GI tract (bowel sequestration, fistulae, pancreatitis)

Artifactual/pseudohyponatremia
- Lipids, proteins (e.g., paraproteinemia)
- Solutes (e.g., glucose, mannitol, ethanol)

Neurosurgical hyponatremia

Etiologies
- Excessive hypotonic fluid administration
- SIADH (e.g., pain, nausea, medications)
- Glucocorticoid deficiency
- Cerebral salt wasting
  - Characterized by diuresis and natriuresis of unknown etiology
  - Associated with traumatic brain injury, particularly subarachnoid hemorrhage
  - Best distinguished from SIADH by hypovolemic status

Classification and clinical features

See Table 28.1 for classification.
- Hyponatremia clinically manifests with neurological symptoms from osmotic fluid shifts and brain edema.
- Symptoms range from asymptomatic to severe depending on the extent of hyponatremia and the rate of development (acute, <48 hours). Acute symptoms include headaches, fatigue, anorexia, nausea, vomiting, altered sensorium, seizure, coma, respiratory arrest and death.

Table 28.1 Pituitary hormone replacement regimens

Classification	Clinical features	<20	>20
Hypovolemic	Dry mucous membranes, poor skin turgor, hypotension, tachycardia	Nonrenal losses	Renal losses
Euvolemic	Mild volume overload in SIADH is usually not clinically apparent.	SIADH + fluid restriction	SIADH
Hypervolemic	Peripheral edema, ascites, increased JVD, pulmonary edema	Cirrhosis CHF	Renal failure CHF + diuretics

CHF, congestive heart failure; JVD, jugular venous distension.

Investigations

- Assess volume status
- Serum osmolality (normal in pseudohyponatremia from hyper-lipidemia/paraproteinemia)
- Urine sodium level (spot)
- Other investigations as indicated (e.g., urine osmolality, cortisol, thyroid function tests, renal/liver biochemistry and B-type natriuretic peptide [BNP] levels).

Hyponatremia treatment

Hypovolemic hyponatremia

- Treat underlying condition (e.g., diarrhea, vomiting, nephropathy).
- IV normal saline and increased dietary salts

Traditional formula for calculating sodium deficit

- Na+ required = Total Body Water (TBW) × Na(desired - current)
- TBW = lean body weight × 0.5 (females) and × 0.6 (males)
- Rate of Na+ normalization (mmol/h) varies by extent and acuity of hyponatremia.
  - Overly rapid correction of severe, chronic hyponatremia can lead to osmotic demyelination syndrome.
  - In general, limit the rise of plasma sodium concentration by <8–12 mmol/L in the first 24 hours, and <18–24 mmol/L in the first 48 hours.

Euvolemic hyponatremia/SIADH

📖 See Syndrome of inappropriate ADH (SIADH) (p. 159).

Hypervolemic hyponatremia

- Treatment of underlying disorder (e.g., CHF, liver disease)
- Diuretics
- Fluid restriction

Artifactual/pseudohyponatremia

Treat underlying disorder only (e.g., normalize hyperglycemia).

Further reading

Moore K, Thompson C, Trainer R (2003). Disorders of water balance. *Clin Med* 3:28–33.

Sterns RH, Nigwekar SU, Hix, JK (2009). The treatment of hyponatremia. *Semin Nephrol* 29:282–299.

Syndrome of inappropriate ADH (SIADH)

Definition

SIADH is a syndrome of sustained AVP release or response in the absence of appropriate hyperosmotic or hypovolemic stimuli.

Features

- SIADH clinically manifests with neurological symptoms from hyponatremia caused by osmotic fluid shifts and brain edema.
- Symptoms range from mild to severe depending on the extent of hyponatremia and the rate of development (acute, <48 hours). Symptoms include headaches, fatigue, anorexia, nausea, vomiting, altered sensorium, seizure, coma, respiratory arrest and death.
- Mild chronic hyponatremia is common in the elderly because of ineffective suppression of ADH.

Criteria for diagnosis

- Hyponatremia and hypotonic plasma (osmolality <275 mOsm/kg of water)
- Inappropriate urine concentration (>100 mOsm/kg)
- Excessive renal sodium loss (>40 mmol/L), with normal salt intake and exclusion of recent diuretic use
- Euvolemic status
- Normal renal, adrenal and thyroid function

Types of SIADH

- Type AI—erratic excess ADH secretion, unrelated to plasma osmolality (most common)
- Type B—elevated basal secretion of AVP, despite normal regulation by osmolality
- Type C—"reset osmostat," AVP secretion at a lower serum osmolality
- Type D—low vasopressin secretion, possible vasopressin receptor defect

📖 See Box 29.1 for causes of SIADH.

Box 29.1 Causes of SIADH

Malignant diseases
- Small-cell lung carcinoma, thymoma, lymphoma, leukemia, sarcoma, mesothelioma, GI/GU tumors

Pulmonary disorders
- Infections (pneumonia, tuberculosis, empyema)
- Pneumothorax
- Asthma
- Respiratory failure, positive pressure ventilation

CNS disorders
- Infections (meningitis, encephalitis, abscess)
- Vascular disorders (subarachnoid hemorrhage, cerebrovascular accident, traumatic brain injury, hydrocephalus)
- Other (multiple sclerosis, Guillain–Barre, Shy–Drager syndromes, HIV)

Drugs
- Chemotherapy (vincristine, vinblastine, cyclophosphamide)
- Psychiatric drugs (phenothiazines, SSRIs, TCAs)
- Other (carbamazepine, clofibrate, chlorpropamide, nicotine, narcotics, 'ectasy')

Metabolic
- Hypothyroidism
- Glucocorticoid deficiency
- Other (pain, stress, nausea, idiopathic)

Treatment

- Treat underlying cause.
- Fluid restriction to 500–1000 mL/24 hours
- Vasopressin antagonists (e.g., tolvaptan (oral route, V1 specific) and Conivaptan (IV route, V1/V2 antagonism). *Expense currently limits their practical use in most cases*
- Hypertonic saline (3% infusion) for severe symptomatic hyponatremia (eg. seizures or altered mentation). It is important to limit the rate of sodium correction to ≤ 8–12 mmol/L during the first 24 hours to avoid central pontine myelinolysis, particularly if hyponatremia is chronic (>48 hours duration).

Further reading

Ellison DH, Berl T (2007). The syndrome of inappropriate antidiuresis. *N Engl J Med* 356:2064–2071.

Pineal gland

Physiology

The pineal gland lies behind the third ventricle and produces melatonin, which is important for sleep and entraining some pituitary hormones to light–dark cycles.

Pineal and intracranial germ cell tumors

- Incidence: 0.5%–3% intracranial neoplasms
- Epidemiology: more common in children and in males
- Three most common pineal gland tumors: germ cell >> pineal parenchymal > gliomas; 2/3 malignant and 1/3 benign
- Germ cell tumors are classified as germinomas or nongerminomatous.
- Pineal parenchymal tumors and gliomas have histological subtypes that vary from low- to high-grade tumors.

Features

- Obstructive hydrocephalus. ↑ intracranial pressure, headaches, vomiting, ataxia and lethargy
- Parinaud's syndrome (paralysis of upward gaze, convergent nystagmus, Argyll–Robertson pupils)
- Vision disturbances (bitemporal hemianopsia)
- Hypothalamic/pituitary dysfunction: hypopituitarism and DI
- Sexual precocity (if tumor secretes β-hCG which mimics LH)

Investigations and staging

- Imaging of craniospinal axis by MRI/CT
- CSF cytology
- Tumor markers (β-hCG, α-fetoprotein)
- Tumor biopsy
- Pituitary function assessment for hypopituitarism and DI

Management

- Multimodal approach from among surgical resection, radiation therapy and chemotherapy, depending on the tumor type and stage.
- Pure germinomas are very radiosensitive.

Prognosis

The prognosis is excellent for germinomas (90% 5-year survival), but is less favorable for nongerminomatous germ cell tumors (60–70% 5-year survival). Prognosis for pineal parenchymal tumors and gliomas, varies by histological sub-type and disease extent, and trends with tumor grade.

Further reading

Al-Hussaini M, Sultan I, Abuirmileh N, Jaradat I, et al. (2009). Pineal gland tumors: experience from the SEER database. *J Neurooncol* 94:351–358.

Haddock MG, Schild SE, Scheithauer BW, Schomberg, PJ (1997). Radiation therapy for histologically confirmed primary central nervous system germinoma. *Int J Radiat Oncol Biol Phys* 38:915–923.

Rosenblum MK, Nakazato Y, Matsutani M (2007). CNS germ cell tumors. In Louis D, Ohgaki H, Wiestler O, Cavenee WK (eds.), *WHO Classification of Tumours of the Central Nervous System*, 3rd ed. Albany, NY: WHO Publication Center, pp. 197–204.

Part 3

Adrenals

Boris Draznin

Anatomy and physiology

Anatomy

The normal adrenal glands weigh 4–5 g. The cortex represents 90% of the normal gland and surrounds the medulla. The arterial blood supply arises from the renal arteries, aorta, and inferior phrenic artery. Venous drainage occurs via the central vein into the inferior vena cava on the right, and into the left renal vein on the left.

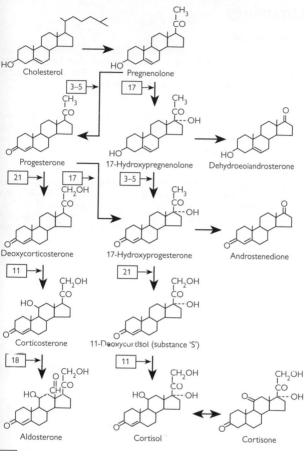

Fig. 31.1 Pathways and enzymes involved in synthesis of glucocorticoids, mineralocorticoids, and adrenal androgens from a cholesterol precursor. Reprinted with permission from Besser M, Thorner GM (1994). *Clinical Endocrinology*, 2nd ed. New York: Elsevier.

Physiology

Glucocorticoids
Glucocorticoid (cortisol 10–20 mg/day) (Table 31.1) production occurs from the zona fasciculata, and adrenal androgens arise form the zona reticularis. Both of these are under control of ACTH, which regulates both steroid synthesis and adrenocortical growth.

Mineralocorticoids
Mineralocorticoid (aldosterone 100–150 mcg/day) (Table 31.1) synthesis occurs in zona glomerulosa predominantly under the control of the renin–angiotensin system (🕮 see Fig 31.2), although ACTH also contributes to its regulation.

Androgens
The adrenal gland (zona reticularis and zona fasciculata) also produces sex steroids, in the form of dehydroepiandrostenedione (DHEA) and androstenedione. The synthetic pathway is under the control of ACTH.

Urinary steroid profiling provides quantitative information on the biosynthetic and catabolic pathways. Profiling can be useful in the following:
- Mineralocorticoid hypertension
- Polycystic ovary syndrome
- Congenital adrenal hyperplasia
- Steroid-producing tumors
- Precocious puberty and virilization
- Hirsutism

Table 31.1 Adrenal cortex steroid production

Adrenal cortex	Cortisol	Aldosterone	DHEA	DHEAS
Production rate/24 hours	10 mg	100 mcg	10 mg	25 mg
t½	80 min	20 min	20 min	9 hr
Control	ACTH	Renin	ACTH	ACTH

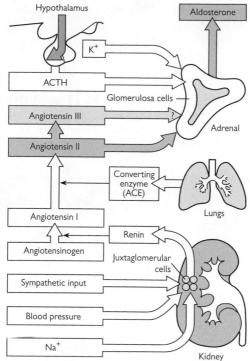

Fig. 31.2 Physiological mechanisms governing the production and secretion of aldosterone. Reprinted with permission from Besser M, Thorner GM (1994). *Clinical Endocrinology*, 2nd ed. New York: Elsevier.

Further reading

Taylor NF (2006). Urinary steroid profiling. *Method Mol Biol* 324:159–175.

Imaging

Computed tomography (CT) scanning

CT is the most widely used modality for imaging the adrenal glands. It is able to detect masses >5 mm in diameter. It can be useful in differentiating between different adrenal cortical pathologies (Fig. 32.1).

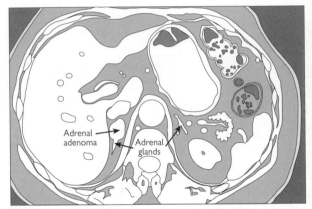

Fig. 32.1 Typical appearance of adrenal adenoma on CT scan.

Magnetic resonance imaging (MRI)

MRI can also reliably detect adrenal masses >5–10 mm in diameter and in some circumstances provides additional information to CT data, e.g., differentiation of cortical from medullary tumors.

Ultrasound (US) imaging

US detects masses >20 mm in diameter, but normal adrenal glands are not usually visible except in children. Body morphology and bowel gas can provide technical difficulties.

Normal adrenal

Normal adrenal cortex is assessed by measuring limb thickness and is considered enlarged at >5 mm, approximately the thickness of the diaphragmatic crus nearby.

Radionucleotide imaging

^{123}Iodine-metaiodobenzylguanidine (MIBG)

This is a guanethidine analog, concentrated in some pheochromocytomas, paragangliomas, carcinoid tumors, and neuroblastomas, and is useful diagnostically. A different isotope, ^{131}I-MIBG, may be used therapeutically, e.g., in malignant pheochromocytomas when the diagnostic imaging shows uptake.

^{75}Se 6β-selenomethyl-19-norcholesterol

This isotope is concentrated in functioning steroid-synthesizing tissue and is used to image the adrenal cortex. It can be used in determining whether a nodule is functioning or not and can be helpful in localizing residual adrenal tissue following failed bilateral adrenalectomy.

However, high-resolution CT and MRI have largely replaced it in localizing functional adrenal adenomas.

Positron emission tomography (PET)

PET can be useful in locating tumors and metastases. Radiopharmaceuticals for specific endocrine tumors are being developed, e.g., [11C] metahydroxyephedrine for pheochromocytoma. Combined with CT (PET-CT) it may offer particular value in localizing occult neuroendocrine tumors.

Venous sampling

Adrenal vein sampling can be useful to lateralize an adenoma or to differentiate an adenoma from bilateral hyperplasia. It is technically difficult—particularly, catheterizing the right adrenal vein because of its drainage into the IVC.

It may also be used to confirm the diagnosis of bilateral pheochromocytoma. It is of particular value in lateralizing small aldosterone-producing adenomas that cannot easily be visualized on CT or MRI.

Further reading

Pacak K, Eisenhofer G, Goldstein DS (2004). Functional imaging of endocrine tumors: role of positron emission tomography. *Endocr Rev* 25(4):568–580.

Peppercorn PD, Grossman AB, et al. (1998). Imaging of incidentally discovered adrenal masses. *Clin Endocrinol* 48:379–388.Reznek RH, Armstrong P (1994). The adrenal gland. *Clin Endocrinol* 40:561–576.

Mineralocorticoid excess

Definitions

Most cases of mineralocorticoid excess are due to excess aldosterone production, which may be primary or secondary, and are typically associated with hypertension and hypokalemia.

Primary hyperaldosteronism is a disorder of autonomous aldosterone hypersecretion with suppressed renin levels.

Secondary hyperaldosteronism occurs when aldosterone hypersecretion occurs secondary to elevated circulating renin levels. This is typical of heart failure, cirrhosis, or nephrotic syndrome, but can also be due to renal artery stenosis and, occasionally, a very rare renin-producing tumor (reninoma).

Other mineralocorticoids may occasionally be the cause of this syndrome (📖 see Box 33.1).

Box 33.1 Causes of mineralocorticoid excess

Primary hyperaldosteronism
- Conn's syndrome (aldosterone-producing adrenal adenoma): 35%
- Bilateral adrenal hyperplasia: 60%
- Glucocorticoid remedial aldosteronism (GRA): <1%
- Aldosterone-producing adrenal carcinoma

Secondary hyperaldosteronism
- Renal artery stenosis
- Renal hypoperfusion
- Cirrhosis
- Congestive cardiac failure
- Nephrotic syndrome
- Renin-secreting tumor

Other mineralocorticoid excess syndromes
- Apparent mineralocorticoid excess (📖 see p. 182)
- Liquorice ingestion (p. 183) (inhibits II β HSOH) ↓ aldosterone, ↓ renin, ↓ K⁺ found in sweets, chewing tobacco, cough mixtures, and herbal medicines
- Deoxycorticosterone and corticosterone (📖 see p. 183)
- Ectopic ACTH secretion (📖 see p. 183)
- Congenital adrenal hyperplasia (📖 see p. 239)
- Exogenous mineralocorticoids

Pseudoaldosteronism due to abnormal renal tubular transport
- 📖 Bartter's syndrome (p. 191)
- 📖 Gitelman's syndrome (p. 190)
- 📖 Liddle's syndrome (p. 190)

Primary aldosteronism

Epidemiology

Primary hyperaldosteronism is present in approximately 5% of hypertensive patients. The most common cause is bilateral adrenal hyperplasia (□ see Table 34.1).

Pathophysiology

Aldosterone causes renal sodium retention and potassium loss. This results in expansion of body sodium content, leading to suppression of renal renin synthesis.

The direct action of aldosterone on the distal nephron causes sodium retention and loss of hydrogen and potassium ions, resulting in a hypokalemic alkalosis, although serum potassium may not be significantly reduced and may be normal in up to 50% of cases.

Aldosterone has pathophysiological effects on a range of other tissues, causing cardiac fibrosis, vascular endothelial dysfunction, and nephrosclerosis.

Clinical features

Moderately severe hypertension occurs, which is often resistant to conventional therapy. There may be disproportionate left ventricular hypertrophy.

Hypokalemia is usually asymptomatic. Occasionally, patients may present with tetany, myopathy, polyuria, and nocturia (hypokalemic nephrogenic diabetes insipidus) due to severe hypokalemia.

Conn's syndrome—aldosterone-producing adenoma

Very high levels of the enzyme aldosterone synthase are expressed in tumor tissue. Although aldosterone production is autonomous, ACTH has a greater stimulatory effect than angiotensin II (aldosterone often displays a diurnal variation that mirrors that of cortisol), although a subtype that remain more responsive to angiotensin II has been described.

Very rarely, Conn's adenomas may be part of the MEN1 syndrome.

Table 34.1 Causes of hyperaldosteronism

Condition	Relative frequency	Age	Sex	Pathology
Aldosteronoma (Conn's adenoma)	35%	3rd–6th decade	Predominant in women	Benign, adenoma, <2.5 cm diameter, yellow because of high cholesterol content
Idiopathic waldosteronism/ adrenal hyperplasia	60%	Older than Conn's	No sex difference	Macronodular or micronodular hyperplasia
Adrenal carcinoma	Rare	5th–7th decade (occasionally young)	More common in women	Tumor >4 cm in diameter, often larger, may be evidence of local invasion
Glucocorticoid suppressible hyperaldosteronism	Rare	Childhood	No sex difference	Bilateral hyperplasia of zona glomerulosa

Bilateral adrenal hyperplasia (bilateral idiopathic hyperaldosteronism)

This is the most common form of primary hyperaldosteronism in adults. Hyperplasia is more commonly bilateral than unilateral and may be associated with micronodular or macronodular hyperplasia. However, CT-demonstrable nodules have a prevalence of 2% in the general population, including hypertensive patients without excess aldosterone production.

The pathophysiology is not known, although aldosterone secretion is very sensitive to circulating angiotensin II. The pathophysiology of bilateral adrenal hyperplasia is not understood; it is possible that it represents an extreme end of the spectrum of low rennin-essential hypertension.

Glucocorticoid-remedial aldosteronism (GRA)

This is a rare autosomal dominantly inherited condition due to the presence of a chimeric gene (8q22) containing the 5´ sequence that determines regulation of the 11β-hydroxylase gene *(CYP11B1)* coding for the enzyme catalyzing the last step in cortisol synthesis, and the 3´ sequence from the aldosterone synthase gene *(CYP11B2)* coding for the enzyme catalyzing the last step in aldosterone synthesis.

This results in expression of aldosterone synthase in the zona fasiculata as well as the zona glomerulosa, and aldosterone secretion becomes under ACTH control. Glucocorticoids lead to suppression of ACTH and suppression of aldosterone production.

- There is early hypertension and family history.
- Hybrid steroids (18OHcortisol and 18oxocortisol) are elevated

Aldosterone-producing carcinoma

This is rare and usually associated with excessive secretion of other corticosteroids (cortisol, androgen, estrogen). Hypokalemia may be profound, and aldosterone levels very high.

Screening

Indications

- Patients resistant to conventional antihypertensive medication (i.e., not controlled on three agents)
- Hypertension associated with hypokalemia (potassium < 3.7 mmol/L, irrespective of thiazide use)
- Hypertension developing before 40 years of age
- Adrenal incidentaloma

Method

False-negative and false-positive results can occur if the test is not performed under controlled circumstances.

- Give oral supplements of potassium to control hypokalemia.
- Stop medication that can interfere with the test using appropriate washout period (Table 34.2).
- Blood pressure (BP) can be controlled using doxazosin or verapamil (rather than other calcium antagonists).
- Measure aldosterone/renin ratio.

Table 34.2 Effects of medication on renin and aldosterone measurement

Drug	Washout	Magnitude of effect	Effect on screening test
Methyl-dopa			False positive
Clonidine	–	–	False positive
β-Blockers, e.g., atenolol	2	62% (±82)	False positive
α-Blockers, e.g., doxazosin	na	–5% (±26)	Little effect
ACE inhibitors, e.g., fosinopril	2	–30% (±24)	False negative
ARB, e.g., irbesartan	2	–43% (±24)	False negative
Ca antagonists, e.g., amlodipine	2	–17% (±32)	False negative
Diuretics	6	–	False negative

NSAIDS may give false positives.

A high ratio is suggestive of primary hyperaldosteronism (aldosterone [ng/dL]/plasma renin activity [ng/mL/h] >30–50). Newer assays that measure renin mass (rather than activity) will require development of different cutoffs. The greater the ratio, the more likely the diagnosis of primary aldosteronism.

A false negative can occur in patients with chronic renal failure due to an inappropriately high plasma renin activity.

Confirmation of diagnosis

Confirmation of autonomous aldosterone production is made by demonstrating failure to suppress aldosterone in the face of sodium/volume loading. This can be achieved through a number of mechanisms after optimizing test conditions as described.

Dietary sodium loading

Patients can be instructed to take a diet with high sodium content (sufficient to raise the sodium intake to 200 mmol/day for 3 days. If necessary, this can be achieved by adding supplemental sodium chloride tablets.

It is important to ensure that potassium is maintained during this period; potassium supplementation may also be required. Failure to suppress 24-hour urinary aldosterone secretion at the end of this period is diagnostic of primary aldosteronism.

Saline infusion test

- Administer 2 L normal saline over 4 hours, preferably between 8 A.M. and noon.
- Measure plasma aldosterone at 0 and 4 hours.
- Aldosterone fails to suppresses to <7.5 ng/mL (7.5–10 equivocal) in 80–90% of primary aldosteronism.

Frequently, this test is followed by measurements of plasma rennin activity (PRA) with upright posture and use of a diuretic (furosemide up to 80 mg). Low PRA under these conditions supports the diagnosis.

Other testing

A number of tests have been described that are said to differentiate between the various subtypes of primary aldosteronism (solitary Conn's adenoma, bilateral adrenal hyperplasia, GRA). However, none of these are sufficiently specific to influence management decisions, and more specific investigations (imaging and adrenal vein sampling) are necessary if there is doubt.

Additional tests, such as postural response of aldosterone and the basal plasma 18-hydroxycorticosterone >100 ng/dL, are suggestive of primary aldosteronism.

Diagnosis of GRA is best made using a specific genetic test rather than on the ability of dexamethasone (0.5 mg q6h for 3 days) to suppress aldosterone.

Other dynamic tests

If these tests are nondiagnostic, then it is usual to proceed to venous sampling rather than dynamic testing. However, such tests can sometimes be helpful.

Captopril suppression test
- Plasma aldosterone is measured in the sitting position, basally, and 60 minutes after captopril 25 mg.
- Inhibition of angiotensin II leads to a fall in aldosterone in patients with idiopathic hyperaldosteronism but not in Conn's syndrome.

Fludrocortisone suppression test
- Give fludrocortisone 100 mcg q6h for 4 days.
- Measure aldosterone basally and on last day.
- Aldosterone is suppressed in hyperplasia but unchanged in adenomas.

Table 34.3 Differential diagnosis of primary hyperaldosteronism

Condition	Test	Upright posture and time	ACE inhibitor	Dexamethasone suppression
Normal	PRA	↑	←	↑
	Aldosterone	↑	→	↑
Aldosterone-producing adenoma	PRA	↑	↑	↑
	Aldosterone	↓	↑	↑
Angiotensin-responsive adenoma (?~20% adenomas)	PRA	↑	←	↑
	Aldosterone	↑	→	↑
Idiopathic adrenal hyperplasia	PRA	↑	←	↑
	Aldosterone	↑	→	↑
Glucocorticoid-suppressible hyperaldosteronism	PRA	↑	↑	←
	Aldosterone	→	↑	→

Localization and confirmation of differential diagnosis

CT/MRI scan

CT and MRI scanning are of value in identifying adrenal adenomas. It should be noted, however, that the frequency of adrenal incidentalomas rises with age and, for this reason, it is prudent to consider adrenal vein sampling in older patients (age >50) with primary aldosteronism who have an apparent solitary adenoma on scanning.

- Identifies most adenomas >5 mm diameter. Bilateral abnormalities or tumors <1 cm in diameter require further localization procedures.
- In bilateral adrenal hyperplasi,a both glands can appear enlarged or normal in size.
- Macronodular hyperplasia may result in identifiable nodules on imaging.
- A mass >4 cm in size is suspicious of carcinoma but is unusual in Conn's syndrome.
- In essential hypertension, nodules are described.

Adrenal vein sampling

Aldosterone measurements from both adrenal veins allow a gradient between the two sides to be identified in the case of unilateral disease. It is the gold standard for differentiation between uni- and bilateral aldosterone production, but cannulating the right adrenal vein is technically difficult, as it drains directly into the inferior vena cava.

Cortisol measurements must also be taken concomitantly with aldosterone to confirm successful positioning within the adrenal veins and should be more than 3× a peripheral sample (central/peripheral ratio >3). The aldosterone/cortisol ratio with an adenoma is >4.1.

Radiolabeled iodocholesterol scanning

This test has low sensitivity and specificity and offers no advantage over a high-resolution CT or MRI with, where necessary, adrenal vein sampling.

Treatment

Surgery

Laparascopic adrenalectomy is the treatment of choice for aldosterone-secreting adenomas and is associated with lower morbidity than open adrenalectomy.

Surgery is not indicated in patients with idiopathic hyperaldosteronism, as even bilateral adrenalectomy may not cure the hypertension.

Presurgical spironolactone treatment may be used to correct potassium stores before surgery.

The BP response to treatment with spironolactone (50–400 mg/day) before surgery can be used to predict the response to surgery of patients with adenomas.

Hypertension is cured in about 70% of patients. If it persists (more likely in those with long-standing hypertension and increased age), it is more amenable to medical treatment.

Overall, 50% become normotensive in 1 month and 70% within 1 year.

Medical treatment

Medical therapy remains an option for patients with a solitary adrenaladenoma who are unlikely to be cured by surgery, who are unfit for operation, or who express a preference for medical management.

The aldosterone antagonist *spironolactone* (50–400 mg/day) has been used successfully for many years to treat the hypertension and hypokalemia associated with bilateral adrenal hyperplasia and idiopathic hyperaldosteronism.

There may be a delay in response of hypertension of 4–8 weeks. However, combination with other antihypertensive agents (ACE inhibitor and calcium channel blockers) is usually required.

Side effects are common, particularly gynecomastia and impotence in men, menstrual irregularities in women, and GI effects.

Eplerenone (50–100 mg/day) is a mineralocorticoid antagonist without antiandrogen effects and greater selectivity than that of spironolactone.

Alternative drugs include the potassium-sparing diuretics *amiloride* and *triamterene*. Amiloride may need to be given in high dose (up to 40 mg/day) in primary aldosteronism, and monitoring of serum potassium is essential. Calcium channel antagonists may also be helpful.

Glucocorticoid-remedial aldosteronism can be treated with low-dose *dexamethasone* (0.5 mg on going to bed). Side effects often limit therapy, and spironolactone or amiloride treatment is often preferred.

For adrenal carcinoma, surgery and postoperative adrenolytic therapy with *mitotane* is usually required, but the prognosis is usually poor (📖 see Treatment, p. 186).

Further reading

Allolio BS, Hahner S, Weismann D, Fassnacht M (2004). Management of adrenocortical carcinoma. *Clin Endocrinol* 60:273–287.

Espiner EA, Ross DG, Yandle TG, Richards AM, Hunt PJ (2003). Predicting surgically remedial primary aldosteronism: role of adrenal scanning, posture testing, and adrenal vein sampling *J Clin Endocrinol Metab* 88(8):3637–3644.

Funder JW, Carey RM, Fardella C, et al. (2008). Case detection, diagnosis, and treatment of patients with primary aldosteronism: an Endocrine Society clinical practice guideline. *J Clin Endocrinol Metab* 93(9):3266–3281.

Ganguly A (1998). Primary aldosteronism. *N Engl J Med* 339:1828–1833. Young WF (2007). Primary aldosteronism—renaissance of a syndrome. *Clin Endocrinol* 66:607–618.

Excess other mineralocorticoids

Epidemiology

Occasionally, the clinical syndrome of hyperaldosteronism is not associated with excess aldosterone, and a process due to another mineralocorticoid is suspected. This can either be due to an increase in an alternative mineralcorticoid or to ↑ mineralocorticoid effect of cortisol. These conditions are rare.

Apparent mineralocorticoid excess

The aldosterone receptor has an equal affinity for cortisol and aldosterone, but there is a 100-fold excess of circulating cortisol over aldosterone. The receptor is usually protected from the effects of stimulation by cortisol by the 11β-hydroxysteroid type 2 dehydrogenase enzyme, which converts cortisol to cortisone.

In this syndrome, there is deficiency of 11β-hydroxysteroid dehydrogenase (HSD) enzyme type 2 encoded on chromosome 16q22. Congenital absence (autosomal recessive) of the enzyme or inhibition of its activity allows cortisol to stimulate the receptor and leads to severe hypertension.

Type 1 is seen predominantly in children, presenting with failure to thrive, thirst, polyuria, and severe hypertension. Patients are not cushingoid as there is intact negative feedback, and circulating cortisol levels are not raised. The urinary terahydrocortisol and allotetrahydrocortisol-to-terahydrocortisone ratio is raised to 10 × normal.

Type 2 is a milder form that may be a cause of hypertension in adolescence or early adulthood. The urinary terahydrocortisol and allo-tetrahydrocortisol-to-terahydrocortisone ratio is normal.

However, multiple mutations have been found in the 11β-HSD2 gene for both types, and some authors believe there is a spectrum of disease: mild forms may present with salt-sensitive hypertension.

Biochemistry

- Suppression of renin and aldosterone
- Hypokalemic alkalosis
- Urinary free cortisol-to-cortisone ratio ↑
- Ratio of urinary tetrahydrocortisol and allotetrahydrocortisol to tetrahydrocortisone is raised (>10 ×) in type 1 but is normal in type 2.
- Confirm with genetic testing.

Treatment

Dexamethasone leads to suppression of ACTH secretion, reduced cortisol concentrations, and lowered BP in 60%. It has a much lower affinity for the mineralocorticoid receptor.

Other antihypertensive agents are often required.

One patient with hypertensive renal failure was cured with a renal transplant.

Licorice ingestion

Licorice contains glycyrrhetinic acid, which is used as a sweetener. It inhibits the action of 11β-HSD, making the aldosterone receptor more sensitive to cortisol.

It is found in candies, chewing tobacco, cough mixtures, and some herbal medicines.

Ectopic ACTH syndrome

📖 See p. 184.

In the syndrome of ectopic ACTH, the 11β-HSD protection is overcome because of high cortisol secretion rates, which saturate the enzyme, leading to impaired conversion of cortisol to cortisone, and thus hypokalemia and hypertension.

Deoxycorticosterone (DOC) excess

Two forms of congenital adrenal hyperplasia (📖 see Part 4 p. 239) are associated with excess production of DOC, which acts as an agonist at the mineralocorticoid receptor, resulting in hypertension with suppression of renin:

- 17α-hydroxylase deficiency
- 11β-hydroxylase deficiency

Glucocorticoid replacement to inhibit ACTH is effective treatment for these conditions.

Adrenal tumors rarely secrete excessive amounts of DOC. Usually this is concomitant with excessive aldosterone production, but occasionally it may occur in an isolated fashion.

Adrenal Cushing's syndrome

Definition and epidemiology

Cushing's syndrome results from chronic excess cortisol and is described in Chapter 18 (📖 Cushing's disease, p. 116).

The causes may be classified as ACTH dependent and ACTH independent. This section describes ACTH-independent Cushing's syndrome, which is due to adrenal tumors (benign and malignant) and is responsible for 10–20% cases of Cushing's syndrome.

Adrenal tumors causing Cushing's syndrome are more common in women. The peak incidence is in the fourth and fifth decades.

Causes and relative frequencies of adrenal Cushing's syndrome in adults are as follows:

- Adrenal adenoma: 12%.
- Adrenal carcinoma: 6%.
- Bilateral micronodular adrenal hyperplasia: 1%.
- Bilateral macronodular hyperplasia: 1%.

Pathophysiology

Benign adenomas are usually encapsulated and <6 cm in diameter. They are usually associated with pure glucocorticoid excess.

Adrenal carcinomas are usually >6 cm in diameter, although they may be smaller, and are often associated with local invasion and metastases at the time of diagnosis. They may be associated with secretion of excess androgen production in addition to cortisol. Occasionally, they may be associated with mineralocorticoid or estrogen secretion.

Carney complex (📖 see Carney complex, p. 496) is an autosomal dominant condition characterized by atrial myxomas, spotty skin pigmentation, peripheral nerve tumors, and endocrine disorders, e.g., Cushing's syndrome due to pigmented adrenal nodular hyperplasia.

Adrenal hyperplasia may be micronodular (<1 cm diameter) or macronodular (>1 cm).

Bilateral macronodular adrenal hyperplasia

Most cases of bilateral macronodular hyperplasia do not have an identifiable cause.

Abnormal gastric inhibitory peptide (GIP), vasopressin, β-agonist, human chorionic gonadotropin\luteinizing hormone, and serotonin receptors have been described.

Several cases of food-dependent Cushing's syndrome have been described that are due to GIP receptor expression.

Clinical features

The clinical features of ACTH-independent Cushing's syndrome are as described in 📖 Clinical features, p. 157 in Chapter 18, Cushing's disease.

It is important to note that in patients with adrenal carcinoma, there may also be features related to excessive androgen production in women, as well as a relatively more rapid time course of development of the syndrome.

Investigations

Once the presence of Cushing's syndrome is confirmed (📖 see Clinical features, p. 157), subsequent investigation of the cause depends on whether ACTH is suppressed (ACTH independent), or measurable or elevated (ACTH dependent).

Patients with ACTH-independent Cushing's syndrome do not suppress cortisol to <50% basal on high-dose dexamethasone testing and fail to show a rise in cortisol and ACTH following administration of CRH. (The latter test is often important when patients have borderline or low ACTH to differentiate pituitary-dependent disease from adrenal diesase.)

ACTH-independent causes are adrenal in origin, and the mainstay of further investigation is adrenal imaging.

CT scanning allows excellent visualization of the adrenal glands and their anatomy.

Adenomas are usually small and homogeneous and usually associated with contralateral gland atrophy.

Adrenal carcinomas are usually >6 cm in diameter, are heterogeneous with calcification and necrosis, and have evidence of local invasion.

Bilateral macronodular adrenal hyperplasia

- Monitor ACTH and cortisol response to a mixed meal, luteinizing hormone releasing hormone (LHRH), and posture.
- ACTH independent
- Medical treatment may be possible, e.g., octreotide, for GIP-dependent disease.

Treatment

📖 See Treatment, p. 356.

Adrenal adenoma

Unilateral adrenalectomy (normally laparoscopic) is curative.

Postoperative temporary adrenal insufficiency ensues because of long-term suppression of ACTH and the contralateral adrenal gland, requiring glucocorticoid replacement for up to 2 years.

Adrenal carcinoma

Surgery is useful to debulk tumor mass, and occasionally adrenalectomy and local clearance leads to cure. However, most patients have distant metastases at the time of diagnosis.

Postoperative drug treatment with the adrenolytic agent *mitotane* (*orthopara* DDD) 3–12 g daily may prolong survival. This may lead to adrenal insufficiency, and glucocorticoid replacement may be required.

Side effects may limit therapy and include nausea and vomiting, dizziness, and diarrhea. Monitoring of drug levels can be helpful to ensure concentrations within the therapeutic range (14–20 mcg/mL) and thus limit unwanted side effects.

Other drugs may be required to control cortisol hypersecretion (e.g., *metyrapone*).

Newer treatments such as *suramin, 5-fluorouracil*, and *gossypol* have also been tried without evidence of benefit.

Bilateral adrenal hyperplasia

Bilateral adrenalectomy is curative. Lifelong glucocorticoid and mineralocorticoid treatment is required.

Medical treatment may be possible for cases with aberrant receptors, e.g., octreotide for GIP-dependent disease.

Prognosis

Adrenal adenomas, which are successfully treated with surgery, have a good prognosis, and recurrence is unlikely. The prognosis depends on the long-term effects of excess cortisol before treatment—in particular, atherosclerosis and osteoporosis.

The prognosis for adrenal carcinoma is very poor, despite surgery. Reports suggest a 5-year survival of 22% and median survival time of 14 months. Age >40 years and distant metastases are associated with a worse prognosis.

Subclinical Cushing's syndrome

This describes a subset of 5–10% of patients with an adrenal incidentaloma with autonomous glucocorticoid production that is insufficient to produce overt Cushing's syndrome.

Urinary free cortisol measurement may be within the normal range, but there is a failure to suppress with low-dose dexamethasone.

An associated ↑ risk of diabetes mellitus, osteoporosis, and hypertension has been reported.

Data are insufficient to indicate the superiority of a surgical or nonsurgical approach to management.

Hypoadrenalism post-adrenalectomy has been reported that is due to suppression of the contralateral adrenal gland. Perioperative steroid cover is therefore required with re-evaluation postoperatively.

Further reading

Allolio B, Fassnacht M (2006). Clinical review: adrenocortical carcinoma: clinical update. *J Clin Endocrinol Metab* 91(6):2027–2037.

Lacroix A, N'Diaye N, Tremblay J, et al. (2001). Ectopic and abnormal hormone receptors in adrenal Cushing's syndrome. *Endocr Rev* 22(1):75–110.

Terzolo M, Angeli A, Fasscacht M, et al. (2007). Adjuvant mitotane treatment for adrenocortical carcinoma. *N Engl J Med* 356(23):2372–2380.

Adrenal surgery

Adrenalectomy

Open adrenalectomy may still be necessary for large and complex pathology. However, laparoscopic adrenalectomy (first performed in 1992) has become the procedure of choice for removal of most adrenal tumors.

Retrospective comparisons with open approaches suggest reduced hospital stay and analgesic requirements and lower postoperative morbidity. However, there are few long-term outcome data on this technique. It is most useful in the management of small (<6 cm) benign adenomas.

Laparoscopic bilateral adrenalectomy, although technically demanding, offers a useful approach to patients with macronodular hyperplasia and in selected patients with ACTH-dependent Cushing's syndrome where alternative therapeutic options are not appropriate.

Preoperative preparation of patients
- Cushing's—metyrapone or ketoconazole (☐ see p. 123)
- Phaeochromocytoma—α- and β-blockade (☐ see p. 218).

Perioperative management
See Box 37.1.

Box 37.1 Perioperative management of patients undergoing adrenalectomy

Management is for adrenal cortical tumors (benign and malignant) and bilateral adrenalectomy for Cushing's syndrome.

Perioperative glucocorticoid cover is required, as even "silent" adenomas may be associated with subclinical excess cortisol secretion and hence suppression of the contralateral adrenal gland.

Hydrocortisone is given as for pituitary surgery—100 mg IM with the premedication, and then continued every 6 hours for 24–48 hours, until the patient can take oral medication and is eating and drinking.

This is changed to oral hydrocortisone at double replacement dose—20 mg on waking, 10 mg at lunchtime and 10 mg at 5 P.M., and mineralocorticoid replacement commenced if bilateral adrenalectomy has been performed (0.1 mg fludrocortisone daily). Electrolytes and BP guide adequacy of treatment. Normal replacement hydrocortisone (20–25 mg/24 hours) can be commenced when the patient is recovered and may be omitted altogether if the patient did not have preoperative evidence of Cushing's syndrome/suppression of the contralateral gland/ bilateral adrenalectomy. Mineralocorticoid replacement is only required in patients who have had bilateral adrenalectomy.

A Cortrosyn® stimulation test (off hydrocortisone for at least 24 hours) is performed after at least 2 weeks to demonstrate adequate function of the contralateral adrenal. However, in patients with ACTH-independent Cushing's syndrome, it may take up to 2 years for full recovery of the contralateral adrenal gland to recover.

The exception is patients undergoing adrenalectomy for mineralocorticoid-secreting tumors. These patients do not usually require perioperative glucocorticoid replacement, but preoperative amiloride or spironolactone allows recovery of potassium stores and control of hypertension prior to surgery.

Further reading

Dudley NE, Harrison BJ (1999). Comparison of open posterior versus transperitoneal laparoscopic adrenalectomy. *Br J Surg* 86:656–660.

McCallum R, Connell JMC (2001). Laparoscopic adrenalectomy. *Clin Endocrinol* 55:435–436.

Wells SA, Merke DP, Cutler GB, et al. (1998). The role of laparoscopic surgery in adrenal disease. *J Clin Endocrinol Metab* 83:3041–3049.

Renal tubular abnormalities

Background

Bartter's syndrome is associated with hypokalemic alkalosis and activation of the renin–angiotensin system, but without hypertension. Liddle's syndrome is associated with hypokalemic alkalosis and hypertension but low renin and aldosterone levels.

Liddle's syndrome

This is a rare autosomal dominant (AD) condition with variable penetrance. Mutations have been localized to genes on chromosome 16.

Cause

A mutation occurs in the gene encoding the β- or γ-subunit of the highly selective epithelial sodium channel in the distal nephron. This leads to constitutive activation of sodium transport independent of circulating mineralocorticoid; secondary activation of the sodium–potassium exchange occurs.

Features
• Hypokalemia and hypertension

Investigation
• Hypokalemic alkalosis
• Suppressed renin and aldosterone levels
• 📖 See Table 38.1

Treatment

Hypertension responds to amiloride (doses up to 40 mg/day) but not spironolactone, because amiloride acts on the sodium channel directly, whereas spironolactone acts on the mineralocorticoid receptor.

Table 38.1 Summary of features of renal tubular abnormalities

Syndrome*	BP	Renin	Aldosterone	Urinary calcium	Other
Bartter's	N	↑	↑	↑	
Gitelman's	N	↑	↑	↓	↓ Mg
Liddle's	↑	↓	↓	N	

*All three conditions have hypokalemic alkalosis.

Bartter's syndrome

Cause

There is loss of function of the bumetanide-sensitive Na–K–2Cl co-transporter in the thick ascending limb of the loop of Henle. Mutations in three genes have been reported to account for the phenotype—these encode regulatory ion channels *(NKCC2, ROMK, CLCNKB)*.

Inactivation of the co-transporter leads to salt wasting, activation of the renin–angiotensin system, and ↑ aldosterone, which leads to ↑ sodium reabsorption at the distal nephron and causes hypokalemic alkalosis. Reabsorption of calcium also occurs in the thick ascending loop and thus inactivation leads to hypercalciuria.

The lack of associated hypertension is thought to be due to ↑ prostaglandin production from the renal medullary interstitial tissue in response to hypokalemia.

Rare (~1/million) autosomal recessive hypokalemic metabolic alkalosis is associated with salt wasting and normal or reduced BP.

The syndrome is usually present at an early age (<5 years).

Features

- Intravascular volume depletion
- Seizures
- Tetany
- Muscle weakness

Investigations

- Hypokalemic alkalosis
- ↑ PRA and aldosterone
- Hypercalciuria

Treatment

Potassium replacement

Potassium-sparing diuretics may help, but they are usually inadequate to correct hypokalemia. Prostaglandin synthase inhibitors (NSAIDS), e.g., indometacin 2–5 mg/kg per day or ibuprofen, may be required.

Further reading

Amirlak I, Dawson KP (2000). Bartter's syndrome. *QJM* 93:207–215.

Furuhashi M. Kitamura K, Adachi M, et al. (2005). Liddle's syndrome caused by a novel mutation in the proline-rich PY motif of the epithelial sodium channel β-subunit. *J Clin Endocrinol Metab* 90(1):340–344.

Mineralocorticoid deficiency

Epidemiology

This deficiency is rare, apart from the hyporeninemic hypoaldosteronism associated with diabetes mellitus.

Causes

Congenital

- *Adrenal hypoplasia:* X-linked failure of development of the adrenal gland. Presents in infancy with salt-losing state. Differentiated from CAH by normal external genitalia and steroid levels
- *Congenital adrenal hyperplasia (CAH):* certain types, most commonly 21-hydroxylase deficiency, are associated with MC deficiency; 📖 see p. 239.
- Rare *inherited disorders* of aldosterone biosynthesis
- *Adrenoleukodystrophy:* X-linked affecting 1/20,000 men, where very long-chain fatty acids cannot be oxidized in peroxisomes and accumulate in tissues. CNS symptoms may be absent but progressive demyelination can lead to hypertonic tetraparesis, dementia, epilepsy, coma, or death.
- *Pseudohypoaldosteronism:* inherited resistance to the action of aldosterone; 📖 see p. 570. Autosomal dominant and recessive forms are described. Usually presents in infancy. Treated with sodium chloride

Acquired

- Adrenal insufficiency: 📖 see p. 193
- *Drugs:* heparin (heparin for >5 days may cause severe hyperkalemia due to a toxic effect on the zona glomerulosa); ciclosporin
- *Hyporeninemic hypoaldosteronism:* interference with the renin–angiotensin system leads to mineralocorticoid deficiency and hyperkalemic acidosis (type IV renal tubular acidosis), e.g., diabetic nephropathy. Treatment is fludrocortisone and potassium restriction. ACE inhibitors may produce a similar biochemical picture, but here the PRA will be elevated as there is no angiotensin II feedback on renin.

Treatment

- Fludrocortisone

Adrenal insufficiency

Definition

Adrenal insufficiency results from inadequate adrenocortical function and may be due to destruction of the adrenal cortex (primary or Addison's disease) or to disordered pituitary and hypothalamic function (secondary).

Epidemiology

- The prevalence of Addison's disease is approximately 93–140/million adults. Incidence is 4.7–6.2 per million in the white population.
- Secondary adrenal insufficiency is most commonly due to suppression of pituitary–hypothalamic function by exogenous glucocorticoid administration.

Causes of secondary adrenal insufficiency

Lesions of the hypothalamus and/or pituitary gland
- Tumors—pituitary tumor, metastases, craniopharyngioma
- Infection—tuberculosis
- Inflammation—sarcoidosis, histiocytosis X, hemochromatosis, lymphocytic hypophysitis
- Iatrogenic—surgery, radiotherapy
- Other—isolated ACTH deficiency, trauma

Suppression of the hypothalamic–pituitary–adrenal axis
- Glucocorticoid administration
- Cushing's disease (after pituitary tumor removal)

Features of secondary adrenal insufficiency

As primary (📖 see Clinical features, p. 198), except:
- Absence of pigmentation—skin is pale
- Absence of mineralocoticoid deficiency
- Associated features of underlying cause, e.g., visual field defects if there is a pituitary tumor
- Other endocrine deficiencies may manifest due to pituitary failure (📖 see p. 352).
- Acute onset may occur due to pituitary apoplexy.

Isolated ACTH deficiency

- Rare
- Pathogenesis is unclear. It may be autoimmune (associated with other autoimmune conditions, and antipituitary antibodies are described in some patients).
- Absent ACTH response to CRH
- POMC mutations and POMC processing abnormalities (e.g., proconvertase PC1).

Pathophysiology

Primary

Adrenal gland destruction or dysfunction occurs from a disease process that usually involves all three zones of the adrenal cortex, resulting in inadequate glucocorticoid, mineralocorticoid, and androgen secretion. Autoimmunity is the main etiologic factor.

The manifestations of insufficiency do not usually appear until at least 90% of the gland has been destroyed and are usually gradual in onset, with partial adrenal insufficiency leading to an impaired cortisol response to stress, and the features of complete insufficiency occurring later.

Acute adrenal insufficiency may occur in the context of acute septicemia (e.g., meningococcal or hemorrhage).

Mineralocorticoid deficiency leads to reduced sodium retention and hypotension with ↓ intravascular volume, in addition to hyperkalemia due to ↓ renal potassium and hydrogen ion excretion.

Androgen deficiency presents in women with reduced axillary and pubic hair and reduced libido. (Testicular production of androgens is more important in men.)

Lack of cortisol negative feedback increases CRH and ACTH secretion. An increase in other POMC-related peptides leads to skin pigmentation and other mucous membranes.

Secondary

Inadequate ACTH results in deficient cortisol production (and ↓ androgens in women).

There is no pigmentation because ACTH and POMC secretion is reduced. Mineralocorticoid secretion remains normal, as it is mainly regulated by the renin–angiotensin system.

The onset is usually gradual with partial ACTH deficiency resulting in reduced response to stress. Prolonged ACTH deficiency leads to atrophy of the zona fasiculata and reduced ability to respond acutely to ACTH.

Investigations

📖 See p. 94 for pituitary/hypothalamic disease and p. 206 for long-term endogenous or exogenous glucocorticoids.

Addison's disease

Causes of primary adrenal insufficiency
- Autoimmune—most common cause in the developed world (approximately 70% cases).
- Autoimmune polyglandular deficiency—type 1 or 2 (see p. 198, 199).

Malignancy
- Metastatic (lung, breast, kidney—adrenal metastases found in ~50% of patients, but symptomatic adrenal insufficiency much less common)
- Lymphoma

Infiltration
- Amyloid
- Hemochromatosis

Infection
- Tuberculosis (medulla more frequently destroyed than cortex)
- Fungal, e.g., histoplasmosis, cryptococcosis
- Opportunistic infections in, e.g., AIDS—CMV, mycobacterium intracellulare, cryptococcus (up to 5% patients with AIDS develop primary adrenal insufficiency in the late stages)

Vascular hemorrhage
- Anticoagulants
- Waterhouse–Friedrichson syndrome in meningococcal septicemia

Infarction
- E.g., secondary to thrombosis in antiphospholipid syndrome

Adrenoleucodystrophy
- Inherited disorder of fatty acid metabolism
- Diagnosed by measuring very long-chain fatty acids
- Presents in childhood
- Progresses to quadraparesis and dementia in association with adrenal failure
- Treat with Lorenzo's oil

Congenital adrenal hyperplasia
- See p. 239

Congenital adrenal hypoplasia
- Rare familial failure of adrenal cortical development due to mutations and deletion of *DAX 1* gene

Iatrogenic
- Adrenalectomy
- Drugs: ketoconazole and fluconazole (inhibit cortisol synthesis), phenytoin, rifampicin (increases cortisol metabolism), etomidate, aminoglutethamide (usually do not cause hypoadrenalism unless reduced adrenal or pituitary reserve)

Autoimmune adrenalitis

This is mediated by humoral and cell-mediated immune mechanisms. Autoimmune insufficiency associated with polyglandular autoimmune syndrome is more common in women (70%).

Adrenal cortex antibodies are present in the majority of patients at diagnosis, and although titers decline and eventually disappear, they are still found in approximately 70% of patients 10 years later. Up to 20% patients/year with positive adrenal antibodies develop adrenal insufficiency. Antibodies to 21-hydroxylase are commonly found, although the exact nature of other antibodies that block the effect of ACTH for example are yet to be elucidated.

Antiadrenal antibodies are found in <2% of patients with other autoimmune endocrine disease (Hashimoto's thyroiditis, diabetes mellitus, autoimmune hypothyroidism, hypoparathyroidism, pernicious anemia). In addition, antibodies to other endocrine glands are commonly found in patients with autoimmune adrenal insufficiency (thyroid microsomal in 50%, gastric parietal cell, parathyroid, and ovary and testis).

Polyglandular autoimmune conditions also occur (📖 see Autoimmune polyglandular syndrome [APS] type 1, p. 198; APS types 2–4, p. 199). The presence of 17-hydroxylase antibodies in association with 21-hydroxylase antibodies is a good marker of patients at risk of developing premature ovarian failure in association with primary adrenal failure.

Patients with type 1 diabetes mellitus and autoimmune thyroid disease only rarely develop autoimmune adrenal insufficiency. Approximately 50% of patients with Addison's disease have other autoimmune or endocrine disorders.

Clinical features

Chronic
- Anorexia and weight loss (>90%)
- Tiredness
- Weakness—generalized, no particular muscle groups
- Pigmentation—generalized, but most common in light-exposed areas and areas exposed to pressure (elbows and knees, and under bras and belts); mucosa and scars acquired after onset of adrenal insufficiency. Look at palmar creases in Caucasians.
- Dizziness and postural hypotension
- GI symptoms—nausea and vomiting, abdominal pain, diarrhea
- Arthralgia and myalgia
- Symptomatic hypoglycemia—rare in adults
- ↓ Axillary and pubic hair and reduced libido in women
- Pyrexia of unknown origin—rarely

Associated conditions
- Vitiligo
- Features of other autoimmune endocrinopathies

Laboratory investigations
- Hyponatremia
- Hyperkalemia
- Elevated urea
- Anemia (normocytic normochromic)
- Elevated ESR
- Eosinophilia
- Mild hypercalcemia—↓ absorption, ↓ renal absorption of calcium

Autoimmune polyglandular syndrome (APS) type 1

- Also known as autoimmune polyendocrinopthy, candidiasis, and epidermal dystrophy (APECED)
- Autosomal recessive with childhood onset
- Chronic mucocutaneous candidiasis
- Hypoparathyroidism (90%), primary adrenal insufficiency (60%)
- Primary gonadal failure
- Primary hypothyroidism
- Rarely hypopituitarism, diabetes insipidus, type 1 diabetes mellitus
- Associated chronic active hepatitis (20%), malabsorption (15%), alopecia (40%), pernicious anemia, vitiligo
- Mutations in the AIRE (autoimmune regulator) gene located on chromosome 21p22.3

APS types 2–4

- Autosomal recessive, autosomal dominant, polygenic
- Adult onset
- Adrenal insufficiency (100%)
- Primary hypothyroidism (69%)
- Type 1 diabetes mellitus (52%)
- Primary gonadal failure (4–10%)
- Rarely diabetes insipidus (<0.1%)
- Associated vitiligo, myasthenia gravis, alopecia, pernicious anemia, immune thrombocytopenic purpura
- APS3—thyroid disease without adrenal insufficiency
- APS4—adrenal insufficiency without thyroid disease

Eponymous syndromes

Schmidt syndrome

- Addison's disease *and*
- Autoimmune hypothyroidism

Carpenter syndrome

- Addison's disease *and*
- Autoimmune hypothyroidism *and/or*
- Type 1 diabetes mellitus

Screening recommendations

- 2.4% of patients with a monoglandular autoimmune endocrinopathy have APS2 on subsequent follow-up.
- Functional screening is recommended every 3 years until the age of 75 years.
  - Serum Na^+, K^+, Ca^{2+}, blood cell count
  - TSH, free T_4
  - FSH, LH, testosterone, or estradiol
  - Fasting morning cortisol and glucose
  - Optional: ACTH stimulation test
- If a second endocrinopathy is diagnosed, measure organ-specific autoantibodies and consider functional screening in first-degree relatives.
  - Islet cells, GAD, IA2
  - TPO, TSH receptor
  - Cytochrome P450 enzymes
  - H^+-K^+-ATPase of the parietal cells, intrinsic factor
  - Transglutaminase, gliadin

Further reading

Dittmar M, Kahaly GJ (2003). Polyglandular autoimmune syndromes: immunogenetics and long-term follow-up. *J Clin Endocrinol Metab* 88(7):2983–2992.

Investigation of primary adrenal insufficiency

Electrolytes
- Hyponatremia is present in 90% and hyperkalemia in 65%.
- Elevated urea

Serum cortisol and ACTH
Undetectable serum cortisol is diagnostic of adrenal insufficiency, but the basal cortisol is usually in the normal range. A cortisol >21 mcg/dL precludes the diagnosis. At times of acute stress, an inappropriately low cortisol is very suggestive of the diagnosis.

Simultaneous 8 A.M. cortisol and ACTH will show an elevated ACTH for the level of cortisol. This is a very sensitive means of detecting Addison's disease.

Drugs causing ↑ cortisol-binding globulin (e.g., estrogens) will result in higher total cortisol concentration measurements.

Response to ACTH

Cortrosyn® stimulation test
Following basal cortisol measurement, 250 mcg Cortrosyn® is administered IM and serum cortisol checked at 30 and 60 minutes.

Serum cortisol should rise to a peak of 21 mcg/dL (note that this cutoff may depend on local assay conditions).

Failure to respond suggests adrenal failure.

Increased plasma renin activity (assessment of mineralocorticoid sufficiency)
This is one of the earliest abnormalities in developing primary adrenal insufficiency.

Thyroid function tests
Reduced thyroid hormone levels and elevated TSH may be due to a direct effect of glucocorticoid deficiency (cortisol inhibits TRH) or to associated autoimmune hypothyroidism. Re-evaluation is therefore required after adrenal insufficiency has been rectified.

Establish cause of adrenal insufficiency

Adrenal autoantibodies

These detect antibodies to adrenal cortex and, more recently, specific antibodies to 21-hydroxylase, side-chain cleavage enzyme, and 17-hydroxylase.

21-hydroxylase antibodies are the major component of adrenal cortex antibodies and are present in 80% of recent-onset autoimmune adrenalitis. Adrenal cortex antibodies (present in 80% patients with recent-onset autoimmune adrenalitis) are not detectable in non-autoimmune primary adrenal failure.

Imaging

Adrenal enlargement with or without calcification may be seen on CT of the abdomen, suggesting tuberculosis, infiltration, or metastatic disease. The adrenals are small and atrophic in autoimmune adrenalitis.

Specific tests

These include serological or microbiological investigations directed at particular infections, or very long-chain fatty acids (adrenoleucodystrophy) in men and women with antibody-negative isolated primary adrenal insufficiency.

Acute adrenal insufficiency

Clinical features

- Shock
- Hypotension (often not responding to measures such as inotropic support)
- Abdominal pain (may present as acute abdomen)
- Unexplained fever
- Often precipitated by major stress such as severe bacterial infection, major surgery, unabsorbed glucocorticoid medication due to vomiting
- Occasionally occurs due to bilateral adrenal infarction

Investigations

- As chronic
- In the acute situation, if the diagnosis is suspected, an inappropriately low cortisol (i.e., <19 mcg/dL) is often sufficient to make the diagnosis.

📖 See Box 41.1 for Emergency management.

Box 41.1 Emergency management of acute adrenal insufficiency

This is a life-threatening emergency and should be treated if there is strong clinical suspicion, rather than waiting for confirmatory test results.

Blood should be taken for urgent analysis of electrolytes and glucose, in addition to cortisol and ACTH.

Fluids

Large volumes of 0.9% saline may be required to reverse the volume depletion and sodium deficiency. Several liters may be required in the first 24–48 hours, but caution should be exercised where there has been chronic hyponatremia; in this circumstance rapid correction of the deficit exposes the patient to risk of central pontine myelinolysis.

If plasma sodium is <120 mmol/L at presentation, aim to correct this by no more than 10mmol/L in the first 24 hours.

Hydrocortisone

A bolus dose of 100 mg hydrocortisone is administered intravenously. Hydrocortisone 100 mg IM is then continued 6-hourly for 24–48 hours or until the patient can take oral therapy. Double replacement dose hydrocortisone (20, 10, and 10 mg orally) can then be instituted until well.

This traditional regimen causes supraphysiological replacement, and some authors suggest lower doses, e.g., 150 mg IV/24 hours.

Specific mineralocorticoid replacement is not required, as the high-dose glucocorticoid has sufficient mineralocorticoid effects (40 mg hydrocortisone ~100 mcg fludrocortisone). Once the dose of glucocorticoid is reduced after a couple of days and the patient is taking food and fluids by mouth, fludrocortisone 100 mcg/day can be commenced.

Glucose supplementation

Occasionally, this is required because of risk of hypoglycemia (low glycogen stores in the liver as a result of glucocorticoid deficiency).

Investigate and treat precipitant

This is often infection.

Monitoring treatment

Monitor electrolytes, glucose, and urea.

Treatment

Maintenance therapy

Glucocorticoid replacement

Hydrocortisone is the treatment of choice for replacement therapy, as it is reliably and predictably absorbed and allows biochemical monitoring of levels.

It is administered 3 × daily 10 mg on waking, 5 mg at midday, and 5 mg at 6 P.M. Some patients can be managed adequately with twice-daily administration of hydrocortisone.

An alternative is prednisone 5 mg once daily. This has the disadvantage that levels cannot be biochemically monitored, but its longer t½ may lead to better suppression of ACTH if pigmentation and markedly elevated morning ACTH levels are a problem. Occasionally, dexamethasone is required for this purpose.

Mineralocorticoid replacement

Fludrocortisone (9-flurohydrocortisone) is given at a dose of 0.1 mg daily. Aim to avoid significant postural fall in BP (>10 mmHg).

Occasionally, lower (0.05 mg) or higher (0.2 mg) doses are required.

A dose of 40 mg hydrocortisone has the equivalent mineralocortisone effects as 0.1 mg fludrocortisone.

Renin activity can help guide adequacy of therapy.

DHEA replacement

Dihydroepiandrosterone (DHEA) is also deficient in hypoadrenalism.

DHEA replacement (25–50 mg/day) may improve mood and well-being (as dietary supplement).

Monitoring of therapy

Clinical

- For signs of glucocorticoid excess, e.g., ↑ weight
- BP (including postural change)

Hypertension and edema suggest excessive mineralocorticoid replacement, whereas postural hypotension and salt craving suggest insufficient treatment.

Biochemical

- Serum electrolytes
- Plasma renin activity (elevated if insufficient fludrocortisone replacement). Very dependent on when the last dose was taken
- Cortisol day curve to assess adequacy of treatment

Monitor ACTH levels prior to and following morning glucocorticoid replacement if the patient develops ↑ pigmentation. If levels are elevated or rising with little suppression following glucocorticoid, obtain an MRI scan to exclude the rare possibility of pituitary hyperplasia or, very rarely, the development of a corticotrope adenoma.

Intercurrent illness

Cortisol requirements increase during severe illness or surgery.

For moderate elective procedures or investigations, e.g., endoscopy or angiography, patients should receive a single dose of 100 mg hydrocortisone before the procedure.

For major surgery, patients should take 20 mg hydrocortisone orally or 100 mg intramuscularly with the premedication and receive:

- 50–100 mg IM hydrocortisone 6-hourly for the first 3 days *or*
- 100–150 mg per 24 hours IV in 5% dextrose before reverting rapidly to a maintenance dose.

To cover severe illness, e.g., pneumonia, patients should receive 50–100 mg IM hydrocortisone q6h until resolution of the illness.

Box 41.2 Adrenal insufficiency in pregnancy

📖 Also see Normal changes during pregnancy (p. 361).
  During normal pregnancy:
- Cortisol-binding globulin gradually increases.
- Free cortisol increases in the third trimester.
- Progesterone increases exerting an antimineralocorticoid effect.
- Renin levels increase.

In Addison's disease, therefore:
- The usual glucocorticoid and mineralocorticoid replacement is continued initially.
- Increase the hydrocortisone 50% in the third trimester.
- Adjust mineralocorticoids to BP and serum potassium (not renin).

Severe hyperemesis gravidarum during the first trimester may require temporary parenteral therapy and patients should be warned about this to avoid precipitation of a crisis.
  During labor and for 24–48 hours:
- Parenteral glucocorticoid therapy is administered (100 mg IM every 6 hours).
- Or hydrocortisone 100 mg IV in 5% dextrose per 24 hours.
- Fluid replacement with IV 0.9% saline may be required.

Drug interactions

Rifampicin
- Increases the clearance of cortisol
- Double usual dose of hydrocortisone

Mitotane
- Increases cortisol binding globulin
- Double usual dose of hydrocortisone

Education of the patient

Patient education is the key to successful management. Patients must be taught never to miss a dose. They should be encouraged to wear a Medic Alert bracelet.

Every patient should know how to double the dose of glucocorticoid during febrile illness and to get medical attention if unable to take the tablets because of vomiting. They should have a vial of 100 mg hydrocortisone with a syringe, diluent, and needle for times when parenteral treatment may be required.

Further reading

Arlt W (2009) The approach to the adult with newly diagnosed adrenal insufficiency. *J Clin Endocrinol Metab* 94(4):1059–1067.

Arlt W, Allolio B (2003). Adrenal insufficiency. *Lancet* 361:1881–93.

Hunt PJ, Gurnell EM, Huppert FA, et al. (2000). Improvement in mood and fatigue after dehydroepi-androsterone replacement in Addison's disease in a randomized, double blind trial. *J Clin Endocrinol Metab* 85(12):4650–4656.

Kong MF, Lawden M, Howlett T (2008). The Addison's disease dilemma—autoimmune or ALD? *Lancet* 371:1970.

Oelkers W (1996). Adrenal insufficiency. *N Engl J Med* 335:1206–1212.

Long-term glucocorticoid administration

Both exogenous glucocorticoid administration and endogenous excess glucocorticoids (Cushing's syndrome) lead to a negative feedback effect on the hypothalamo–pituitary–adrenal (HPA) axis, leading to suppression of both CRH and ACTH secretion and atrophy of the zona fasiculata and reticularis of the adrenal cortex.

Short-term steroids

Any patient who has received glucocorticoid treatment for <3 weeks is unlikely to have clinically significant adrenal suppression, and if the medical condition allows it, glucocorticoid treatment can be stopped acutely. A major stress within a week of stopping steroids should, however, be covered with glucocorticoids.

Exceptions to this are patients who have other possible reasons for adrenocortical insufficiency, who have received >40 mg prednisolone (or equivalent), where a short course has been prescribed within 1 year of cessation of long-term therapy, or evening doses (↑ HPA axis suppression).

Steroid cover

While receiving glucocorticoid treatment and within 1 year of steroid withdrawal, patients should receive standard steroid supplementation (Box 42.1) at times of stress, e.g., major trauma, surgery, and infection (📖 p. 562).

Box 42.1 Steroid equivalents

- 1 mg hydrocortisone
- 1.25 mg cortisone acetate
- 0.25 mg prednisolone
- 0.20 mg prednisone
- 3.75 mcg dexamethasone

4 mg prednisolone ≡ 20 mg hydrocortisone ≡ 75 mcg dexamethasone

---

Box 42.2 Dehydroepiandrosterone (DHEA)

- DHEA is an abundant circulating adrenal androgen with a production rate of 25–50 mg/day. Its levels undergo a progressive decline with ↑ age, and there has been interest in its physiological role.
- Epidemiological data suggest a link between changes in DHEA and age-related changes including an inverse relationship between DHEA and cardiovascular disease, Alzheimer disease, and malignancy.
- Although animal studies have suggested potential therapeutic benefit of DHEA therapy, small studies in humans have so far failed to demonstrate convincing benefit otherwise and apart from short-term improvement in well-being.
- Recent evidence suggests that DHEA replacement in patients with Addison's disease may have beneficial effects on well-being.

Long-term steroids

When patients are receiving supraphysiological doses (>5.0 mg prednisone, or equivalent) of glucocorticoid, dose reduction depends on disease activity. Once a daily equivalent of 5.0 mg prednisone is reached, the rate of reduction should be slower to allow recovery of the HPA axis.

If concerned about disease resolution, the rate of reduction of glucocorticoids is determined by the disease process until 5.0 mg equivalent is reached. If the disease has resolved, the dose can be rapidly reduced to 5.0 mg prednisone by a reduction of 2.5 mg every 3–5 days.

Once the patient is established on 5.0 mg prednisolone, consider changing to hydrocortisone (20 mg in the morning), as this has a shorter t½ and will therefore lead to less prolonged suppression of ACTH.

The daily hydrocortisone dose should be reduced by 2.5 mg every 1–2 weeks or as tolerated until a dose of 10 mg is reached. After 2–3 months, a 9 A.M. cortisol is checked 24 hours after last dose of hydrocortisone. If it is >10 mcg/dL, then hydrocortisone can be stopped and a Cortrosyn® test performed. If the 9 A.M. cortisol is <10 mcg/dL, then continue hydrocortisone 10 mg for another 2–3 months and repeat the 9 A.M. cortisol.

When basal cortisol is >14 mcg/dL, stop regular hydrocortisone and administer in emergency only. Supplemental steroids during intercurrent illness are not required.

Cushing's syndrome

Patients with Cushing's syndrome who are on metyrapone or have recently treated disease, whatever the cause, may also have HPA axis suppression and may therefore need steroid replacement at times of stress.

Further reading

Baulieu E (1996). DHEA: a fountain of youth? *J Clin Endocrinol Metab* 81:3147–3151.Nippoldt TB, Nair KS (1998). Is there a case for DHEA replacement? *Balli're Clin Endocrinol Metab* 12:507–520.

Adrenal incidentalomas

Definition and epidemiology

A true *incidentaloma* is an incidentally detected lesion with no pathophysiological significance. It needs to be differentiated from incidentally detected but clinically relevant masses.

The incidental detection of an adrenal mass is becoming more common as ↑ numbers of imaging procedures are performed and with technological improvements in imaging.

Autopsy studies suggest an incidence of adrenal adenomas of 1–6%. Imaging studies suggest an incidence of approximately 3.5%.

Importance

It is important to determine whether the incidentally discovered adrenal mass is
- Malignant
- Functioning and associated with excess hormonal secretion

Differential diagnosis of an incidentally detected adrenal nodule

- Cortisol-secreting adrenal adenoma causing Cushing's syndrome or subclinical Cushing's syndrome (5.2%)
- Mineralocorticoid-secreting adrenal adenoma
- Androgen-secreting adenoma
- CAH
- Adrenal carcinoma (12%)
- Metastasis (2%)
- Pheochromocytoma (11%)
- Adrenal cysts (5%)
- Lipoma
- Myelolipoma (8%)
- Hematoma
- Ganglioneuroma (4%)

Investigations

- Clinical assessment for symptoms and signs of excess hormone secretion and signs of extra-adrenal carcinoma
- Urinary free cortisol and overnight dexamethasone suppression test
- Urinary free catecholamines/metadrenalines
- Plasma free metanephrines if available (📖 see p. 215)
- Aldosterone/renin ratio if hypertensive or hypokalemic
- A homogeneous mass with a low attenuation value (<10 HU) on CT scan is likely to be a benign adenoma.

Additional tests if adrenal carcinoma suspected:
- 24-hour urinary excretion of corticosteroid metabolites
- DHEA, 17α OH progesterone
- 17α estradiol (in males only)
- Testosterone, androstendione (in virilizing tumors)

Management

Up to 20% of patients may develop hormonal excess during follow-up. This is unlikely if the tumor is <3 cm. Cortisol is the most common excess hormone.

Surgery is indicated if there is the following:
- Evidence of a syndrome of hormonal excess attributable to the tumor
- Biochemical evidence of pheochromocytoma
- Mass diameter >4 cm (↑ likelihood of malignancy and definitely if >6 cm in diameter)
- Imaging features suggestive of malignancy (e.g., lack of clearly circumscribed margin, vascular invasion)

Nonsurgical management includes the following:
- Repeat MRI at 6 and 12 months
- Repeat biochemical screening annually
- In patients with tumors that remain stable on two imaging studies carried out at least 6 months apart and do not exhibit hormonal hypersecretion over 4 years, further follow-up may not be warranted.

Further reading

Chidiac RM, Aron DC (1997). Incidentalomas. *Endocrinol Metab Clin North Am* 26:233–253.

Kloos RT, Gross MD, Francis IR, et al. (1995). Incidentally discovered adrenal masses. *Endocr Rev* 16:460–484.

Mansmann G, Lau J, Balk E, et al. (2004). The clinically inapparent adrenal mass: update in diagnosis and management. *Endocr Rev* 25(2):309–340.

Newell-Price J, Grossman A (1996). Adrenal incidentaloma. *Postgrad Med J* 72:207–210.

Turner HE, Moore NR, Byrne JV, et al. (1998). Pituitary, adrenal and thyroid incidentalomas. *Endocr Rel Cancer* 5:131–150.

Young WF Jr (2007). Clinical practice. The incidentally discovered adrenal mass. *N Engl J Med* 356(6):601–610.

Pheochromocytomas and paragangliomas

Definition

Pheochromocytomas are adrenomedullary catecholamine-secreting tumors

Paragangliomas are tumors arising from extra-adrenal medullary neural crest derivatives, e.g., organ of Zuckerkandl (sympathetic) or carotid body, aorticopulmonary, intravagal, or jugulotympanic (parasympathetic). They are usually in the head and neck, and only 25% are secretory.

Incidence

These are rare tumors, accounting for <0.1% of causes of hypertension. However, it is a very important diagnosis because of the following:

• The development of potentially fatal hypertensive crises
• The reversibility of all its manifestations after surgical removal of the tumor
• The lack of long-term efficacy of medical treatment
• The appreciable incidence of malignancy

Epidemiology

There is equal sex distribution, and tumors most commonly present in the third and fourth decades. Up to 50% may be diagnosed postmortem.

Tumors may be bilateral, particularly where part of an inherited syndrome (Table 44.1).

Table 44.1 Syndromes associated with pheochromocytomas

Familial pheochromocytomas	Isolated autosomal dominant trait
MEN-IIa and b ⬚ see p. 503	Mutation in RET proto-oncogene (chromosome 10)
	Hyperparathyroidism and medullary thyroid carcinoma associated with pheochromocytoma
	MEN IIb also associated with marfanoid phenotype ⬚ see p. 505
Von Hippel–Lindau syndrome ⬚ see p. 493	Mutation of VHL tumor suppressor gene (chromosome 3)
	Renal cell carcinoma, cerebellar hemangioblastoma, retinal angioma, renal and pancreatic cysts
	Pheochromocytomas in 25%
Neurofibromatosis (NF) ⬚ see p. 490	Autosomal dominant condition caused by mutations of *NF1* gene on chromosome 17
	Phechromocytomas in 0.5–1.0%
Familial carotid body tumor	Dominantly inherited disorder characterized by vascular tumors in the head and neck, most frequently at the carotid and bifurcation
	Succinate dehydrogenase gene (subunit D)
Familial paraganglionoma	Succinate dehydrogenase (subunits B,C,D)

Pathophysiology

Sporadic tumors are usually unilateral and <10 cm in diameter. Tumors associated with familial syndromes (see Box 44.1) are more likely to be bilateral and associated with pre-existing medullary hyperplasia.

Box 44.1 Who should be screened for the presence of a pheochromocy-toma?

- Patients with a family history of MEN, VHL, neurofibromatosis (NF), or SDH gene mutations
- Patients with paroxysmal symptoms
- Young patients with hypertension
- Patient developing hypertensive crisis during general anesthesia or surgery
- Patients with unexplained heart failure
- Patients with an adrenal incidentaloma

Malignancy

Approximately 15–20% are malignant, and these are characterized by local invasion or distant metastasis rather than capsular invasion.

Differentiating benign and malignant tumors is difficult and based mainly on presence of metastases, although chromosomal ploidy may be useful. Paragangliomas are more likely to be malignant and to recur.

Typical sites for metastases are retroperitoneum, lymph nodes, bone, liver, and mediastinum.

Secretory products

Catecholamine secretion is usually adrenaline or noradrenaline and may be constant or episodic. Phenylethanolamine-N-methyl transferase (PNMT) is necessary for methylation of noradrenaline to adrenaline and is cortisol dependent.

Paragangliomas (except organ of Zuckerkandl) secrete noradrenaline only, as they lack PNMT. Small adrenal tumors tend to produce more adrenaline, whereas larger adrenal tumors produce more noradrenaline, as a proportion of their blood supply is direct rather than corticomedullary and therefore lower in cortisol concentrations.

Pure dopamine secretion is rare and may be associated with hypotension. These tumors are more likely to be malignant.

Other non-catecholamine secretory products may also be produced, including VIP, neuropeptide Y, ACTH (associated with Cushing's syndrome), parathyroid hormone (PTH), and PTH-related peptide (PTHrP).

Clinical features

Sustained or episodic *hypertension* is often resistant to conventional therapy.

General
- Sweating and heat intolerance >80%
- Pallor or flushing
- Feeling of apprehension
- Pyrexia

Neurological
- Headache (throbbing or constant) (65%), paresthesiae, visual disturbance, seizures

Cardiovascular
- Palpitations (65%), chest pain, dyspnea, postural hypotension

GI
- Abdominal pain, constipation, nausea

Complications

- *Cardiovascular*—left ventricular failure, dilated cardiomyopathy (reversible), dysrhythmias
- *Respiratory*—pulmonary edema
- *Metabolic*—carbohydrate intolerance, hypercalcemia
- *Neurological*—cerebrovascular, hypertensive encephalopathy

Factors precipitating a crisis
- Straining
- Exercise
- Pressure on abdomen—tumor palpation, bending over
- Surgery

Drugs
- Anesthetics
- Unopposed β-blockade
- IV contrast agents
- Opiates
- Tricyclic antidepressants
- Phenothiazines
- Metoclopramide
- Glucagon

Investigations

Demonstrate catecholamine hypersecretion

A 24-hour urine collection is the standard test for screening for a pheo-chromocytoma. In a patient with suggestive symptoms, this is usually sufficient to confirm or exclude the diagnosis.

False negatives are more common when patients are asymptomatic and early in the disease. Particular care is needed in familial cases, incidentalomas, and those in whom a general anesthetic has precipitated a hypertensive episode.

Metadrenalines (either urine or plasma) offer more specific diagnostic tools than measurement of unmetabolized catecholamines and provide the best biochemical tests for diagnosing pheochromocytoma.

24-hour urine collection for vanillylmandelic acid (VMA)/catecholamines/metadrenalines (📖 see Table 44.2)
Urine is collected into bottles containing acid (warn patient).

Because of the episodic nature of catecholamine secretion, at least 2 × 24-hour collections should be performed. It is useful to perform a collection while a patient is having symptoms if episodic secretion is suspected.

Table 44.2 Substances interfering with urinary catecholamine levels

Increased catecholamines	Decreased catecholamines	Variable effect
α-Blockers	Mono-amine oxidase inhibitors	Levodopa
β-Blockers	Clonidine	Tricyclic antidepressants
Levodopa	Guanethidine and other adrenergic neuron blockers	Phenothiazines
Drugs containing catecholamines, e.g., decongestants		Calcium channel inhibitors
Metoclopramide		ACE inhibitors
Domperidone		Bromocriptine
Hydralazine		
Diazoxide		
Glyceryltrinitrate		
Sodium nitroprusside		
Nicotine		
Theophylline		
Caffeine		
Amphetamine		

The sensitivity of urinary VMAs (Table 44.3) is somewhat less than free catecholamines or metadrenalines and also influenced by dietary intake.

Tricyclic antidepressants (TCAs) and labetalol interfere with adrenaline measurements and should be stopped for 4 days.

Plasma catecholamine measurement

Intermittent secretion, and the short t½ of catecholamines, makes this test of limited use in screening. Plasma metadrenalines may be more useful as their t½ is longer and offer high specificity.

Normal levels drawn during an episode are strongly against the diagnosis. Routine measurement requires controlled conditions—supine and cannulated for 30 minutes, 10 mL blood drawn into a lithium heparin tube and cold spun.

Plasma catecholamines are elevated by renal failure, caffeine, nicotine, exercise, and some drugs.

Plasma catecholamines 3 × the upper limit of normal are suspicious of a pheochromocytoma in symptomatic individuals.

Catecholamine levels in asymptomatic individuals investigated for an adrenal incidentaloma or due to a familial condition are often diagnosed at an earlier stage and may therefore have lower catecholamines.

Suppression tests (📖 see Box 44.2)

These tests may be used to differentiate patients who have borderline catecholamine levels but may offer little advantage over the screening tests already described.

- *Clonidine 300 mcg orally*—failure of suppression of plasma catecholamines into normal range at 120 and 180 minutes is suggestive of tumor

Provocative tests

These are not used routinely as they do not enhance diagnostic accuracy and are potentially dangerous.

Table 44.3 Sensitivity and specificity of tests

Test	Sensitivity	Specificity
Plasma free metanephrines	99%	89%
2 × 24-hour urinary free catecholamines	96%	95%
Urinary metanephrines	93%	93%
Urinary VMA	65%	95%
Clonidine suppression test	97%	
MRI	98%	70%
CT	93%	70%
MIBG	80%	95%

Box 44.2 Test procedures

Clonidine suppression test
- Patient supine and cannulated for 30 minutes
- Clonidine 300 mcg orally
- Plasma catecholamines measured at time 0, 120, and 180 minutes
- Failure to suppress into the normal range is suggestive of a tumor.
- 1.5% false-positive rate in patients with essential hypertension

Localization of tumor

Imaging
These are large tumors, in contrast to Conn's syndrome, and not easily missed with good-quality imaging to the bifurcation of the aorta. Approximately 98% will be detected in the abdomen.

Less than 2% are in the chest and 0.02% are in the head.

Adrenal imaging with nonionic contrast should be performed initially, then body imaging (ideally MRI) if tumor is not localized in adrenal.
- *MRI:* bright hyperintense image on T2
- *CT:* less sensitive and specific—less good at distinguishing between different types of adrenal tumors

^{123}I-MIBG scan (📖 see Box 44.3)
Meta-Iodobenzylguanidine is a chromaffin-seeking analog. Imaging using MIBG is positive in 60–80% pheochromocytomas and may locate tumors not visualized on MRI, e.g., multiple and extra-adrenal tumors. Specificity is nearly 100%.

An MIBG scan is performed preoperatively to exclude multiple tumors.

Phenoxybenzamine may lead to false-negative MIBG imaging, so these scans should be preformed before commencing this drug.

Box 44.3 Drugs interfering with MIBG uptake in pheochromocytoma*

- Opioids
- Cocaine
- Tramadol
- Tricyclic antidepressants
  - Amitriptyline
  - Imipramine
- Sympathomimetics
  - Phenylpropanolamine, pseudoephedrine, amphetamine, dopamine, salbutamol
- Antihypertensives/cardiovascular agents
  - Labetalol, metoprolol, amiodarone, reserpine, guanethidine, calcium channel blockers nifedipine and amlodipine, ACE inhibitors captopril and enalapril

*Should be discontinued 7–14 days prior to scan.

18F fluorodopamine PET scanning is superior to MIBG in localizing metastatic disease. No K$^+$ iodide is necessary to block thyroid uptake.

Positron emission tomography (PET)

[18F]fluorodeoxyglucose (FDG) and the norepinephrine analog [11C]metahydroxyephedrine (mHED) have both been used as radionucleotides.

Current data are insufficient to determine which radionucleotide has the greatest sensitivity and specificity.

Sensitivity is better than MIBG and approaches 100%, but specificity is worse with false positives being reported.

Venous sampling

This is used to localize a pheochromocytoma/paraganglioma if imaging is unhelpful.

Caution: α- and β-blockade should be administered before the procedure.

Reversal of the ratio of noradrenaline to adrenaline (N <1) in the adrenal vein is suggestive of a pheochromocytoma.

Screening for associated conditions

Up to 24% of patients with apparently sporadic pheochromocytomas may have a familial disorder. Therefore, high-risk patients should be screened for the presence of associated conditions, even if asymptomatic. Screening can be performed either by looking for associated clinical manifestations or by genetic testing.

Genetic testing in nonsyndromic pheochromocytoma has shown a hereditary predisposition in 24%, of which 45% had germ-line mutations in VHL, 20% had mutations in RET, 18% mutations in SDHD, and 17% mutations in SDHB.

MEN (p. 504)

- Serum calcium
- Serum calcitonin (pheochromocytomas precede medullary thyroid carcinoma in 10%)

VHL (p. 494)

- Opthalmoscopy—retinal angiomas are usually the first manifestation
- MRI posterior fossa and spinal cord
- US of kidneys—if not adequately imaged on MRI of adrenals

NF1 (see p. 490)

- Clinical examination for café-au-lait spots and cutaneous neuromas

Indications for screening for genetic conditions as a cause for a pheochromocytoma

- Bilateral tumors
- Extra-adrenal tumor including head and neck
- Age of onset (<50 years 45% positive, >40 years 7% positive, >50 years 1% positive)
- Malignancy

Management

Medical

It is essential that any patient be fully prepared with α- and β-blockade before receiving IV contrast or undergoing a procedure such as venous sampling or surgery.

α-Blockade must be started before β-blockade to avoid precipitating a hypertensive crisis due to unopposed α-adrenergic stimulation.

- α-*blockade*—begin phenoxybenzamine, as soon as diagnosis is made. Start at 10 mg 2 × day by mouth, and increase up to 20 mg 4 × day.
- β-*blockade*—use a β-blocker such as propranolol 20–80 mg q8h by mouth 48–72 hours after starting phenoxybenzamine and with evidence of adequate α-blockade blockade (generally noted by a postural fall in BP).

Treatment is started in the hospital. Monitor BP, pulse, and hematocrit. The goal is a BP of 130/80 or less sitting and 100 mg systolic standing, pulse 60–70 sitting and 70–80 standing. Reversal of α-mediated vasoconstriction may lead to hemodilution (check Hb preoperatively).

To ensure complete blockade before surgery, IV phenoxybenzamine (1 mg/kg over 4 hours in 100 mL 5% dextrose) is administered on the 3 days before surgery. There is less experience with competetive α-adrenergic blockade such as prazosin.

Surgical

Surgical resection is curative in most patients, leading to normotension in at least 75%.

Mortality from elective surgery is <2%. It is essential that the anesthetic and surgical teams have expertise of management of phechromocytomas perioperatively.

Surgery may be laparoscopic if the tumor is small and apparently benign. Careful perioperative anesthetic management is essential, as tumor handling may lead to major changes in BP and also occasionally cardiac arrythmias.

Phentolamine, nitroprusside, or *IV nicardipine* are useful to treat perioperative hypertension, and *esmolol* or *propranolol* for perioperative arrythmias. Hypotension (e.g., after tumor devascularization) usually responds to volume replacement, but occasionally requires inotropic support.

Follow-up

Cure is assessed by 24-hour urine free catecholamine measurement, but since catecholamines may remain elevated for up to 10 days following surgery, these should not be performed until 2 weeks postoperatively.

Lifelong follow-up is essential to detect recurrence of a benign tumor, or metastasis from a malignant tumor, as it is impossible to exclude malignancy on a histological specimen.

Chromogranin A is also a useful marker (falsely elevated with proton pump therapy, steroids, and renal failure).

Malignancy

Malignant tumors require long-term α- and β-blockade. The tyrosine kinase inhibitor α-*methylparatyrosine* may help control symptoms.

High-dose ^{131}I MIBG can be used to treat metastatic disease.

Chemotherapy with *cyclophosphamide, vincristine, adriamycin,* and *dacarbazine* has been associated with symptomatic improvement.

Radiotherapy can be useful palliation in patients with bony metastases.

Prognosis

Hypertension may persist in 25% patients who have undergone successful tumor removal.

- 5-year survival for benign tumors is 96%, and the recurrence rate is <10%.
- 5-year survival for malignant tumors is 44%.
- SHB gene mutation is associated with a shorter survival.

Further reading

Astuti D, Latif F, Dallol A, et al. (2001). Gene mutations in the succinate dehydrogenase subunit SDHB cause susceptibility to familial pheochromocytoma and to familial paraganglioma. *Am J Hum Genet* 69:49–54.

Erickson D, Kudva YC, Ebersold MJ, et al. (2001). Benign paragangliomas: clinical presentation and treatment outcomes in 236 patients. *J Clin Endocrinol Metab* 86(11):5210–5216.

Gimm O, Armanios M, Dziema H, et al. (2000). Somatic and occult germ-line mutations in SDHD, a mitochondrial complex II gene, in nonfamilial pheochromocytoma. *Cancer Res* 60(24):6822–6825.

Ilias I, Yu J, Carrasquillo JA, et al. (2003). Superiority of 6-[18F]-fluorodopamine positron emission tomography versus [131I]-metaiodobenzylguanidine scintigraphy in the localization of metastatic pheochromocytoma. *J Clin Endocrinol Metab* 88(9):4083–4087.

Kudva YC, Sawka AM, Young WF Jr (2003). The laboratory diagnosis of adrenal pheochromocytoma: the Mayo Clinic experience. *J Clin Endocrinol Metab* 88(10):4533–4539.

Lenders JWM, Pacak K, Walther MM, et al. (2002) Biochemical diagnosis of pheochromocytoma: Which test is best? *JAMA* 287(11):1427–1434.

Neumann HP, Bausch B, McWhinney SR, et al. (2002). Germ-line mutations in nonsyndromic pheochromocytoma. *N Engl J Med* 346(19):1459–1466.

Part 4

Reproductive endocrinology

Margaret E. Wierman

Hirsutism

Definition

Hirsutism (not a diagnosis in itself) is the presence of excess hair growth in females as a result of ↑ androgen production and ↑ skin sensitivity to androgens. 📖 See Table 45.1 for causes.

Physiology of hair growth

Before puberty, the body is covered with fine, unpigmented vellus hairs. During adolescence, androgens convert vellus hairs into coarse, pigmented terminal hairs in androgen-dependent areas. The extent of terminal hair growth depends on the concentration and duration of androgen exposure as well as on the sensitivity of the individual hair follicle.

The reason different body regions respond differently to the same androgen concentration is unknown but may be related to the number of androgen receptors in the hair follicle.

Genetic factors play an important role in the individual susceptibility to circulating androgens, as evidenced by racial differences in hair growth.

Table 45.1 Causes of hirsutism

Ovarian	• Polycystic ovary syndrome (PCOS) • Androgen-secreting tumors
Adrenal	• Congenital adrenal hyperplasia • Cushing's syndrome • Androgen-secreting tumors • Acromegaly • Severe insulin resistance

Androgen production in women

In females, testosterone (T) is secreted primarily by the ovaries and adrenal glands, although a significant amount is produced by the peripheral conversion of androstenedione and dehydroepiandrosterone (DHEA). Ovarian androgen production is regulated by lutenizing hormone (LH), whereas adrenal production is ACTH dependent.

The predominant androgens produced by the ovaries are T and androstenedione, and DHEA sulfate (DHEAS) by the adrenal glands. Circulating T is mainly bound to sex hormone binding globulin (SHBG) and it is the free T that is biologically active.

Testosterone is converted to dihydrotestosterone (DHT) in the skin by the enzyme 5α-reductase. Androstenedione and DHEA are not significantly protein-bound. See Fig. 45.1.

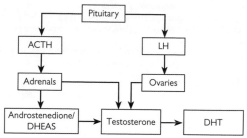

Fig. 45.1 Regulation of androgen production in females.

Evaluation

Androgen-dependent hirsutism

Normally, this develops at puberty. Hairs are coarse and pigmented and typically grow in a male pattern. It is often accompanied by other evidence of androgen excess, such as acne, oily skin and hair, and male-pattern alopecia. Virilization refers to severe hirsuitism associated with male pattern balding, anabolic phenotype and clitoromegaly and is associated with very high androgen levels. For signs of virilization, indicating hyperandrogenism, see Box 45.1.

History

- *Age and rate of onset of hirsutism:* Slowly progressive hirsutism following puberty suggests a benign cause, whereas rapidly progressive hirsutism of recent onset requires further immediate investigation to rule out an androgen-secreting neoplasm.
- *Menstrual history:* ?oligomenorrheic or amenorrhea
- Presence of other evidence of *hyperandrogenism*, e.g., acne or bitemporal hair recession
- *Drug history:* Some progestins used in oral contraceptives may be androgenic (e.g., norethisterone. levonorgestryl).

Physical examination

Distinguish between androgen-dependent and androgen-independent hair growth.

Assess the extent and severity of hirsutism. The Ferriman–Gallwey score (◻ see Table 45.2) is used to assess the degree of hair growth in 11 regions of the body. This provides a semi-objective method of monitoring disease progression and treatment outcome.

Virilization should be looked for, as this indicates severe hyperandrogenism and should be further investigated (see Box 45.1).

Acanthosis nigricans is indicative of insulin resistance of any cause.

Rare causes of hyperandrogenism, such as Cushing's syndrome and acromegaly, should be ruled out.

Laboratory investigation

Serum testosterone should be measured in all females presenting with hirsutism. If this is <150 ng/dL the risk of a tumor is low.

Further investigations and management of the individual disorders will be discussed in the following chapters.

Box 45.1 Signs of virilization

- Frontal balding
- Deepening of voice
- ↑ Muscle size
- Clitoromegaly

Table 45.2 Assessment of hir-suitism—Ferriman–Gallway score*

Site	Grade	Definition
Upper lip	1	A few hairs at outer margin
	2	A small moustache at outer margin
	3	A moustache extending halfway from outer margin
	4	A moustache extending to midline
Chin	1	A few scattered hairs
	2	Scattered hairs with small concentrations
	3	Complete cover, light
	4	Complete cover, heavy
Chest	1	Circumareolar hairs
	2	With midline hair
	3	Fusion of these areas
	4	Complete cover
Upper back	1	A few scattered hairs
	2	More, but still scattered
	3	Complete cover, light
	4	Complete cover, heavy
Lower back	1	Sacral tuft of hair
	2	Some lateral extension
	3	Three-quarters cover
	4	Complete cover
Upper abdomen	1	A few midline hairs
	2	More than this, still midline
	3	Half cover
	4	Full cover
Lower abdomen	1	A few midline hairs
	2	A midline streak of hair
	3	A midline band of hair
	4	An inverted V-shaped growth
Arm	1	Sparse growth affecting not more than a quarter of the limb surface
	2	More than this, cover still incomplete
	3	Complete cover, light
	4	Complete cover, heavy
Forearm	1, 2, 3, 4	Complete cover of dorsal surface, 2 grades of light and 2 grades of heavy growth
Thigh	1, 2, 3, 4	As for arm
Leg	1, 2, 3, 4	As for arm
Total score		

*Reproduced with permission from Ferriman D, Gallwey JD (1961). Clinical assessment of body hair growth in women. *J Clin Endocrinol and Metab* 21(11):1440–1447.

Box 45.2 Androgen-independent hair growth

Excess vellus hairs are over the face and trunk, including forehead. It does not respond to antiandrogen treatment.

Causes of androgen-independent hair growth
- Drugs, e.g., phenytoin, ciclosporin, glucocorticoids
- Anorexia nervosa
- Hypothyroidism
- Familial

Further reading

Martin KA, Chang JR, Ehrmann DA, et al (2008). Evaluation and treatment of hirsutism in pre-menopausal woman: an Endocrine Society clinical practice guideline. *J Clin Endocrinol Metab* 93:1105–1120.

Polycystic ovary syndrome (PCOS)

Definition

PCOS is a heterogeneous genetic clinical syndrome characterized by hyperandrogenism (both ovarian and/or adrenal), ovulatory dysfunction, and hyperinsulinemia, in which other causes of androgen excess have been excluded (📖 see Box 46.1).

The diagnosis is further supported by the presence of characteristic ovarian morphology on ultrasound (US).

> **Box 46.1 2003 Joint European Society of Human Reproduction and Embryology and American Society of Reproductive Medicine consensus on the diagnosis criteria for PCOS (Rotterdam criteria)**
>
> At least two out of three of the following are present:
> • Oligo- or amenorrhea
> • Hyperandrogenism (clinical or biochemical)
> • Polycystic ovaries on US and exclusion of other disorders

Epidemiology

PCOS is the most common endocrinopathy in women of reproductive age.

The estimated prevalence of PCOS ranges from 5 to 10% on clinical criteria. Polycystic ovaries on US alone are present in 20–25% of women of reproductive age.

Other causes of hyperandrogenic anovulation

- Congenital adrenal hyperplasia
- Acromegaly
- Cushing's syndrome
- Testosterone-secreting tumors
- Obesity-induced hyperandrogenic anovulation

Pathogenesis

The fundamental pathophysiological defect is unknown, but both genetic and environmental factors contribute to the disorder.

Genetic

- Familial aggregation of PCOS in 50% of women. A family history of type 2 diabetes mellitus is also more common in women with PCOS.
- PCOS is probably a polygenic disorder.
- Insulin synthesis genes, steroid enzyme biosynthesis genes, and genes involved in reproduction and metabolism are possible candidates, e.g., *INS*, *VNTR*, and *CYP11* genes; also FTO gene.

Hyperandrogenism

The main sources of hyperandrogenemia are the ovaries and adrenals.

The biochemical basis of ovarian dysfunction is unclear. Studies suggest an abnormality of cytochrome P-450c17 α activity. However, this is unlikely to be the primary event, rather, an index of ↑ steroidogenesis by ovarian theca cells.

There is also an increase in the frequency and amplitude of GnRH pulses, resulting in ↑ LH concentrations (high LH/FSH ratio), which is characteristic of the syndrome. This may be secondary to anovulation and low progesterone levels.

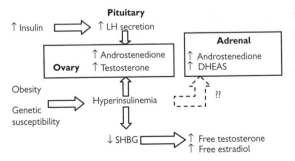

Fig. 46.1 Abnormalities of hormone secretion in PCOS.

Hyperinsulinemia

The overwhelming majority of women with PCOS are insulin resistant. The defect in insulin sensitivity appears to be selective, mainly affecting the metabolic effects of insulin (effects on muscle and liver) rather than its mitogenic actions (e.g., effects on ovaries). Hyperinsulinemia is further exacerbated by obesity.

Women with PCOS have insufficient β-cell response to a glucose challenge, which is known to be a precursor to type 2 diabetes mellitus.

Insulin and IGF-1 receptors are found in abundance in the ovarian stroma, and it has been shown that insulin, in the presence of LH, stimulates ovarian production of androgens. This is exaggerated in PCOS ovaries.

Insulin also inhibits SHBG synthesis by the liver with a consequent rise in free androgen levels.

Features

- *Onset of symptoms:* Symptoms begin at puberty, often with early menarche.
- *Oligo- and amenorrhea* (70%): Due to anovulation. These women are usually well-estrogenized, so there is little risk of osteoporosis, unlike other causes of amenorrhea.
- *Hirsutism* (66%)
  - 25% of women also suffer from acne or male-pattern alopecia. Virilization is not a feature of PCOS.
  - There is often a family history of hirsutism or irregular periods. Hirsutism secondary to adrenal or ovarian tumors, in contrast, is usually rapidly progressive, associated with virilization and higher testosterone concentrations.
  - Rarely, hirsute women have nonclassical congenital adrenal hyperplasia (🕮see Classic presentation, p. 241). This should be excluded, particularly in women with a family history .? Not all CAH women have high T levels
- *Obesity* (50%): Symptoms worsen with obesity, as it is accompanied by ↑ testosterone concentrations as a result of the associated hyperinsulinemia. Acanthosis nigricans is common in insulin-resistant women with PCOS.
- *Infertility* (30%): PCOS accounts for 75% of cases of anovulatory infertility. The risk of spontaneous miscarriage is also thought to be higher than that in the general population

Rule out an androgen-secreting tumor

If there is the following:
- Evidence of virilization
- Testosterone >200 ng/dL
- Rapidly progressive hirsutism
- MRI or CT of adrenals and US of ovaries detecting tumors >1 cm

Selective venous sampling has not been shown to be useful in detecting tumors.

Risks associated with PCOS

Type 2 diabetes mellitus

Type 2 diabetes mellitus is 2–4×more common in women with PCOS. Impaired glucose tolerance affects 10–30% of women with PCOS, and gestational diabetes is also more prevalent.

The prevalence of diabetes mellitus is ↑ in women with PCOS independent of weight but is highest in the obese group.

Dyslipidemia

Several studies have shown an ↑ risk of hypercholesterolemia, hypertriglyceridemia, and low high-density lipoprotein (HDL) cholesterol in women with PCOS.

Cardiovascular disease

There is evidence that atherosclerosis develops earlier in women with PCOS. For example, women with PCOS have been found to be twice as likely to have coronary artery atherosclerosis compared with controls.

However, in epidemiological studies, women with PCOS have not been found to have ↑ mortality from ischemic heart disease despite their multiple cardiovascular risk factors. No prospective studies are available.

Endometrial hyperplasia and carcinoma

In anovulatory women, endometrial stimulation by unopposed estrogen results in endometrial hyperplasia.

Several studies have also shown that this results in a 2- to 4-fold excess risk of endometrial carcinoma in women with PCOS. However, larger prospective studies are required to confirm this excess risk.

Laboratory evaluation

Selected lab tests are used to confirm the diagnosis, to exclude serious underlying disorders, and to screen for complications.

Confirmation of diagnosis

Testosterone concentration
- Performed to confirm biochemical hyperandrogenism and to exclude other causes of hyperandrogenism

LH concentration
- Raised in 50–70% of anovulatory patients with high LH/FSH ratio.

SHBG
- Low in 50% of women with PCOS owing to the hyperinsulinemic state, with a consequent increase in circulating free androgens
- Indirect marker of insulin resistance

Free androgen index (FAI)
This is used as a surrogate for free T levels.

$$FAI = \frac{100 \times (\text{total testosterone})}{SHBG}$$

Pelvic US of ovaries and endometrium
- 91% sensitivity in experienced hands, with transvaginal ultrasound giving the highest yield
- Ultrasonic diagnosis of PCOS is made by the presence of >12 follicular cysts between 2 and 9 mm in diameter or ovarian volume >10 cm^3.
- Measurement of endometrial thickness is also useful in the diagnosis of endometrial hyperplasia in the presence of anovulation. Endometrial hyperplasia is diagnosed if the endometrial thickness is >10 mm.
- Transvaginal US will also identify 90% of ovarian virilizing tumors.

Exclusion of other disorders

Serum prolactin
This is used in the presence of infertility or oligoamenorrhea.
- Mild hyperprolactinemia may be present in up to 30% of women with PCOS, and dopamine agonist treatment of this may be necessary if pregnancy is desired.

17 OH (17OHP) progesterone level
- Used to exclude late-onset congenital adrenal hyperplasia
- Indicated in those with family history
- One may also conduct a Cosyntropin stimulation test looking for an exaggerated rise in 17OHP 30 minutes after ACTH in the presence of nonclassic 21-hydroxylase deficiency (📖 see Clinical presentation, p. 192).

- If the patient is ovulating, all 17OHP measurements should be taken during the follicular phase of the cycle since androgen levels are higher at midcycle and in the luteal phase.

DHEAS and androstenedione concentrations

- Both can be moderately raised in PCOS. DHEAS is a useful adrenal marker of hyperandrogenism. In cases of suspected tumors, levels are usually in excess of 800 ng/mL.
- Useful as a marker of adrenal hyperandrogenism

Other

- Depending on clinical suspicion, e.g., 1) urinary free cortisol or overnight dexamethasone suppression test if Cushing's syndrome is suspected or 2) IGF-1 if acromegaly suspected, but not routinely

Screening for complications

- *Serum lipids, blood glucose, and hemoglobin A1C:* All women with PCOS should have an annual fasting glucose hemoglobin A1C and fasting lipid profile.
- All women with PCOS who become pregnant should be screened for gestational diabetes.

Management

Weight loss

Studies have uniformly shown that weight reduction in obese women with PCOS will improve insulin sensitivity and significantly reduce hyperandrogenemia. Obese women are less likely to respond to antiandrogens and infertility treatment.

With weight loss, women with PCOS show improvement in hirsutism and restoration of menstrual regularity and fertility.

Metformin

In obese and lean insulin-resistant women with PCOS, metformin (1 g, 2 × daily) improves insulin sensitivity with a corresponding reduction in serum androgen and LH concentrations and an increase in SHBG levels.

Metformin may regulate menstruation by improving ovulatory function and thus inducing fertility. Frequency of menstruation may be improved within 3 months of starting therapy. Metformin does not seem to improve response rates to ovulation induction using clomifene or gonadotropins.

Experience of metformin in pregnancy is limited, so it should be discontinued once pregnancy has been confirmed until further data accrue. However, it does not appear to be teratogenic.

The effects of metformin seem to be independent of weight reduction, although the benefits are greatest in obese women when weight reduction occurs. The effect of metformin on weight loss remains unclear.

There have been few long-term studies looking at the effect of metformin on hirsutism, but it appears that its effects are modest at best, and most women with significant hirsutism will require an antiandrogen.

Women should be warned of its gastrointestinal (GI) side effects. To minimize these, patients should be started on a low dose (500 mg once daily) that may be ↑ gradually to a therapeutic dose. A low-fat diet will decrease side effects and improve response.

Other insulin sensitizers

Troglitazone is a thiazolidinedione, another insulin sensitizer that showed encouraging effects on menstruation and hyperinsulinemia in women with PCOS. However, it was withdrawn from the market because of liver toxicity.

In the future, other thiazolidinediones may be used in the treatment of PCOS, but currently there is insufficient evidence for their use in PCOS.

The thiazolidinediones are associated weight gain and are potentially teratogenic. Their use is therefore not recommended in women seeking fertility.

Hirsutism

Pharmacological treatment of hirsutism is directed at slowing the growth of new hair but has little impact on established hair. It should be combined with mechanical methods of hair removal, such as electrolysis and laser therapy. Therapy is most effective when started early.

There is slow improvement over the first 6–12 months of treatment. Patients should be warned that facial hair is slow to respond, treatment is prolonged, and symptoms may recur after discontinuation of drugs.

Adequate contraception is mandatory during pharmacological treatment of hirsutism because of possible teratogenicity.

Ovarian androgen suppression

Oral contraceptive pill (OCP)

The estrogen component increases SHBG levels and thus reduces free androgen concentrations; the progestin component inhibits LH secretion and thus ovarian androgen production.

A birth control pill with a nonandrogenic progestin is recommended (norgestryl norgestrel ?or similar progestin).

The effect of the OCP alone on hair growth is improved with combination with an antiandrogen.

GnRH analogs

These suppress gonadotropin secretion and thus ovarian androgen production.

They are rarely used. They cause estrogen deficiency so have to be combined with "add-back" estrogen treatment. Also, they are expensive and require parenteral administration.

Use is confined to women with severe hyperandrogenism in whom antiandrogens have been ineffective or not tolerated.

Androgen receptor blockers

These are most effective when combined with oral contraceptives. All are contraindicated in pregnancy.

They act by competitively inhibiting the binding of testosterone and dihydrotestosterone to the androgen receptor.

Spironolactone

- Antiandrogen of choice
- Dose: 50–200 mg/day
- Side effects: irregular menstrual bleeding if not combined with the OCP. A fifth of women complain of GI symptoms when on high doses of spironolactone. Potassium levels should be monitored if the dose is 100 mg/day or greater, and other potassium-sparing drugs should be avoided.

Eflornithine

This agent irreversibly blocks the enzyme ornithine decarboxylase, which is involved in growth of hair follicles.

It is administered as a topical cream on the face; its long-term use reduces new hair growth. Studies have shown its efficacy in the management of mild facial hirsutism following at least 8 weeks of treatment.

Treatment should be discontinued if there is no benefit at 4 months. It is not a depilatory cream and so must be combined with mechanical methods of hair removal.

Side effects include skin irritation with burning or pruritus, acne, hypersensitivity.

Amenorrhea

A minimum of a withdrawal bleed every 3 months minimizes the risk of endometrial hyperplasia.

Treatment
- OCP with nonandrogenic progestin
- Desogestrel is a relatively new progesterone-only contraceptive pill with minimal androgenic properties. It may be used to minimize endometrial hyperplasia in amenorrhoeic women with PCOS.
- Metformin (up to 1 g bid)

Alternatives
A progestin may be added for the latter half of the cycle. However, there is a risk of exacerbating hirsutism. Less androgenic progestins include medroxyprogesterone, e.g., 5–10 mg 12 day/month.

Infertility

Ovulation induction regimens are indicated. Obesity adversely affects fertility outcome with poorer pregnancy rates and higher rates of miscarriage, so weight reduction should be strongly encouraged.

Metformin
Use remains controversial but probably does not improve ovulation and pregnancy rates in insulin-resistant, particularly overweight women with PCOS. There are no reported teratogenic or neonatal complications.
- *Dose:* 500 mg od before meals to be ↑ gradually to 1 g bid. If ovulation is restored following 6 months of treatment, then continue for up to 1 year. If pregnancy does not occur, consider other treatments.
- *Side effects:* nausea, bloating, diarrhea, vomiting

Clomifene citrate
This inhibits estrogen negative feedback, ↑ FSH secretion, and thus stimulating ovarian follicular growth.
- *Dose:* 25–150 mg/day from days 5 to 9 of menstrual cycle
- *Response rates:* 80% of women with PCOS will ovulate, although the pregnancy rate is only 67% and live births are lower. Recent studies have shown that treatment with metformin may improve response to clomifene in resistant cases.
- *Complications:* 8% twins, 0.1% higher-order multiple pregnancy. Risk of ovarian neoplasia following prolonged clomifene treatment remains unclear, so limit treatment to a maximum of 6 cycles.

Gonadotropin preparations
(human menopausal gonadotropin [hMG] or FSH)
These are used in those unresponsive to clomifene. Low-dose regimes show better response rates and less complications, e.g., 75 IU/day for 2 weeks then increase by 37.5 IU/day every 7 days as required.
- 94% ovulation rate and 40% conception rate after 4 cycles
- *Complications:* hyperstimulation, multiple pregnancies
- Close ultrasonic monitoring is essential.

Surgery
Surgery is particularly effective in slim women with PCOS and high LH concentrations.
- *Complications:* surgical adhesions, although usually mild

In vitro fertilization (IVF)
- In women who fail to respond to ovulation induction
- 60–80% conception rate after 6 cycles

Acne

Treatment for acne should be started as early as possible to prevent scarring. All treatments take up to 12 weeks before significant improvement is seen. All treatments other than benzoyl peroxide are contraindicated in pregnancy.

Mild to moderate acne
Topical benzoyl peroxide 5% has bactericidal properties. It may be used in conjunction with oral antibiotic therapy to reduce the risk of developing resistance to antibiotics
- *Side effects:* skin irritation and dryness. Add oral antibiotics if no improvement is seen after 2 months of treatment.

Moderate to severe acne
Topical retinoids, e.g., tretinoin, isotretinoin, are useful alone in mild acne or in conjunction with antibiotics in moderately severe acne. Continue as maintenance therapy to prevent further acne outbreaks.
- *Side effects:* irritation, photosensitivity. Apply high factor sunscreen before sun exposure. Avoid in acne involving large areas of skin.

Oral antibiotics, e.g., tetracycline 500 mg bid, doxycycline 100 mg od or minocycline 100 mg OD can also be used. Response is usually seen by 6 weeks and full efficacy by 3 months. Continue antibiotics for 2 months after control is achieved. Prescription is usually given for a 3- to 6-month course. Continue topical retinoids and/or benzoyl peroxide to prevent further outbreaks.

Spironolactone and birth control pills containing nonandrogenic progestins will improve acne.

Severe acne
Isotretinoin is very effective in women with severe acne or acne that has not responded to other oral or topical treatments. Used early it can minimize scarring in inflammatory acne. However, it is highly toxic and can only be prescribed by a dermatologist.

Further reading
Dunaif A (1997). Insulin resistance and polycystic ovary syndrome: mechanism and implications for pathogenesis. *Endocr Rev* 18(6):774–800.

Ehrmann DA (2005). Polycystic ovary syndrome. *N Engl J Med* 352:1223–1236.

Ehrmann DA, Rychlik D (2003). Pharmacological treatment of polycystic ovary syndrome. *Semin Reprod Med* 21(3):277–283.

Ledger WL, Clark T (2003). Long-term consequences of polycystic ovary syndrome. *Royal College of Obsterics and Gynaecology* Guideline number 33.

Lord JM, Flight IHK, Norman RJ (2003). Insulin-sensitizing drugs for polycystic ovary syndrome. *Cochrane Database Syst Rev* 2003(3):CD003053.

Neithardt AB, Barnes RB (2003). The diagnosis and management of hirsutism. *Semin Reprod Med* 21(3):285–293.

Nestler JE (2008) Metformin for the treatment of the polycystic ovary syndrome. *N Engl J Med* 358(1):47–54.

Pierpoint T, McKeigue PM, Isaacs AJ, et al. (1998). Mortality of women with polycystic ovary syndrome at long-term follow-up. *J Clin Epidemiol* 51(7):581–586.

Rotterdam ESHRE/ASRM-sponsored PCOS Consensus Workshop Group (2004). Revised 2003 consensus on diagnostic criteria and long-term health risks related to polycystic ovary syndrome. *Hum Reprod* 19:41–47.

Tsilchorozidou T, Overton C, Conway GS (2004). The pathophysiology of polycystic ovary syndrome. *Clin Endocrinol* 60(1):1–17.

Congenital adrenal hyperplasia (CAH) in adults

Definition

CAH is an inherited group of disorders characterized by a deficiency of one of the enzymes necessary for cortisol biosynthesis. More than 90% of cases are due to 21α-hydroxylase deficiency.

There is a wide clinical spectrum, from presentation in the neonatal period with salt wasting and virilization to nonclassic CAH in adulthood.

CAH is inherited in an autosomal recessive manner.

Epidemiology

- Wide racial variations, most common in those of Jewish origin
- Carrier frequency of classic CAH: 1:60 in white people
- Carrier frequency of nonclassic CAH: 19% in Ashkenazi Jews, 13.5% in Hispanics, 6% in Italians, and 3% in other Caucasian populations

Pathogenesis

Genetics

CYP21 encodes for the 21α-hydroxylase enzyme, located on the short arm of chromosome 6 (chromosome 6p21.3). In close proximity is the *CYP21* pseudogene, with 90% homology but no functional activity.

21α-Hydroxylase deficiency results from gene mutations, partial gene deletions, or gene conversions in which sequences from the pseudogene are transferred to the active gene, rendering it inactive.

There is a correlation between the severity of the molecular defect and the clinical severity of the disorder. Nonclassic CAH is usually due to a point mutation (single base change); missense mutations result in simple virilizing disease, whereas a gene conversion or partial deletion usually results in presentation in infancy with salt wasting or severe virilization.

Biochemistry

📖 See Fig. 47.1.

21α-Hydroxylase deficiency results in aldosterone and cortisol deficiency. There is ACTH oversecretion because of the loss of negative feedback, and this causes adrenocortical hyperplasia and excessive accumulation of 17-hydroxy progesterone (17OHP) and other steroid precursors. These are then shunted into androgen synthesis pathways, resulting in testosterone and androstenedione excess.

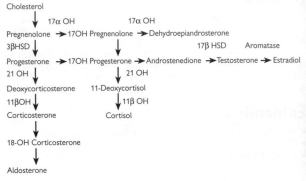

Fig. 47.1 Adrenal steroid biosynthesis pathway.

Clinical presentation

Classic CAH

Most patients are diagnosed in infancy; their clinical presentation is discussed elsewhere (see Congenital adrenal hyperplasia, p. 239).

Problems persisting into adulthood include sexual dysfunction and subfertility in women, particularly in salt wasters. Reconstructive genital surgery is required in the majority of women who were virilized at birth to create an adequate vaginal introitus. With improvement of medical and surgical care, pregnancy rates have improved. Fertility rates of 60–80% have been reported in women with classic CAH.

In men, high levels of adrenal androgens suppress gonadotropins and thus testicular function. Spermatogenesis may therefore be affected if CAH is poorly controlled.

Suboptimally controlled CAH in men also predisposes them to developing testicular adrenal rests. These are always benign but may be misdiagnosed as testicular tumors.

Nonclassic CAH

Nonclassic CAH is due to partial deficiency of 21α-hydroxylase. Glucocorticoid and aldosterone production are normal, but there is overproduction of 17OHP and, thus, androgens.

Patients present with hirsutism (60%), acne (33%), and oligomenorrhea (54%), often around the onset of puberty. Only 13% of women present with subfertility.

One-third of women have polycystic ovaries on US, and adrenal incidentalomas or hyperplasia is seen in 40%.

The nonclassic form is asymptomatic in men. The effect of nonclassic CAH on men fertility is unknown.

Laboratory evaluation

Because of the diurnal variation in adrenal hormonal secretion, all investigations should be performed in the morning.

Diagnosis of non-classic CAH—17OHP measurement

Timing of measurement

- Screen in the follicular phase of the menstrual cycle. 17OHP is produced by the corpus luteum, so false-positive results may occur if measured in the luteal phase of the cycle.
- Must be measured A.M. to avoid false-negative results, as 17OHP has a diurnal variation similar to that of ACTH

ACTH stimulation test

- Measure 17OHP 30 minutes after ACTH administration.
- An exaggerated rise in 17OHP is seen in nonclassic CAH.
- 17OHP level <1000 ng/dL post-ACTH excludes the diagnosis.
- Most patients have levels >1500 ng/dL.
- Levels of 1000–1500 ng/dL suggest heterozygosity or nonclassic CAH.
- Cortisol response to ACTH stimulation is usually low to normal.

Other investigations

Androgens

In poorly controlled classic CAH in women, testosterone and androstenedione levels may be in the adult male range. Dehydroepiandrosterone sulfate levels are usually only mildly, and not consistently, elevated in CAH.

Circulating testosterone and, particularly androstenedione, are elevated in nonclassic CAH, but there is a large overlap with levels seen in PCOS so serum androgen concentrations cannot be used to distinguish between the disorders.

Renin

Plasma renin levels are markedly elevated in 75% of patients with inadequately treated classic CAH, reflecting deficient aldosterone production.

A proportion of women with nonclassic CAH may also have mildly elevated renin concentrations.

ACTH

- Greatly elevated in poorly controlled classic CAH
- Usually normal levels in nonclassic CAH

📖 See Table 47.1 for a list of enzyme deficiencies in CAH.

Table 47.1 Enzyme deficiencies in CAH

Enzyme deficiency	Incidence (per births)	Clinical features
Classic 21α-hydroxylase	1:10 000–1:15 000	Salt wasting, ambiguous genitalia in females, precocious pubarche in males
Nonclassic 21α-hydroxylase (partial deficiency)	1:27–1:1000	Hirsutism, oligomenorrhea in pubertal girls, asymptomatic in boys
11β-hydroxylase	1:100 000	Ambiguous genitalia, virilization, hypertension
3β-hydroxylase	Rare	Mild virilization, salt wasting in severe cases
17α-hydroxylase	Rare	Delayed puberty in females, pseudohermaphroditism in males, hypertension, hypokalemia

Management

The aims of treatment of CAH in adulthood are as follows:
- To maintain normal energy levels and weight and avoid adrenal crises in all patients
- To minimize hyperandrogenism and to restore regular menses and fertility in women
- To avoid glucocorticoid over-replacement
- To treat stress with adequate extra glucocorticoid

Classic CAH

Prednisone

A total dose is 5–7.5 mg/day. This is given in one dose, either in the morning or at bedtime depending on the authority. There are no controlled studies comparing the two regimens. The evening dosing is to suppress the early-morning peak of ACTH and thus androgen secretion. The optimum dose is the minimum dose required to normalize serum androgens.

Occasional patients who are not controlled on prednisone may be treated with nocturnal dexamethasone instead (0.25–0.5 mg).

Other therapies

As with other forms of adrenal insufficiency, glucocorticoid doses should be doubled during illness, as discussed in detail elsewhere (📖 p. 337, 363).

Three-quarters of patients are salt wasters and thus require mineralocorticoid replacement therapy. Fludrocortisone in a dose of 50–200 mcg/day is given as a single daily dose. The aim is to keep plasma renin levels in the mid-normal range.

Bilateral adrenalectomy may very occasionally be considered in patients with severe virilization resistant to conventional therapy.

Experimental therapies

Trials have been performed using a combination of low-dose hydrocortisone, fludrocortisone, testolactone (an aromatase inhibitor), and flutamide (antiandrogen) in children. This 4-drug regimen appears to improve final height and minimize glucocorticoid side effects with no significant adverse effects. However, long-term effects are currently unknown.

Pregnancy

Screen the patient and her partner prior to pregnancy and give genetic advice. If the partner is a carrier, there is a 50% risk of having an affected child (1 in 63 is a carrier of the 21OH gene).

Nonclassic CAH

Oligo- and amenorrhea are treated with glucocorticoid therapy—e.g., noctural dexamethasone 0.25–0.5 mg or prednisone 2.5–5 mg/day, may be used. Slightly higher doses may be required to normalize ovulatory function.

If fertility is not desired, symptoms may be treated with OCPs and antiandrogen.

Hirsutism and acne may be treated using OCPs (📖 see Management, p. 237). Spironolactone should be avoided because of the potential risk of salt wasting and thus hyperreninemia.

If the plasma renin level is elevated, then fludrocortisone given in a dose sufficient to normalize renin concentrations may improve adrenal hyperandrogenism.

Men do not usually require treatment. The occasional man may need glucocorticoids to treat subfertility.

Management of pregnancy in CAH

Indications for prenatal treatment

- *Maternal classic CAH:* Screen patient and partner using basal ± ACTH-stimulated 17OHP levels (📖 see Investigations, p. 242). If levels are elevated, proceed to genotyping. If heterozygote, then prenatal treatment of the fetus is recommended.
- Previous child from same partner with CAH

Aims of prenatal treatment (📖 see Fig. 47.2)

The aim is to prevent virilization of an affected female fetus.

Treatment (commenced before 10 weeks gestation)

Dexamethasone (20 mcg/kg maternal body weight) in 3 divided doses a day crosses the placenta and reduces fetal adrenal hyperandrogenism.

Discontinue treatment if the fetus is male.

Outcome

From 50 to 75% of affected women do not require reconstructive surgery.

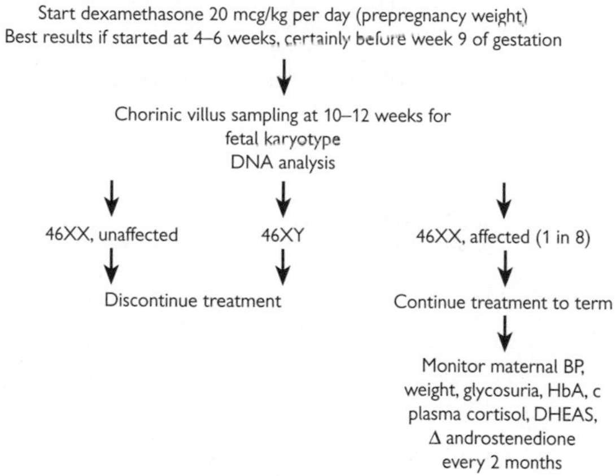

Start dexamethasone 20 mcg/kg per day (prepregnancy weight)
Best results if started at 4–6 weeks, certainly before week 9 of gestation

⬇

Chorinic villus sampling at 10–12 weeks for
fetal karyotype
DNA analysis

46XX, unaffected	46XY	46XX, affected (1 in 8)
⬇	⬇	⬇
Discontinue treatment		Continue treatment to term
		⬇
		Monitor maternal BP, weight, glycosuria, HbA, c plasma cortisol, DHEAS, Δ androstenedione every 2 months

Fig. 47.2 Prenatal treatment protocol.

Complications

There are no known fetal congenital malformations or neonanatal complications from dexamethasone treatment.

Subtle effects of glucocorticoids on neuropsychological function are unknown. No significant long-term follow-up studies on treated children have been published to date.

Maternal complications of glucocorticoid excess include mood swings, weight gain, gestational diabetes, and hypertension. Monitor maternal weight, blood pressure, fasting plasma glucose, and urinary glucose.

There is debate about whether women with nonclassic CAH should be offered prenatal treatment with dexamethasone. There have been no cases of women with nonclassic CAH giving birth to a virilized female.

Additionally, the estimated risk of conceiving an infant with classic CAH is 1:1000. As the risk of fetal virilization is therefore low, dexamethasone treatment of this group of women seems unwarranted. However, these infants should be screened in the neonatal period by measuring 17OHP levels.

Monitoring of treatment

Annual follow-up is usually adequate in adults.
- *Clinical assessment:* Look for evidence of hyperandrogenism and glucocorticoid excess. Amenorrhea in women usually suggests inadequate therapy. Measure BP.
- *17OHP:* Aim for a mildly elevated level (about 2–4×normal). Normalizing 17OHP will result in complications from supraphysiological doses of glucocorticoids.
- *Plasma rennin:* Aim for renin in mid-normal range. Hyperandrogenism will be difficult to control if the patient is mildly salt depleted (ACTH production stimulated by hypovolemia).
- *Androgens:* Aim to normalize serum testosterone/androstenedione taken before A.M. steroids.
- *Consider bone density,* which may be reduced by supraphysiological steroid doses.

In females:
- Good control ensures fertility.
- Testes should be intermittently checked for masses—adrenal cell rests.

Prognosis

Adults with treated CAH have a normal life expectancy. Improvement in medical and surgical care has also improved quality of life (QoL) for most sufferers. However, there are a few unresolved issues.

Height

Despite optimal treatment in childhood, patients with CAH are, on average, significantly shorter than their predicted genetic height. Studies suggest that this may be due to overtreatment with glucocorticoids during infancy.

Fertility

Fertility remains reduced in women with CAH, particularly in salt wasters, from factors including inadequate vaginal introitus and anovulation secondary to both hyperandrogenism and high 17OHP levels.

Fertility may also be affected in men with poorly controlled classic CAH.

Adrenal incidentalomas and testicular adrenal rest tumors

Benign adrenal adenomas have been reported in up to 50% of patients with classic CAH. Men with CAH may develop adrenal rests. These are ACTH-responsive and should be treated by optimizing glucocorticoid therapy.

Occasionally, adults with nonclassic CAH develop adrenal adenomas or testicular rests and should then be started on steroids.

Further reading

Cabrera MS, Vogiatzi MG, New MI (2001). Long-term outcome in adult males with classic congenital adrenal hyperplasia. *J Clin Endocrinol Metab* 86(7):3070–3078.

Joint LWPES/ESPE CAH Working Group (2002). Consensus statement on 21-hydroxylase deficiency from the Lawson Wilkins Paediatric Endocrine Society and the European Society for Paediatric Endocrinology. *J Clin Endocrinol Metab* 87(9):4048–4053.

Merke DP (2008). Approach to the adult with congenital adrenal hyperplasia due to 21-hydroxylase deficiency. *J Clin Endocrinol Metab* 93:653–660.

New MI (2006). Extensive clinical experience: nonclassical 21-hydroxylase deficiency. *J Clin Endocrinol Metab.* 91(11):205–214.

New MI, Carlson A, Obeid J, et al. (2001). Prenatal diagnosis for congenital adrenal hyperplasia in 532 pregnancies. *J Clin Endocrinol Metab* 86(12):5651–5757.

Ogilvie CM, Crouch NS, Rumsby G, et al. (2006). Congenital adrenal hyperplasia in adults: a review of medical, surgical and psychological issues. *Clin Endocrinol* 64:2–11.

Premawaradhana LDKE, Hughes IA, Read GF, et al. (1997). Longer term outcome in females with congenital adrenal hyperplasia: the Cardiff experience. *Clin Endocrinol* 46:327–332.

Speiser PW, White PC (2003). Congenital adrenal hyperplasia. *N Engl J Med* 349(8):776–788.

Ehrmann DA, Rychlik D (2003). Pharmacological treatment of polycystic ovary syndrome. *Semin Reprod Med* 21(3):277–283.

Ledger WL, Clark T (2003). Long-term consequences of polycystic ovary syndrome. *Royal College of Obstetrics and Gynaecology* Guideline number 33.

Lord JM, Flight IHK, Norman RJ (2003). Insulin-sensitizing drugs for polycystic ovary syndrome. *Cochrane Database Syst Rev* 2003(3):CD003053.

Neithardt AB, Barnes RB (2003). The diagnosis and management of hirsutism. *Semin Reprod Med* 21(3):285–293.

Nestler JE (2008) Metformin for the treatment of the polycystic ovary syndrome. *N Engl J Med* 358(1):47–54.

Pierpoint T, McKeigue PM, Isaacs AJ, et al. (1998). Mortality of women with polycystic ovary syndrome at long-term follow-up. *J Clin Epidemiol* 51(7):581–586.

Rotterdam ESHRE/ASRM-sponsored PCOS Consensus Workshop Group (2004). Revised 2003 consensus on diagnostic criteria and long-term health risks related to polycystic ovary syndrome. *Hum Reprod* 19:41–47.

Tsilchorozidou T, Overton C, Conway GS (2004). The pathophysiology of polycystic ovary syndrome. *Clin Endocrinol* 60(1):1–17.

Androgen-secreting tumors

Definition

These rare tumors of the ovary or adrenal gland may be benign or malignant and cause virilization in women through androgen production.

Epidemiology and pathology

Androgen-secreting ovarian tumors

Three-quarters develop before the age of 40 years. They account for 0.4% of all ovarian tumors. 20% are malignant.

Tumors are variable in size. The larger they are, the more likely they are to be malignant. They are rarely bilateral. There are two major types:
- Sex cord stromal cell tumors often contain testicular cell types.
- Adrenal-like tumors often contain adrenocortical or Leydig cells.

Other tumors, e.g., gonadoblastomas and teratomas, may also on occasion present with virilization.

Androgen-secreting adrenal tumors

Half of these tumors develop before the age of 50 years. Larger tumors, particularly >6 cm, are more likely to be malignant.

Clinical features

Onset of symptoms
- Usually recent onset of rapidly progressive symptoms

Hyperandrogenism
- Hirsutism of varying degree, often severe (Ferriman–Gallwey score) (□ see Table 45.2, p. 225). Male-pattern balding and acne are also common.
- Usually oligo- or amenorrhea
- Infertility may be a presenting feature.

Virilization (□ Box 45.1, p. 224)
- Indicates severe hyperandrogenism is associated with clitoromegaly and is present in 98% of women with androgen-producing tumors. Not usually a feature of PCOS

Other
- Abdominal pain
- Palpable abdominal mass
- Ascites
- Symptoms and signs of Cushing's syndrome are present in 50% of females with adrenal tumors.

Laboratory evaluation

□ See Fig. 48.1.

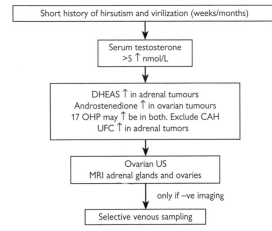

Fig. 48.1 Investigation of androgen-secreting tumors.

Management

Surgery
- Adrenalectomy or ovarian cystectomy/oophorectomy
- Curative in benign lesions

Adjunctive therapy
Malignant ovarian and adrenal androgen-secreting tumors are often resistant to chemotherapy and radiotherapy.

Prognosis

Benign tumors
Prognosis is excellent. Hirsutism improves postoperatively, but clitoromegaly, male-pattern balding, and deep voice may persist.

Malignant tumors
- *Adrenal tumors:* 20% 5-year survival. Most patients have metastatic disease at the time of surgery
- *Ovarian tumors:* 30% disease-free survival; 40% overall 5-year survival

Further reading
Hamilton-Fairley D, Franks S (1997). Androgen-secreting tumours. In Sheaves R, Jenkins PJ, Wass JAH (Eds.), *Clinical Endocrine Oncology.* Oxford: Blackwell Science, pp. 323–329.

Menstrual function disorders

Definitions

Oligomenorrhea is defined as the reduction in the frequency of menses to <9 periods a year.

Primary *amenorrhea* is the failure of menarche by the age of 16 years. Prevalence is ~0.3%

Secondary amenorrhea refers to the cessation of menses for >6 months in women who had previously menstruated. Prevalence is ~3–6%.

Many disorders may present with either primary or secondary amenorrhea.

The normal menstrual cycle is presented in Fig. 48.1.

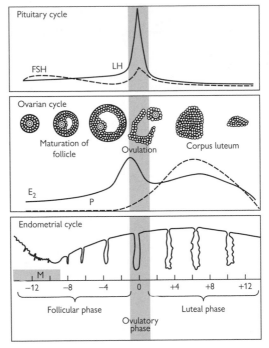

Fig. 49.1 The normal menstrual cycle.

Clinical evaluation

History
- Estrogen deficiency, e.g., hot flushes, reduced libido, and dyspareunia.
- Hypothalamic dysregulation, e.g., exercise and nutritional history, body weight changes, emotional stress, recent or chronic physical illness
- In primary amenorrhea—history of breast development, history of cyclical pain, age of menarche of mother and sisters
- In secondary amenorrhea—duration and regularity of previous menses, family history of early menopause, or familial autoimmune disorders, or galactosemia
- Anosmia may indicate Kallmann syndrome from GnRH deficiency.
- Hirsutism or acne
- Galactorrhea
- History suggestive of pituitary, thyroid, or adrenal dysfunction
- Drug history—e.g., causes of hyperprolactinemia, chemotherapy, hormonal contraception, recreational drug use
- Obstetric and surgical history

Physical examination
- Height, weight, body mass index (BMI)
- Features of Turner's syndrome or other dysmorphic features
- Secondary sex characteristics
- Galactorrhea
- Evidence of hyperandrogenism or virilization
- Evidence of thyroid dysfunction
- Anosmia, visual field defects

For causes, 📖 see Box 49.1.

Box 49.1 Causes of amenorrhea

Physiological
- Pregnancy and lactation
- Postmenopause

Iatrogenic
- Depomedroxyprogesterone acetate
- Levonorgestrel-releasing intrauterine device
- Progesterone-only pill
- Pathological—primary
- Chromosomal abnormalities—50%
  - Turner's syndrome
  - Other X chromosomal disorders
- Secondary hypogonadism—25%
  - Kallmann's syndrome
  - Pituitary disease
  - Hypothalamic amenorrhea
- Genitourinary malformations—15%
  - Imperforate hymen
  - Congenital absence of uterus, cervix, or vagina
- Other—10%
  - Androgen insensitivity syndrome
  - CAH
  - PCOS
  - Galactosemia

Most causes of secondary amenorrhea can cause primary amenorrhea.
- Pathological—secondary
- Ovarian—70%
  - PCOS
  - Premature ovarian failure
- Hypothalamic—15%
  - Weight loss
  - Excessive exercise
  - Physical or psychological stress
  - Craniopharyngioma
  - Infiltrative lesions of the hypothalamus
  - Drugs e.g., opiates
- Pituitary—5%
  - Hyperprolactinemia
  - Hypopituitarism
  - Isolated gonadotropin deficiency
- Uterine—5%
  - Intrauterine adhesions
- Other endocrine disorders—5%
  - Thyroid dysfunction
  - Cushing's syndrome
    - Other causes of hyperandrogenism

Laboratory evaluation

📖 See Fig. 49.2.

Is it primary or secondary ovarian dysfunction?
• FSH, LH, estradiol, prolactin

Transvaginal US:
• Ovarian and uterine morphology—exclude anatomical abnormalities, PCOS, and Turner's syndrome
• Endometrial thickness to assess estrogen status

Other tests, depending on clinical suspicion, are as follows:
• Induce withdrawal bleed with progesterone (e.g., 5–10 mg medroxyprogesterone acetate daily for 7 days). If a bleed occurs, there is adequate estrogen priming and endometrial development.
• Serum testosterone in the presence of hyperandrogenism
• Thyroid function tests if any evidence of hyper- or hypothyroidism
• Karyotype in ovarian failure or if Turner's syndrome or androgen insensitivity syndrome suspected.
• MRI of the pituitary if LH, FSH low or in the presence of hyperprolactinemia.

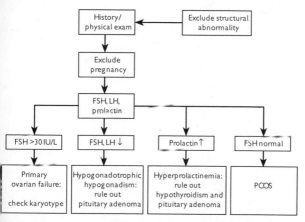

Fig. 49.2 Investigation of amenorrhea.

Management

Treat underlying disorder, e.g.:
- Dopamine agonists for prolactinomas
- Pituitary surgery for pituitary tumors
- Weight gain in anorexia nervosa

Treat estrogen deficiency with low-dose estrogen/progestogen preparations or OCPs.

Treat infertility—see p. 236

Further reading

Baird DT (1997). Amenorrhoea. *Lancet* 350:275–279.

Beswick SJ, Lewis HM, Stewart PM (2002). A recurrent rash treated by oophrectomy. *QJM* 95(9),:636–637.

Hickey M, Balen A (2003). Menstrual disorders in adolescence: investigation and management. *Hum Reprod Update* 9(5):493–504.

Premature ovarian insufficiency (POI)

Definition

POI is a disorder characterized by amenorrhea, estrogen deficiency, and elevated gonadotropins developing in women <40 years as a result of loss of ovarian follicular function.

Epidemiology

Incidence is 0.1% of women <30 years and 1% of those <40 years. POI accounts for 10% of all cases of secondary amenorrhea.

Causes of POI

- Chromosomal abnormalities (60%) (see Table 50.1)
  - Turner's syndrome (see Box 50.1)
  - Fragile × syndrome
  - Other × chromosomal abnormalities
- Gene mutations
  - β subunit of FSH
  - FSH receptor
  - LH receptor
- Autoimmune disease (20%)
- Iatrogenic
  - Chemotherapy
  - Radiotherapy
  - Hysterectomy
- Other
  - Familial ovarian failure
  - Galactosemia
  - Enzyme deficiencies, e.g., 17-hydroxylase deficiency.
  - Infections, e.g., mumps, CMV, HIV, *Shigella*
- Idiopathic
  - ?Environmental toxin

Table 50.1 Correlation of karyotype with phenotype

Karyotype	Phenotype
45,X (50%)	Most severe phenotype High incidence of cardiac and renal abnormalities
46,Xi(Xq) (20%)	↑ Prevalence of thyroiditis, inflammatory bowel disease, and deafness
45,X/46,XX (10%)	Least severe phenotype ↑ Mean height Spontaneous puberty and menses in up to 40%
46,Xr(X) (10%)	Spontaneous menses in 33% Congenital abnormalities uncommon Cognitive dysfunction in those with a small ring chromosome
45,X/46,XY (6%)	↑ Risk of gonadoblastoma
Other (4%)	

Box 50.1 Turner's syndrome

📖 Also see Turner's syndrome (p. 442).
- Most common X-chromosome abnormality in females, affecting 1:2500 live female births.
- Result of complete or partial absence of one X chromosome.
- *Clinical features:* short stature and gonadal dysgenesis. 90% of affected women have POI.
- *Characteristic phenotype:* webbed neck, micrognathia, low-set ears, high arched palate, widely spaced nipples, and cubitus valgus
- *Other associated abnormalities:* aortic coarctation and other left-sided congenital heart defects, hypothyroidism, osteoporosis, skeletal abnormalities, lymphedema, celiac disease, congenital renal abnormalities, and ear, nose, throat (ENT) abnormalities
- *Diagnosis:* lymphocyte karyotype

Management in adults
- Sex hormone replacement therapy
- Treat complications

Follow-up
- Baseline renal US, thyroid autoantibodies
- Annual BMI, BP, TFT, lipids, fasting blood glucose liver function
- 3- to 5-yearly echocardiogram and bone densitometry
- Hearing loss every 5 years

Pathogenesis

Failure of normal ovarian follicular response to gonadotropins leads to consequent failure of ovarian steroidogenesis. POI is the result of either ovarian follicle depletion or failure of the follicles to function (resistant ovary syndrome). It may be distinguished by ovarian US or histologically by ovarian biopsy.

Treatment options are the same, so invasive techniques looking for the presence of follicles are not indicated.

POI is usually permanent; however, more data show a variable intermittent pattern of hormone production. Additionally, <50% of karyotypically normal women with established disease produce estrogen intermittently and up to a 1/5 of women may ovulate despite high gonadotropin levels. Spontaneous pregnancy has been reported in 5%.

Clinical presentation

Amenorrhea
- May be primary, particularly in those with chromosomal abnormalities

Symptoms of estrogen deficiency
- Not present in those with primary amenorrhea
- 75% of women who develop secondary amenorrhea report hot flushes, night sweats, mood changes, fatigue, or dyspareunia; symptoms may precede the onset of menstrual disturbances.

Autoimmune disease
- Screen for symptoms and signs of associated autoimmune disorders.

Other
- Past history of radiotherapy, chemotherapy, or pelvic surgery
- Positive family history in 10% of patients

Box 50.2 Autoimmune diseases and POI

Autoimmune disease is responsible for 20% of all cases of POI. A second autoimmune disorder is present in 10–40% of women with autoimmune POI:
- Addison's disease (10%)
- Autoimmune thyroid disease (25%)
- Type 1 diabetes mellitus (2%)
- Myaesthenia gravis (2%)
- B_{12} deficiency
- Systemic lupus erythematosus (SLE) is also more common

POI is present in the following:
- 60% of 5 with autoimmune polyglandular syndrome type 1 (📖 p. 198)
- 25% of 5 with autoimmune polyglandular syndrome type 2 (📖 p. 199)

Steroid cell antibodies are positive in 60–100% of patients with Addison's disease in combination with POI. Presence of positive steroid cell antibodies in women with Addison's disease confers a 40% risk of ultimately developing POI. Other ovarian antibodies have no predictive value.

Laboratory evaluation

Serum gonadotropins

- Diagnosis is confirmed by serum FSH >40 mIU/L (actual level depends on the assay) on at least two occasions at least 1 month apart associated with a low estradiol.
- Disease may have a fluctuating course with high FSH levels returning to normal and later regaining of ovulatory function.
- LH is also elevated; FSH is usually disproportionately higher than LH.

Serum estradiol levels

- Usually low

Karyotype

- All women below age 40 presenting with hypergonadotropic amenorrhea should have karyotyping performed.
- Women with Y-chromosomal material should be referred for bilateral gonadectomy to prevent the development of gonadoblastoma.

Pelvic US

- To identify normal ovarian and uterine morphology

Transvaginal US

- Ovarian volume and blood flow
- Uterine size and anatomy

Bone mineral density

- Risk of osteoporosis

Screen for autoimmune disease

- Thyroid and adrenal cortex autoantibodies. If positive, this increases the risk of progression to overt adrenal or thyroid insufficiency.
- Ovarian antibodies are of no proven clinical value.
- TSH and fasting blood glucose, FBC
- Cosyntropin stimulation test only if adrenal insufficiency is suspected clinically
- Other tests as clinically indicated

Ovarian biopsy

- Not indicated

Annual assessment of women with POI

Assess adequacy of sex hormone replacement therapy:
- Tolerance and compliance
- Side effects and complications
- Persistent symptoms of sex hormone deficiency

Address fertility issues.

Screen for other autoimmune disease (in autoimmune POI):
- Clinical evaluation
- TSH and fasting blood glucose
- Cosyntropin stimulation test if clinically indicated.

Screen for complications:
- Osteoporosis
- Cardiovascular disease

Management

Sex hormone replacement therapy

Exogenous estrogens (hormone replacement therapy [HT]) are required to alleviate symptoms and prevent the long-term complications of estrogen deficiency—osteoporosis and possibly cardiovascular disease (📖 see Table 50.2).

In non-hysterectomized women, a progestagen should be added for 12–14 days a month to prevent endometrial hyperplasia.

Low-dose androgen replacement therapy may improve persistent fatigue and poor libido despite adequate estrogen replacement.

Oral contraceptives are an alternative convenient approach to HT in younger women with POI.

Fertility

A minority of women with POI and a normal karyotype will recover spontaneously. There is a 5% spontaneous fertility rate.

Oocyte donation and in vitro fertilization offer these women their best chance of fertility. Results are promising, with a pregnancy rate of 35% per patient. Results are less good in women with chemotherapy-induced gonadal damage or after pelvic radiotherapy.

Ovulation induction therapy has been tried, but the results have been poor. Glucocorticoid therapy has been used in autoimmune POI, but efficacy is poor.

Table 50.2 Hormone replacement therapy in POI

Hormone replacement	Dose
Estrogen	
Conjugated estrogens	1.25 mg daily
Estradiol valerate	2–4 mg daily
Transdermal estradiol	100 mcg twice a week
Progestagen	12–14 days a month:
Norethisterone	1 mg
Medroxyprogesterone	10 mg
Testosterone	
IM testosterone	50–100 mg/month
Testosterone SC implants	50–100 mg every 6 months

There is currently much research into the removal of functioning ovarian tissue in women prior to undergoing cancer chemotherapy followed by its cryopreservation with the aim of reimplantation at a later stage when fertility is required.

Research into this technique is still in its infancy so if considered, patients and their families must be counseled about the uncertainty of future success rates associated with ovarian cryopreservation.

Recent improvements in methods of oocyte cryopreservation using rapid freezing in liquid nitrogen (vitrification) have allowed women with high chance of POI (e.g., before chemo- or radiotherapy) to store oocytes collected after superovulation. However, this is also experimental, and quoted success rates are 20–30% per patient and depend on age and egg quality at the time of collection.

📖 See Chapter 51, Menopause, p. 264–274, for a full review of hormone therapy.

Prognosis

Mortality of women with POI left untreated may be ↑ 2-fold.

Estrogen deficiency leads to the following:
- ↑ Risk of cardiovascular and cerebrovascular disease
- ↑ Risk of osteoporosis. Up to 2/3 of women with POI and a normal karyotype have ↓ bone mineral density (BMD), with a z score of −1 or less despite at least intermittent HT. This may be due to a combination of factors, including an initial delay in initiating HT, poor compliance with HT, and estrogen "underdosing."

Further reading

Barlow DH (1996). Premature ovarian failure. *Baillière Clin Obstet Gynecol* 10(3):361–384.

Kalantaridou SN, Davis SR, Nelson LM (1998). Premature ovarian failure. *Endocrinol Metab Clin* 27(4):989–1006.

Welte, CK (2008). Primary ovarian insufficiency: a more accurate term for premature ovarian failure. *Clin Endocrinol* 68:499–509.

Menopause

Definition

The *menopause* is the permanent cessation of menstruation as a result of ovarian failure (see Box 51.1) and is a retrospective diagnosis made after 12 months of amenorrhea. The average age of women at the time of the menopause is ~50 years, although smokers reach the menopause ~2 years earlier.

The *perimenopause* encompasses the menopause transition and the first year following the last menstrual period.

Box 51.1 Physiology

The physiology of the menopause remains poorly understood. Ovaries have a finite number of germ cells, with maximal numbers at 20 weeks of intrauterine life. Thereafter, there is a gradual reduction in the number of follicles until the perimenopause when there is an exponential loss of oocytes until the store is depleted at the time of the menopause. Table 51.1 summarizes hormonal changes during the menopausal transition.

Inhibin B and anti-Müllerian hormone (AMH) are ovarian glycoprotiens produced by follicles as they develop from pre-antral to antral stages. Both may participate in ovarian paracrine regulation and, with other molecules, regulate the rate of attrition of follicles. Inhibin B and AMH fall with ovarian aging, before any detectable rise in FSH, and are thus early markers of incipient ovarian failure and onset of perimenopause.

In the early perimenopausal period, FSH levels fluctuate, but the gradual rise in FSH levels maintains estradiol production by the ovarian follicles. So, contrary to previous belief, average serum estradiol levels may be high at the onset of the meno-pause transition, falling only toward the end as the follicles are depleted.

Table 51.1 Hormonal changes during the menopausal transition

	Premenopause (from age 36 years)	Early perimenopause	Advanced perimenopause	Menopause
Menstrual cycle	Regular, ovulatory	Irregular, often short cycles, increasingly anovulatory	Oligomenorrhea	Amenorrhea
FSH	Rising but within normal range	Intermittently raised, especially in follicular phase	Persistently ↑	↑↑
Inhibin B	Declining	Low	Low	Very low
E2	Normal>	Normal	Normal/low	Low

Long-term consequences

- *Osteoporosis:* During the perimenopausal period there is an accelerated loss of BMD, with postmenopausal women being more susceptible to osteoporotic fractures.
- *Ischemic heart disease (IHD):* Postmenopausal women are 2–3× more likely to develop IHD than are premenopausal women, even after age adjustments. The menopause is associated with an increase in risk factors for atherosclerosis, including less favorable lipid profile, ↓ insulin sensitivity, and an ↑ thrombotic tendency.
- *Dementia:* Women are 2–3× more likely to develop Alzheimer disease than men. It is suggested that estrogen deficiency may play a role in the development of dementia.

Clinical presentation

There are marked cultural differences in the frequency of symptoms related to the menopause. In particular, vasomotor symptoms and mood disturbances are more commonly reported in Western countries.

Menstrual disturbances (90%)
Cycles gradually become increasingly anovulatory and variable in length from about 4 years prior to the menopause. Oligomenorrhea often precedes permanent amenorrhea. In 10% of women, menses cease abruptly with no preceding transitional period.

Hot flashes (40%)
These are often associated with sweats and skin flushing. They are highly variable and thought to be related to fluctuations in estrogen concentrations. They tend to resolve spontaneously within 5 years of menopause.

Urinary symptoms (50%)
There is atrophy of urethral and bladder mucosa after the menopause and ↓ sensitivity of α-adrenergic receptors of the bladder neck in the perimenopausal period. This may result in urinary incontinence and an ↑ risk of urinary tract infections.

Sexual dysfunction (40%)
Vaginal atrophy may result in dyspareunia and vaginal dryness. Additionally, falling androgen levels may reduce sexual arousal and libido.

Mood changes (25–50%)
Anxiety, memory problems, difficulty in concentration, and irritability have all been attributed to the menopause. Women with a history of affective disorders are at ↑ risk of mood disturbances in the perimenopausal period.

Evaluation (if HT is being considered)

History
- Perimenopausal symptoms and their severity
- Assess risk factors for cardiovascular disease and osteoporosis.
- Assess risk factors for breast cancer and thromboembolic disease.
- History of active liver disease

Examination
- BP
- Breasts
- Pelvic examination, including cervical smear

Investigations

FSH levels fluctuate markedly in the perimenopausal period and correlate poorly with symptoms. A raised FSH in the perimenopausal period may not necessarily indicate infertility, so contraception, if desired, should continue until the menopause.

Mammography is indicated prior to starting estrogen replacement therapy and then following national guidelines.

Endometrial biopsy does not need to be performed routinely but is used in women with abnormal uterine bleeding and an abnormal US.

Hormone replacement therapy (HT)

The aim of treatment of postmenopausal women is to alleviate menopausal symptoms. HT is no longer indicated for the prevention of chronic disease in postmenopausal women.

However, women who have POI should receive HT unless there is an absolute contraindication, until the age of 50 years.

Benefits of HT

Hot flashes

These respond well to estrogen therapy in a dose-dependent manner. Start with a low dose and increase gradually as required to control symptoms. Higher doses may be required after hysterectomy, particularly in younger women.

For 75% of women, vasomotor symptoms are resolved, so the dose is tapered to the lowest one to control symptoms. The dose of HT should be gradually reduced over weeks, as sudden withdrawal of estrogen may precipitate the return of vasomotor symptoms.

In women with a contraindication to HT or who are intolerant of it, nonhormonal therapies are available, summarized in Table 51.2.

Urinary symptoms

A trial of HT, local or systemic, may improve stress and urge incontinence as well as the frequency of cystitis.

Table 51.2 Alternatives to HT

Symptom	Management
Vasomotor symptoms	Venlafaxine (75 mg od), paroxetine (20 mg od), and fluoxetine (20 mg od) have been shown to significantly reduce the frequency and severity of hot flashes, with minimal side effects.
	Gabapentin (300 mg tid) has also been shown to reduce the frequency and severity of hot flashes. Side effects include dizziness, somnolescence, and weight gain.
	Megestrol acetate in a dose of 20 mg bid also reduces hot flashes by up to 70%, but its use is limited by side effects, particularly weight gain.
	Clonidine is less effective, reducing the occurrence of flushes by 20%, and is often associated with disabling side effects such as dizziness, drowsiness, and dry mouth.
Genitourinary symptoms	Vaginal lubri-cants, e.g., Replens®
Osteoporosis	Selective estrogen receptor modulators (SERMs), e.g., raloxifene; however, these may exacerbate vasomotor symptoms if present.
	Bisphosphonates, e.g., alendronic acid and risedronate

Vaginal atrophy

Systemic or local estrogen therapy improves vaginal dryness and dyspareunia. A maximum of 6 months' use of vaginal cream is recommended unless combined with a progestin, as systemic absorption may increase the risk of endometrial hyperplasia.

An estradiol vaginal ring (Estring®) has little stimulatory effect on endometrial tissue and does not increase serum estradiol concentrations. Concomitant progestin therapy is therefore not necessary. If estrogens are contraindicated, then vaginal moisturizers, e.g., Replens®, may help.

Osteoporosis

HT has been shown to increase BMD in the lumbar spine by 3–5%/year and at the femoral neck by about 2%/year by inhibiting bone resorption. There is an associated 30–50% reduction in fracture risk, protection being highest in women on HT for at least 10 years.

The Women's Health Initiative trial (WHI) confirmed that HT reduces the risk of both hip and vertebral fractures by a third. Timing of initiation of treatment to achieve maximal bone protection remains controversial.

Evidence suggests that initiation of HT soon after the menopause is associated with the lowest hip fracture risk, but discontinuation of HT ultimately results in bone loss to pretreatment levels.

Colorectal cancer

Observational studies have shown that HT may protect against colon cancer. This has been confirmed by WHI, which showed a 20% reduction in the incidence of colon cancer in HT users. However, HT should currently not be prescribed solely to prevent colorectal cancer.

Risks of HT (see Box 51.2)

Breast cancer

No personal or family history of breast cancer

There is an ↑ risk of breast cancer in HT users, which is related to the duration of use. The risk increases by 35% following 5 years of use and falls to never-used risk 5 years after discontinuing HT.

For women aged 50 not using HT, about 45 in every 1000 will have cancer diagnosed over the following 20 years, that is, up to age 70. This number increases to 47/1000 women using HT for 5 years, 51/1000 using

---

Box 51.2 Summary of contraindications to HT

Absolute
- Undiagnosed vaginal bleeding
- Pregnancy
- Active DVT
- Active endometrial cance
- Breast cancer

Relative-seek advice
- Past history of endometrial cancer
- Family or past history of thromboembolism
- Ischemic heart disease
- Cerebrovascular disease
- Active liver disease.
- Hypertriglyceridemia

HT for 10 years, and 57/1000 after 15 years of use. The risk is highest in women on combined HT compared with estrogens alone.

Mortality has not been shown to be ↑ in breast cancer developing in women on HT.

Family history of breast cancer

Risk of breast cancer may be ↑ 4-fold as a result of family history, but there is little evidence that the risk is ↑ further by the use of HT. HT may be used short term at lower doses in these women if severe vasomotor symptoms are present, after counseling regarding the above risks.

Past history of breast cancer

Avoid HT in women with a past history of breast cancer.

Venous thromboembolism (DVT)

HT increases the risk approximately 3-fold, resulting in an extra 2 cases/10,000 woman-years. The risk is highest in the first year of use of HT and has been shown to be halved by aspirin or statin therapy.

This risk is ↑ in women who already have risk factors for DVT, including previous DVT, cardiovascular disease, and within 90 days of hospitalization. Many suggest discontinuation of HT with any hospitalization.

Low-risk women

• Absolute risk remains small—30 per 100,000 women.
• Stop HT during immobilization or use prophylactic anticoagulation.

Family history of DVT

If HT is being considered because of severe vasomotor symptoms, do a thrombophilia screen. If positive, then avoid HT or use it with anticoagulation therapy.

Women with a positive family history of thromboembolism are still at a slightly ↑ risk themselves, even if the results of the thrombophilia screen are negative, so prescribe HT with caution after counseling the patient. Transdermal E2 may be preferable.

Past history of DVT/PE

Risk of recurrence is 5% per year, so avoid HT unless the patient is on long-term warfarin therapy.

Cerebrovascular disease

HT has been shown to increase the risk of ischemic stroke in older women, particularly in the presence of atrial fibrillation. HT should therefore not be used in women with a history of cerebrovascular disease or atrial fibrillation unless they are anticoagulated.

Endometrial cancer

There is no ↑ risk in women taking continuous com-bined HT preparations. Women using sequential combined preparations do not appear to have an ↑ risk of endometrial cancer initially, but the risk of endometrial hyperplasia does increase with long-term use (>5 years) despite regular withdrawal bleeds, so these women need regular follow-up.

Women with cured stage I tumors may safely take HT.

Ovarian cancer

It is unclear if HT may be associated with an ↑ risk of ovarian cancer. A couple of large casecontrol studies have shown anrisk of ovarian cancer in long-term (>10 years) users of unopposed estrogen replacement therapy.

There are few data available on the risk of ovarian cancer in women taking combined HT. However, studies have also shown that HT does not have a negative effect in ovarian cancer survivors.

Gallstones

The risk of gallstones is ↑ 2-fold in HT users.

Migraine

Migraines may increase in severity and frequency in HT users. A trial of HT is still worthwhile if indications are present, providing there are no focal neurological signs associated with the migraine. Modification in the dose of estrogen or its preparation may improve symptoms.

Endometriosis and uterine fibroids

The risk of recurrence of endometriosis or of growth of uterine fibroids is low on HT.

Liver disease

Use transdermal estrogens to avoid hepatic metabolism and monitor liver function in women with impaired liver function tests. Do not use HT in the presence of active liver disease or liver failure.

Areas of uncertainty with HT

Cardiovascular disease (CVD)

Data from >30 observational studies suggest that HT may reduce the risk of developing CVD by up to 50%. However, randomized placebo-controlled trials, e.g., the Heart and Estrogen-Progestin Replacement Study (HERS) and the WHI trial, have failed to show that HT protects against CVD.

Currently, HT should not be prescribed to prevent cardiovascular disease. Analysis of the WHI showed that women 50–59 had cardiac protection on HT, whereas older women had increased risk. These data support the primary prevention hypothesis.

Alzheimer disease

Recent evidence suggests that the risk of developing Alzheimer disease may be reduced by up to 50% in women receiving HT, particularly if started early in the menopause.

However, in women with established Alzheimer disease, there is no evidence to suggest reversal of cognitive dysfunction following initiation of HT. There is currently insufficient evidence to recommend the use of HT to prevent Alzheimer disease.

In postmenopausal women without dementia, HT may improve certain aspects of cognitive function.

Mood disturbances
There has been a strongly held belief that HT improves well-being and QoL in perimenopausal and post-menopausal women. However, in recent trials in which QoL was assessed, notably HERS and WHI, in women many years after menopause, the improvement in QoL and improved sleep was only seen in women with vasomotor symptoms.

Side effects commonly associated with HT

Breast tenderness usually subsides within 4–6 months of use. If troublesome, use a lower estrogen dose and increase it gradually.

Mood changes commonly associated with progestin therapy can be managed by changing the dose or preparation of progestin.

Irregular vaginal bleeding may be a problem in women on a continuous combined preparation. It usually subsides after 6–12 months of treatment. Spotting persists in 10%; patients may change to a cyclic preparation. 📖 See Box 51.3.

Summary of WHI trial

- WHI was a ran-domized, controlled trial of effects of continuous combined conjugated estrogen and medroxyprogesterone acetate on healthy postmenopausal women, with a mean follow-up 5.2 years.
- Mean age was 63 years, with 66% of women >60 years of age.
- 70% of partici-pants were overweight or obese and 50% were current or past smokers.
- Absolute risk was highest in the older age group (>65 years).

Box 51.3 **Whom and how to investigate for irregular uterine bleeding**

Sequential cyclical HT
- Three or more cycles of bleeding before the ninth day of progestin therapy or change in the duration or intensity of uterine bleeding

Continuous combined HT
- In first 12 months if bleeding is heavy or extended, if it continues after 12 months of use, or if it starts after a period of amenorrhea

Endometrial assessment
- Essential in women with irregular uterine bleeding. Vaginal US, looking at endometrial thickness, is a sensitive method of detecting endometrial disease.

Endometrial thickness of <5 mm excludes disease in 96–99% of cases, a sensitivity similar to that of endometrial biopsy.

However, specificity is poor, so if the endometrium is >5 mm (as it will be in 50% of postmenopausal women on HT), endometrial biopsy will be required to rule out carcinoma

- Results of WHI cannot be extrapolated to younger HT users (<55 years of age).
- It is unclear whether different HT preparations or routes of administration would necessarily have the same benefit/risk pro-file.

Dietary phytoestrogens

Phytoestrogens are found in foods such as soybeans, cereals, and seeds. Although they have estrogen-like activity, data from clinical trials are conflicting. It appears that the effect of phytoestrogens on vasomotor symptoms is modest at best.

Research does suggest that soy protein has a favorable effect on plasma lipid concentrations and may reduce the risk of cardiovascular disease. However, the actual daily dose required is unclear.

Finally, data regarding the effect of phytoestrogens on bone loss and breast cancer risk are inconclusive. Phytoestrogen supplements cannot therefore be recommended for the prevention of chronic disease in peri- and postmenopausal women until they are adequately evaluated in clinical trials.

HT regimens

Estrogen preparations

See Table 51.3. Only symptomatic women should be treated with HT and dose tapered to the lowest dose to control symptoms.

Route of administration

Oral route is the most popular. Disadvantages are as follows:
- First-pass hepatic metabolism means that plasma estrogen levels are variable.
- Transdermal patches avoid the first-pass effect and are thus ideal in women with liver disease or hypertriglyceridemia. Additionally, patches provide constant systemic hormone levels. However, 10% of women develop skin reactions. Patients should try to avoid moisture and rotate patch sites to limit side effects.
- Gels have the advantages of patches, but skin irritation is less common.

Progestin preparations

See Table 51.4. These must be added in non-hysterectomized women to avoid endometrial hyperplasia and subsequent carcinoma.

Sequential cyclical regimen

Give progestin for a minimum of 12 days a month. It is usually given for the first 12 days of each calendar month. As the estrogen dose is tapered,

Table 51.3 Estrogen preparations

Preparation	Dose
Conjugated estrogens (PO)	0.625–1.25 mg daily
Transdermal estro-gen/progestin	Daily or intermittently

Table 51.4 Estrogen preparations

Progestin	Cyclical dose (days 1–12)	Continuous daily dose
Medroxyprogesterone acetate (least androgenic)	5 mg	2.5 mg

intermittent progestin 4 × a year may be feasible. However, the risk of endometrial hyperplasia on such a regimen is unknown.

Ninety percent of women have a monthly withdrawal bleed; 10% may be amenorrheic with no harmful consequences. Bleeding should start after the ninth day of progestin therapy.

Continuous combined regimen

Lower doses of progestin are given on a daily basis. Uterine bleeding is usually light in amount but timing is unpredictable. Bleeding should stop in 90% of women within 12 months, in the majority in 6 months.

This regimen is suggested for older women who do not want monthly withdrawal bleeds, but in the WHI trial continuous combined therapy was associated with ↑ risk of breast cancer.

The impact of other forms of HT is unknown.

Further reading

Arlt W (2006). Androgen therapy in women. *Eur J Endocrinol* 154:1–11.

Davis SR, et al. (2008). Testosterone for low libido in postmenopausal women not taking estrogen. *N Engl J Med* 359:2005–2017.

Humphries KH, Gill S (2003). Risks and benefits of hormone replacement therapy: the evidence speaks. *CMAJ* 168:1001–1010.

Million Women Study Collaborators (2003). Breast cancer and hormone-replacement therapy in the Million Women Study. *Lancet* 362:419–423.

Rymer J, Wilson R, Ballard K (2003). Making decisions about hormone replacement therapy. *BMJ* 326:322–326.

Writing Group for Women's Health Initiative Investigators (2002). Risks and benefits of estrogen plus progestin in healthy postmenopausal women: principal results from the Women's Health Initiative randomized controlled trial. *JAMA* 288:321–333.

Oral contraceptive pill (OCP)

Introduction

The OCP is very effective contraception, with approximately 5 per 100 users becoming pregnant per year.

Ethinylestradiol (EE2)

- The standard dose is 30 mcg, but in older women or those with possible cardiovascular risk factors, 20 mcg EE2 may be appropriate.
- A dose of 50 mcg EE2 may be indicated in patients on antiepileptic medication but is otherwise associated with an excess risk of arterial and venous thromboembolism.

Progestin

- Commonly used OCPs contain second-generation progestagens, such as levonorgestrel (150–250 mg) and norethisterone or norithindrone (1 mg).
- OCPs containing third-generation progestagens (e.g., norgestimate and desogestrel) are less androgenic; however, they may be associated with an ↑ risk of thromboembolism.
- Yasmin® contains a new progestagen, drospirenone, which is derived from spironolactone. It therefore has antimineralocorticoid activity. It may have antiandrogenic properties.

For a list of OCP preparations see Box 52.1.

OCP side effects

- Breakthrough bleeding
- Mood changes
- Nausea
- Fluid retention and weight gain
- Breast tenderness and enlargement
- Headache
- Reduced libido
- Chloasma

Box 52.1 OCP preparations

First generation
• Norinyl-1®

Second generation
• BiNovum®
• Brevinor®
• Loestrin 20/30®
• Logynon®
• Microgynon 30/30 ED®
• Norimin®
• Ovranette®
• Ovysmen®
• Synphase®
• TriNovum®

Third generation
• Cilest®
• Femodene/ED®
• Femodette®
• Katya 30/75®
• Marvelon®
• Mercilon®
• Sunya 20/75®
• Triadene®

Fourth generation
• Yasmin®

Benefits

Ovarian cancer

The risks of ovarian cancer are halved in women who have been taking the OCP for 5 years or more. This risk reduction persists long after discontinuation of the OCP.

Acne

The OCP reduces free testosterone concentrations by suppressing ovarian production of androgens and by ↑ hepatic SHBG production. OCP with low androgenic progestins often result in an improvement in acne.

Menstrual disorders

OCPs are associated with reduced menstrual flow and can therefore improve menorrhagia. They also reduce dysmenorrhea.

Risks

Venous thromboembolism

The risk of venous thromboembolism in nonpregnant women (5 per 100,000 women per year) is ↑ 3-fold in women on the OCP. The risk is highest in the first year of use, increases with age, and is ↑ in obese women.

The risk of venous thromboembolism appears to be higher in women taking OCPs containing desogestrel or gestodene.

Women with a family history of thromboembolism should undergo a thrombophilia screen before starting the OCP (see Table 52.1 for contraindications).

Arterial thrombosis

There is a 10-fold excess risk of IHD in female smokers over the age of 35 years who are on the OCP. The risk of IHD does not seem to be significantly ↑ in nonsmokers who take a low-dose OCP.

The relative risk of ischemic stroke is only slightly ↑ in women taking a low-dose OCP. The risk is ↑ in women over the age of 35 years, smokers

Table 52.1 OCP contraindications*

Absolute	Relative
History of heart disease, ischemic or valvular	Migraine
Pulmonary hypertension	Sickle cell disease
History of arterial or venous thrombosis	Gallstones
History of cerebrovascular disease	Inflammatory bowel disease
High risk of thrombosis, e.g., factor V Leiden, antiphospholipid antibodies	Hypertension
Liver disease	Hyperlipidemia
Migraine if severe or associated with focal aura	Diabetes mellitus
Breast or genital tract cancer	Obesity
Pregnancy	Smokers
Presence of two or more relative contraindications	
Age >35 years and a smoker	Otosclerosis
	Family history of thrombosis
	Family history of breast cancer

*Consider using a progesterone-only pill in women with contraindications to the combined OCP.

or women with hypertension. The risk of hemorrhagic stroke does not seem to be ↑ by taking the OCP.

Risk of either arterial or venous thrombosis returns to normal within 3 months of discontinuing the OCP.

Hypertension

Hypertension may be caused by the OCP, and if already present, may be more resistant to treatment.

Hepatic disease

Raised hepatic enzymes may be seen in women on the OCP. The incidence of benign hepatic tumors is also increased.

Gallstones

The risk of developing gallstones is slightly increased by taking the OCP (RR = 1.2).

Breast cancer (controversial)

There may be a slightly ↑ risk of breast cancer in women using the OCP (RR = 1.3), particularly in those who began taking the OCP in their teens.

The risk does not seem to be related to the duration of exposure to the OCP nor to the EE2 dose.

The relative risk of developing breast cancer returns to normal 10 years after discontinuing the OCP.

Cervical cancer

Use of the OCP appears to be associated with an excess risk of cervical cancer in women who are human papillomavirus (HPV) positive. The risk increases with the duration of OCP use. It is not known whether the risk falls again following discontinuation of the OCP.

Thrombophilia screen

- Antithrombin III
- Protein C
- Protein S
- Factor V Leiden

Hormonal emergency contraception

This refers to contraception that a woman can use after unprotected sexual intercourse to prevent pregnancy.

A single 1.5 mg dose of the progestin levonorgestrel is highly efficacious with a pregnancy rate of 2–4% if taken within 72 hours of sexual intercourse. It is most effective the earlier it is taken. The dose is repeated if vomiting occurs within 3 hours of taking the pill.

The mechanism of action is not clear but is thought to be due to inhibition of ovulation as well as an ↓ likelihood of endometrial implantation.

Side effects include nausea in up to 60% of women, vomiting in 10–20%. Consider antiemetic 1 hour before taking contraception. Other side effects are breast tenderness, fatigue, and dizziness.

Contraindication is pregnancy. Women should be advised to use barrier contraception until their next period.

98% of women menstruate within 3–4 weeks of taking levonorgestrel. They should be encouraged to seek medical advice if they do not bleed in that time.

If pregnancy does occur, levonorgestrel is not known to be teratogenic.

Practical issues

Age and the OCP

Women with no risk factors for arterial or venous thrombosis may continue to use the combined OCP until the age of 50 years.

Those with risk factors for thromboembolism and IHD should avoid the OCP after the age of 35 years, particularly if they are smokers.

All women on the OCP after the age of 35 years should be on the lowest effective estrogen dose (e.g., 20 mcg EE2).

Regarding contraception after the menopause, assume that the woman is fertile for the first year after the last menstrual period if >50 years.

Breakthrough bleeding

Causes include the following:
- Genital tract disease
- Insufficient estrogen dose
- Inappropriate progestin
- Missed pill
- Taking 2 packets continuously
- Gastroenteritis
- Drug interactions, e.g., antibiotics, hepatic enzyme inducers

Antibiotics and the OCP

Broad-spectrum antibiotics interfere with intestinal flora, thereby reducing bioavailability of the OCP. Additional methods of contraception should be used.

OCP and surgery

Stop the OCP at least 4 weeks before major surgery and any surgery to the legs. Resume after mobile for at least 2 weeks.

With emergency surgery, stop the OCP and start antithrombotic prophylaxis

Further reading

Petitti DB (2003). Combination oestrogen-progestin oral contraceptives. *N Engl J Med* 349:1443–1450.

Testicular physiology

Anatomy

Normal adult male testicular volume is 15–30 mL. Testicular temperature is 2°C lower than the rest of body because of the scrotal location. This is necessary for normal spermatogenesis.

There are two main units with differing functions:

- *Interstitial cells:* Comprised of Leydig cells, which are found in between the seminiferous tubules and close to the blood vessels. These cells produce testosterone.
- *Seminiferous tubules:* Make up 90% of testicular volume. Spermatogenesis occurs here, in the presence of high intratesticular concentrations of testosterone. They are made up of germ cells and Sertoli cells. Sertoli cells support spermatogenesis and secrete various hormones, including inhibin and, in the embryo, Müllerian inhibitory factor (AMH). The former inhibits FSH secretion from the pituitary gland and the latter is responsible for suppressing female sex organ development during sexual differentiation in utero.

See Fig. 53.1 for testosterone biosynthesis.

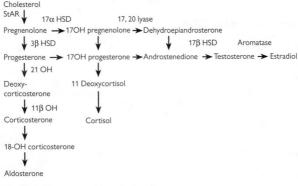

Fig. 53.1 Testosterone biosynthesis pathway.

Regulation of testicular function

Regulation of androgen production

Hypothalamic hormones

Gonadotropin-releasing hormone (GnRH) is secreted by thehypothalamus in a pulsatile manner in response to sex hormones and gonadal peptides, neurotransmitters, and neuropeptides (kisspeptin, leptin, etc.).

Episodic GnRH secretion is present at birth, is inhibited across midchildhood, and then is augmented initially during sleep in early puberty and then throughout the day in adulthood. It stimulates the secretion of *luteinizing hormone* (LH) and *follicle-stimulating hormone* (FSH) by the pituitary gland.

The pattern of GnRH secretion is crucial for normal gonadotropin secretion. Faster pulse frequencies are essential for LH secretion, whereas slower frequencies favor FSH secretion. Continuous administration of GnRH abolishes both LH and FSH secretion.

Pituitary hormones

LH binds to Leydig cell receptors and stimulates the synthesis and secretion of testosterone.

FSH binds to Sertoli cell receptors and stimulates the production of seminiferous tubule fluid as well as a number of substances thought to be important for spermatogenesis.

Their secretion is regulated by GnRH pulses and through negative feedback from testicular hormones and peptides.

Testis

Testosterone is the main androgen produced by the Leydig cells of the testis. Small amounts of androstenedione, DHEA, and dihydrotestosterone (DHT) are also produced. Testosterone has a circadian rhythm with maximum secretion at around 8 A.M. and minimum at around 9 P.M.

Small amounts of estradiol are also produced in the testis by the conversion from testosterone. Additionally, most of the circulating estradiol in men occurs as a result of aromatization of androgens in adipose tissue.

FSH, in the presence of adequate testosterone levels, stimulates the secretion of inhibin B by Sertoli cells. This in turn acts as a potent inhibitor of FSH secretion.

The secretion of pituitary gonadotropins is tightly regulated by testicular function. LH secretion is inhibited by testosterone and its metabolites whereas, FSH secretion is controlled by both inhibin B and testosterone. High concentrations of testosterone or of inhibin B results in a negative feedback inhibition of FSH secretion (□ see Fig. 53.2).

Testicular function is also under paracrine control. Inhibin and insulin-like growth factor-1 (IGF-1) act with LH to enhance testosterone production, whereas cytokines inhibit Leydig cell function.

Regulation of spermatogenesis

📕 See Fig. 53.2.

Both FSH and LH are required for the initiation of spermatogenesis at puberty. LH, by stimulating Leydig cell activity, plays an important part in the early phases of sperm production, when high intratesticular concentrations of testosterone are essential. FSH, through its action on the Sertoli cells, is vital for sperm maturation.

The whole process of spermatogenesis takes approximately 74 days, followed by another 12–21 days for sperm transport through the epididymis. This means that events that may affect spermatogenesis may not be apparent for up to 3 months.

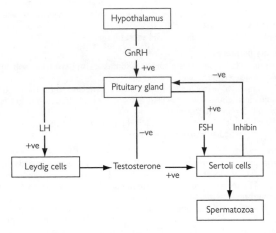

Fig. 53.2 Regulation of spermatogenesis.

Physiology

Testosterone transport

From 2 to 4% of circulating testosterone is free and therefore biologically active. The rest is bound to proteins, particularly albumin and sex hormone binding globulin (SHBG).

Testosterone metabolism

Testosterone is converted in target tissues to the more potent androgen DHT in the presence of the enzyme 5α reductase. There are multiple 5α-reductase isoenzymes; type 2 is the isoenzyme responsible for DHT synthesis in the genitalia, genital skin, and hair follicles. It is therefore essential for normal male virilization and sexual development.

Both testosterone and DHT exert their activity by binding to androgen receptors, the latter more avidly than testosterone. The androgen receptor is encoded by a gene found on the long arm of the X chromosome (Xq).

Testosterone may alternatively be converted into estradiol through the action of the aromatase enzyme, found in greatest quantities in the testes and adipose tissue.

Testosterone and its metabolites are inactivated in the liver and excreted in the urine.

Androgen action

- Male sexual differentiation during embryogenesis
- Development and maintenance of male secondary sex characteristics after puberty
- Normal male sexual function and behavior
- Spermatogenesis
- Regulation of gonadotropin secretion

Estrogen metabolism in males

- Estradiol daily production rate in men: 35–45 mcg
- Source of circulating estradiol:
- Peripheral aromatization of testosterone (60%)
- Testes (20%)
- Peripheral conversion from estrone (20%)
- 2–3% free estradiol that is biologically active; the rest is bound to SHBG

Estrogen action in males

- Pubertal growth and fusion of the epiphyses
- Maintenance of bone density
- Regulation of gonadotropin secretion.

Further reading

De Ronde W, Pols HAP, Van Leeuwen JPTM, et al. (2003). The importance of oestrogens in males. *Clin Endocrinol* 58(5):529–542.

Male hypogonadism

Definition

Male hypogonadism is the failure of testes to produce adequate amounts of testosterone, spermatozoa, or both.

Epidemiology

Klinefelter's syndrome (XXY) (see p. 289–290) is the most common congenital cause and is thought to occur with an incidence of 1:500 live births.

Acquired hypogonadism is even more common, affecting 1:200 men.

Evaluation of male hypogonadism

Presentation
- Failure to progress through puberty
- Sexual dysfunction
- Infertility
- Nonspecific symptoms, e.g., lethargy, reduced libido, mood changes, weight gain

The clinical presentation depends on the following:
- Age of onset (congenital vs. acquired)
- Severity (complete vs. partial)
- Duration (functional vs. permanent)

Secondary hypogonadism (hypogonadotropic hypogonadism)

Definition

This is hypogonadism as a result of hypothalamic or pituitary dysfunction.

Diagnosis

- Low serum testosterone
- Low–normal or low LH and FSH (normal inhibin B and anti-Müllerian hormone)

Causes

📖 See Box 54.1.

Idiopathic hypogonadotropic hypogonadism (IHH)

- The congenital form is indistinguishable from Kallmann syndrome apart from the absence of anosmia. >90% of patients are men.
- GnRH receptor gene mutation is an uncommon cause of IHH.

Box 54.1 Causes of secondary hypogonadism

Idiopathic

- Kallmann syndrome.
- Other genetic causes, e.g., mutations of *GnRH-R* or *GPR54* genes
- Idiopathic hypogonadotropic hypogonadism (IHH)
- Fertile eunuch syndrome
- Congenital adrenal hypoplasia (*DAX-1* gene mutation)

Functional

- Exercise
- Weight changes
- Anabolic steroids
- Stress—physical or psychological
- Systemic illness
- Medication and recreational drugs

Structural

- Tumors, e.g., pituitary adenoma, craniopharyngioma, germinoma
- Infiltrative disorders, e.g., sarcoidosis, hemochromatosis
- Head trauma
- Radiotherapy
- Surgery to the pituitary gland or hypothalamus

Miscellaneous

- Hemochromatosis
- Prader–Willi syndrome
- Laurence–Moon–Biedl syndrome

- Men with acquired IHH may go through normal puberty and have normal testicular size, but present with infertility or poor libido and potency. It may be temporary, with normalization of gonadal function after stopping GnRH or testosterone therapy.

Fertile eunuch syndrome
- Incomplete GnRH deficiency. Enough to maintain normal spermatogenesis and testicular growth but insufficient for adequate virilization
- May require testosterone/hCG for fertility

Congenital adrenal hypoplasia (CAH)
- Rare X-linked or autosomal recessive disease caused by mutation of the *DAX* gene, located on the X chromosome
- Presents with primary adrenal failure in infancy
- Hypothalamic hypogonadism is also present.

Structural
- Usually associated with other pituitary hormonal deficiencies
- In children, craniopharyngiomas are the most common cause. Cranial irradiation for leukemia or brain tumors may also result in secondary hypogonadism.
- The most common lesions in adulthood are prolactinomas.

Kallmann syndrome
This genetic disorder is characterized by failure of episodic GnRH secretion ± anosmia. It results from failure of the proper migration of GnRH-producing neurons into the hypothalamus.

Epidemiology
- Incidence of 1 in 10,000 men
- ♂:♀ ratio = 4:1.

Diagnosis
- Anosmia in 75%
- ↑ Risk of cleft lip and palate, sensorineural deafness, cerebellar ataxia, and renal agenesis
- Low testosterone, LH, and FSH levels
- Rest of pituitary function is normal
- Normal MRI pituitary gland and hypothalamus; absent olfactory bulbs may be seen on MRI
- Normalization of pituitary and gonadal function in response to physiological GnRH replacement

Genetics
- Most commonly a result of an isolated gene mutation
- May be inherited in an X-linked *(KAL1)*, autosomal dominant *FGFR1* mutation/*KAL2*, or recessive trait
- *KAL1* gene mutation responsible for some cases of X-linked Kallmann syndrome is located on Xp22.3. It has a more severe reproductive phenotype.

- Mutations of *FGFR1* (fibroblast growth factor receptor 1) gene, located on chromosome 8p11, is associated with the autosomal dominant form of Kallmann syndrome. Affected men have an ↑ likelihood of undescended testes at birth.
- 12–15% incidence of delayed puberty in families of subjects with Kallmann syndrome compared with 1% general population
- Men with autosomal dominant form (*FGFR1* mutation): 50% transmitted to offspring.

Management
- Androgen replacement therapy
- When fertility is desired, testosterone is stopped and exogenous gonadotropins are administered (🕮 see p. 294).

Systemic illness
Severe illness of any kind may cause hypogonadotropic hypogonadism (🕮 see Box 54.2).

Obstructive sleep apnea may present with low normal testosterone levels and erectile dysfunction together with metabolic syndrome.

Drugs
Anabolic steroids, cocaine, and narcotic drugs may all result in secondary hypogonadism.

All drugs causing hyperprolactinemia (🕮 see Box 16.1, p. 105) will also cause hypogonadism.

Prader–Willi syndrome
This is a congenital syndrome affecting 1:25000 births caused by loss of an imprinted gene on paternally derived chromosome 15q11–13.

It should be suspected in infancy in the presence of characteristic facial features (almond eyes, down-turned mouth, strabismus, thin upper lip), severe hypotonia, poor feeding, and developmental delay. The child then develops hyperphagia due to hypothalamic dysfunction, resulting

---

Box 54.2 Systemic illness resulting in hypogonadism

- Any acute illness (e.g., myocardial infarction, sepsis, head injury)
- Severe stress
- Hemochromatosis
- Endocrine disease (Cushing's syndrome, hyperprolactinemia)
- Liver cirrhosis
- Chronic renal failure
- Chronic anemia (thalassemia major, sickle cell disease)
- GI disease (celiac disease, Crohn's disease)
- AIDS
- Rheumatological disease (rheumatoid arthritis)
- Respiratory disease (e.g., chronic obstructive airways disease, cystic fibrosis)
- Cardiac disease (e.g., congestive cardiac failure)

in severe obesity. Other characteristic features include short stature, hypogonadotropic hypogonadism, and learning disability.

Diabetes mellitus type II occurs in 15–40% of adults.

Laurence–Moon–Biedl syndrome

This congenital syndrome is characterized by severe obesity, gonadotropin deficiency, retinal dystrophy, polydactyly, and learning disability.

Primary hypogonadism (hypergonadotropic hypogonadism)

This condition is due to testicular failure with normal hypothalamus and pituitary function.

Diagnosis

- Low serum testosterone
- Elevated LH and FSH (low inhibin B and anti-Müllerian hormone)

Causes

Genetic: Klinefelter's syndrome

This is the most common congenital form of primary hypogonadism. It is thought that a significant number of men with Klinefelter's syndrome are not diagnosed. Clinical manifestations will depend on the age of diagnosis. Patients with mosaicism tend to have less severe clinical features.

Adolescence

- Small firm testes (mean 5 mL)
- Gynecomastia
- Tall stature ($\uparrow$ leg length)
- Other features of hypogonadism
- Cognitive dysfunction

Adulthood

- Reduced libido and erectile dysfunction
- Gynecomastia
- Reduced facial hair
- Obesity
- Infertility

Risks

- Type 2 diabetes mellitus
- Osteoporosis
- Thromboembolism
- Malignancies e.g., extragonadal germ cell tumors

Diagnosis

- Karyotyping: 47,XXY in 80%; higher-grade chromosomal aneuploidies (e.g., 48,XXXY) or 46,XY/47,XXY mosaicism in the remainder
- Low testosterone, elevated FSH and LH
- Elevated SHBG and estradiol
- Azoospermia

Management

- Lifelong androgen replacement
- May need surgical reduction of gynecomastia

- Fertility: Intracytoplasmic sperm injection (ICSI, 📖 see Chapter 59, Infertility, pp. 316–331) using testicular spermatozoa from men with Klinefelter's syndrome has resulted in successful pregnancies. However, couples should be counseled about the ↑ risk of chromosomal abnormalities in offspring.

Genetic: Other chromosomal disorders

XX males
- Due to an X to Y translocation with only a part of the Y present in one of the X chromosomes
- Incidence is 1:10,000 births
- Similar clinical and biochemical features to Klinefelter's syndrome. In addition, short stature and hypospadias may be present.

XX/X0 (mixed gonadal dysgenesis)
- Occasionally, phenotypically men with hypospadias and intra-abdominal dysgenetic gonads
- Bilateral gonadectomy is essential because of the risk of neoplasia, followed by androgen replacement therapy.

XYY syndrome
- Taller than average, but often have primary gonadal failure with impaired spermatogenesis

Y chromosome microdeletions:
- Causes oligo- and azoospermia. Testosterone levels are not usually affected.

Noonan's syndrome
- Autosomal dominant disorder with an incidence of 1:1000 to 1:2500 live births
- 46,XY karyotype and secondary external genitalia. However, several stigmata of Turner's syndrome (short stature, webbed neck, ptosis, low-set ears, lymphedema) and ↑ risk cardiac anomalies (valvular pulmonary stenosis and hypertrophic cardiomyopathy). Most have cryptorchidism and primary testicular failure.

Cryptorchidism
- 10% of secondary neonates have undescended testes, but most of these will descend into the scrotum eventually, so that the incidence of postpubertal cryptorchidism is < 0.5%.
- 15% of cases have bilateral cryptorchidism.

Consequences
- 75% of males with bilateral cryptorchidism are infertile.
- 10% risk of testicular malignancy, highest risk in those with intra-abdominal testes
- Low testosterone and raised gonadotropins in bilateral cryptorchidism

Treatment
- *Orchidopexy*: best performed before 18 months, certainly before age 5 years, to reduce risk of later infertility
- *Gonadectomy*: in patients with intra-abdominal testes, followed by androgen replacement.

Orchitis
- 25% of males who develop mumps after puberty have associated orchitis and 25–50% of these will develop primary testicular failure.
- HIV infection may also be associated with orchitis.
- Primary testicular failure may occur as part of an autoimmune disease.

Chemotherapy and radiotherapy
Cytotoxic drugs, particularly alkylating agents, are gonadotoxic. Infertility occurs in 50% of patients following chemotherapy for most malignancies, and a significant number of males require androgen replacement therapy because of low testosterone levels.

The testes are radiosensitive, so hypogonadism can occur from scattered radiation during the treatment of Hodgkin's disease, for example.

If fertility is desired, sperm should be cryopreserved prior to cancer therapy.

Other drugs
Sulfasalazine, colchicine, and high-dose glucocorticoids may reversibly affect testicular function.

Alcohol excess will also cause primary testicular failure.

Chronic illness
Any chronic illness may affect testicular function, in particular chronic renal failure, liver cirrhosis, and hemochromatosis.

Testicular trauma
Testicular torsion is another common cause of loss of a testis, and it may also affect the function of the remaining testis.

Box 54.3 Testicular dysfunction—clinical characteristics of male hypogonadism

Testicular failure occurring before onset of puberty
- Testicular volume <5 mL
- Penis <5 cm long
- Lack of scrotal pigmentation and rugae
- Gynecomastia
- High-pitched voice
- Central fat distribution
- Eunuchoidism
- Arm span 1 cm greater than height
- Lower segment > upper segment
- Delayed bone age
- No male escutcheon
- ↓ Body and facial hair

Testicular failure occurring after puberty
- Testes soft, volume <15 mL.
- Normal penile length
- Normal skeletal proportions
- Gynecomastia
- Normal male hair distribution but reduced amount
- Pale skin, fine wrinkles
- Central fat distribution
- Osteoporosis
- Anemia (mild)

Clinical assessment

History

- *Developmental history*: congenital urinary tract abnormalities, e.g., hypospadias, late testicular descent, or cryptorchidism
- Delayed or incomplete puberty
- Infections, e.g., mumps, orchitis
- Abdominal or genital trauma
- Testicular torsion
- Anosmia
- *Drug history*: e.g., sulfasalazine, antihypertensives, chemotherapy, cimetidine, radiotherapy; alcohol and recreational drugs also important
- *General medical history*: chronic illness, particularly respiratory, neurological, and cardiac
- *Gynecomastia*: common (□ see Chapter 56, Gynecomastia, pp. 301) during adolescence. If recent-onset gynecomastia in adulthood, must rule out estrogen-producing tumor
- *Family history*: Young syndrome (□ p. 321), cystic fibrosis, Kallmann's syndrome
- *Sexual history*: erectile function, frequency of intercourse, sexual techniques. Absence of morning erections suggests an organic cause of erectile dysfunction.

Physical examination

- Body hair distribution
- Muscle mass and fat distribution
- Eunuchoidism
- Gynecomastia

Genital examination

- Pubic hair normal male escutcheon
- Phallus normal >5 cm length and >3 cm width
- Testes size (using Prader orchiometer) and consistency (normal >15 m and firm)
- Look for nodules or areas of tenderness.
- Look for evidence of systemic disease.
- Assess sense of smell and visual fields
  - Reflexes
  - Peripheral pulses
  - Rectal examination

Hormonal evaluation of testicular function

Serum testosterone

There is diurnal variation in circulating testosterone, with peak levels occurring in the early morning. A 30% variation occurs between the highest and lowest testosterone levels, so morning plasma testosterone is useful. If the level is low, this should be repeated.

Sex hormone binding globulin (SHBG)

Only 2–4% of circulating testosterone is unbound; 50% is bound to SHBG and the rest to albumin.

Concentrations of SHBG should be taken into account when interpreting a serum testosterone result. SHBG levels may be affected by a variety of conditions (📖 see Table 54.1).

Gonadotropins

Raised FSH and LH levels occur in primary testicular failure and are inappropriately low in pituitary or hypothalamic hypogonadism. One should always exclude hyperprolactinemia in secondary hypogonadism.

Estradiol

Estradiol results from the conversion of testosterone and androstenedione by aromatase. 📖 See Table 54.2 for causes of elevated estradiol. Request serum estradiol level if gynecomastia is present or a testicular tumor is suspected.

Table 54.1 Factors affecting SHBG concentrations

Raised SHBG	Low SHBG
Androgen deficiency	Hyperinsulinemia
GH deficiency	Obesity
Aging	Acromegaly
Thyrotoxicosis	Androgen treatment
Estrogens	HypothyroidismLiver
Liver cirrhosis	Cushing's syndrome/glucocorticoid therapy
	Nephrotic syndrome

Table 54.2 Causes of raised estogens in men

Neoplasia
• Testicular
• Adrenal
• Hepatoma
Primary testicular failure
Liver disease
Thyrotoxicosis
Obesity
Androgen resistance syndromes
Antiandrogen therapy

Inhibin B and AMH
Gonadal glycoproteins secrete into the circulation. These are useful markers of normal testicular functions. They are low if there is primary testicular failure and normal with pituitary or hypothalamic dysfunction.

Other investigations
- Scrotal US (testicular volume/blood flow with Doppler/presence of hydrocele, etc.)
- Semen analysis (A normal semen analysis is indicative of gonadal health. Men with low sperm count should consider sperm cryopreservation to preserve fertility.)

Dynamic tests
These are of limited clinical value and are rarely performed routinely.

hCG stimulation test
- Diagnostic test for examining Leydig cell function
- hCG 2000 IU IM given on days 0 and 2; testosterone measured on days 0, 2, and 4
- In prepubertal boys with absent scrotal testes, a response to hCG indicates intra-abdominal testes. Failure of testosterone to rise after hCG suggests absence of functioning testicular tissue. An exaggerated response to hCG is seen in secondary hypogonadism.

Clomifene stimulation test
- Used to assess integrity of the hypothalamic–pituitary testicular axis
- Normal response to 3 mg/kg (max 200mg) clomifene daily for 7 days is a 2-fold increase in LH and FSH measured on days 0, 4, 7, and 10.
- A subnormal response indicates hypothalamic or pituitary hypogonadism but does not differentiate between the two.

Further reading

AACE Hypogonadism Task Force. (2002). American Association of Clinical Endocrinologists Medical Guidelines for clinical practice for the evaluation and treatment of hypogonadism in adult male patients–2002 update. *Endocr Pract* 8(6):439–456.

Lanfranco F, Kamischke A, Zitzmann M, et al. (2004). Klinefelter's syndrome. *Lancet* 364:273–283.

AQ: We couldn't locate this content in the text. Please advise.

Androgen therapy

Treatment goals

• *Improve libido and sexual function*
Testosterone therapy will induce virilization in the hypogonadal males and restores libido and erectile function.

• *Improve mood and well-being*
Most studies show an improvement in mood, well-being, and QoL following physiologic testosterone therapy.

• *Improve muscle mass and strength*
Testosterone has direct anabolic effects on skeletal muscle and has been shown to increase muscle mass and strength when given to hypogonadal men. Lean body mass is also ↑ with a reduction in fat mass.

• *Prevent osteoporosis*
Hypogonadism is a risk factor for osteoporosis. Testosterone inhibits bone resorption, thereby reducing bone turnover. Its administration to hypogonadal men has been shown to improve bone mineral density and reduce risk of developing osteoporosis. Few fracture data are available.

• *Fertility*
Fertility is inhibited by testosterone therapy. Men with secondary hypogonadism who desire fertility may be treated with gonadotropins to initiate and maintain spermatogenesis (📖 see p. 296). Prior testosterone therapy will not affect fertility prospects but should be stopped before initiating gonadotropin treatment.

Men with primary hypogonadism will not respond to gonadotropin or GnRH therapy.

Indications for treatment

- Men with established primary or secondary hypogonadism of any cause
- 📖 See Box 55.1 for contraindications.

Pretreatment evaluation

Clinical evaluation

History or symptoms of the following:

- Prostatic hypertrophy
- Breast or prostate cancer
- Cardiovascular disease
- Sleep apnea

Examination

- Rectal examination of prostate
- Breasts

Laboratory evaluation

- Prostatic specific antigen (PSA) (PSA is often low in hypogonadal men, rising to normal age-matched levels with androgen replacement)
- Hemoglobin and hematocrit
- Serum lipids

Box 55.1 Contraindications to androgen replacement therapy

Absolute

- Prostate cancer
- Breast cancer

Relative

- Benign prostate hyperplasia
- Polycythemia
- Sleep apnea

Box 55.2 Monitoring of therapy

Monitor 3 months after initiating therapy and then every 6–12 months:

- Clinical evaluation—relief of symptoms of androgen deficiency and exclude side effects
- Serum testosterone
- Rectal examination of the prostate (if >45 years)
- PSA (if >45 years)
- Hemoglobin and hematocrit
- Serum lipids

Risks and side effects

Prostatic disease

Androgens stimulate prostatic growth, and testosterone replacement therapy may therefore induce symptoms of bladder outflow obstruction in men with prostatic hypertrophy.

It is unlikely that testosterone increases the risk of developing prostate cancer, but it may promote the growth of an existing cancer.

Polycythemia

Testosterone stimulates erythropoiesis. Androgen replacement therapy may increase hemoglobin levels, particularly in older men. It may be necessary to reduce the dose of testosterone in men with clinically significant polycythemia.

Cardiovascular disease

Testosterone replacement therapy may cause a fall in both LDL and HDL cholesterol levels, the significance of which remains unclear. The effect of androgen replacement therapy on the risk of developing coronary heart disease is unknown.

Other (see Table 55.1)

- Acne
- Gynecomastia is occasionally enhanced by testosterone therapy, particularly in peripubertal boys. This is the result of the conversion of testosterone to estrogens.
- Fluid retention may result in worsening symptoms in those with underlying congestive cardiac failure or hepatic cirrhosis.
- Obstructive sleep apnea may be exacerbated by testosterone therapy.
- Hepatotoxicity may be induced by oral androgens, particularly the 17α alkylated testosterones.
- Mood swings

Table 55.1 Testosterone preparations

Preparation	Dose	Advantage	Problems
IM testosterone esters	250 mg every 2–3 weeks Monitor predose serum testosterone (should be above the lower limit of normal)	2- to 3-week dosage Effective and cheap	Painful IM injection Contraindicated in bleeding disorders Wide variations in serum testosterone levels between injections that may be associated with symptoms.
'Nebido'®	1 g q3 months (after loading dose)	Convenience of infrequent injection	
Testosterone implants	100–600 mg every 3–6 months Monitor predose serum testosterone	Physiological testosterone levels achieved. 3- to 6-month dosing	Minor surgical procedure. Risk of infection and pellet extrusion (3–10%). Must remove pellet surgically if complications of androgen replacement therapy develop.
Transdermal gel (1%)	5–10 g gel daily	Physiological testosterone levels achieved. Convenience	Skin reactions (rare). Possible person-to-person transfer through direct skin contact
Transdermal patch	2.5–7.5 mg daily	Physiological testosterone levels achieved.	Skin reactions are common.
Oral, e.g., testosterone undecanoate and mesterolone	40 mg tid 25 mg tid	Oral preparations	Highly variable efficacy and bioavailability. Rarely achieves therapeutic efficacy. Multiple daily dosing. 17A alkylated testosterones are not used because of risk of hepatotoxicity.
Buccal testosterone	30 mg bid	Physiological testosterone levels achieved	Local discomfort. Gingivitis. Bitter taste Twice-daily dosing

Further reading

Handelsman DJ, Zajac JD (2004). Androgen deficiency and replacement therapy in men. *Med J Aust* 180:529–535.

Nieschlag E, Behre HM, Bouchard P, et al. (2004). Testosterone replacement therapy: current trends and future directions. *Hum Reprod Update* 10(5):409–419.

Rhoden EL, Morgentaler A (2004). Risks of testosterone replacement therapy and recommendations for monitoring. *N Engl J Med* 350:482–492.

Gynecomastia

Definition

Gynecomastia is enlargement of the male breast as a result of hyperplasia of the glandular tissue to a diameter of >2 cm. 📖 See Fig 56.1.

This condition is common, present in up to 1/3 of males <30 years and in up to 50% of men >45 years. 📖 See Box 56.1 for causes.

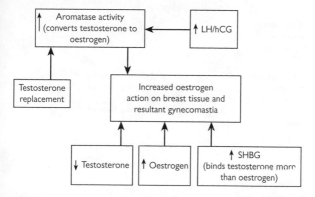

Fig. 56.1 Hormonal influences on gynecomastia

Box 56.1 Causes of gynecomastia

Physiological
- Neonatal
- Puberty: ~50% of boys develop transient gynecomastia
- Idiopathic: ~25% of all cases

Drugs
Possible mechanisms include estrogen-containing agents, androgen receptor blockers, and inhibition of androgen production:
- Estrogens, antiandrogens, testosterone
- Spironolactone, ACE inhibitors, calcium antagonists, digoxin
- Alkylating agents
- Alcohol, marijuana, heroin, methadone
- Cimetidine
- Ketoconazole, metronidazole, antituberculous agents, tricyclic antidepressants, dopamine antagonists, opiates, benzodiazepines
- Antiretroviral drugs
- Imatinib (chronic myeloid leukemia)

Hypogonadism
- Primary
- Secondary

Tumors
- Estrogen or androgen-producing testicular or adrenal tumors
- Human chorionic gonadotropin-producing tumors, usually testicular, e.g., germinoma; occasionally ectopic, e.g., lung
- Aromatase-producing testicular or hepatic tumors

Endocrine
- Thyrotoxicosis
- Cushing's syndrome
- Acromegaly
- Androgen-insensitivity syndromes

Systemic illness
- Liver cirrhosis
- Chronic renal failure
- HIV infection
- Malnutrition

Evaluation

History

- Duration and progression of gynecomastia
- Further investigation is warranted if there is the following:
  - Rapidly enlarging gynecomastia
  - Recent-onset gynecomastia in a lean postpubertal male.
  - Painful gynecomastia
- Exclude underlying tumor, e.g., testicular cancer
- Symptoms of hypogonadism: reduced libido, erectile dysfunction
- Symptoms of systemic disease, e.g., hepatic, renal, endocrine disease
- Drug history, including recreational drugs, e.g., alcohol

Physical examination

Breasts

- Pinch breast tissue between the thumb and forefinger—distinguish it from fat.
- Measure glandular tissue diameter; gynecomastia if >2 cm
- If diameter is >5 cm, hard, or irregular, investigate further to exclude breast cancer.
- Look for galactorrhea.

Testicular palpation

- Exclude tumor
- Assess testicular size—?atrophy

Other

- Secondary sex characteristics
- Look for evidence of systemic disease, e.g., chronic liver or renal disease, thyrotoxicosis, Cushing's syndrome, or chronic cardiac or pulmonary disease.

Investigations (see Fig. 56.2)

Baseline investigations

- Serum testosterone
- Serum estradiol
- LH and FSH
- Prolactin
- SHBG
- hCG
- Liver function tests

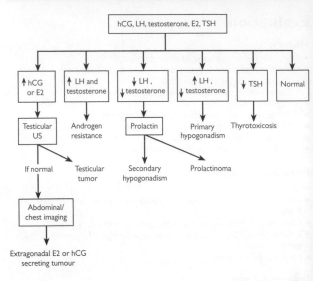

Fig. 56.2 Investigation of gynecomastia .

Additional investigations
- If testicular tumor is suspected, e.g., elevated estradiol/hCG: testicular US
- If adrenal tumor is suspected, e.g., markedly raised estradiol: dehydroepiandrosterone sulfate (DHEAS); abdominal CT or MRI scan
- If breast malignancy is suspected: mammography; FNAC/tissue biopsy
- If lung cancer is suspected, e.g., raised hCG: chest radiograph
- Other investigations depending on clinical suspicion, e.g., renal or thyroid function

Management

Treat underlying disorder when present. Withdraw offending drugs where possible.

Reassurance is adequate treatment in the majority of idiopathic cases. The condition often resolves spontaneously.

Treatment may be required for cosmetic reasons or to alleviate pain and tenderness.

Drug treatment is only partially effective. It may be of benefit in treating gynecomastia of recent onset.

Medical

📖 See Table 56.1.

Surgical

Reduction mammoplasty may be required in males with severe and persistent gynecomastia.

Table 56.1 Medical treatment of gynecomastia

Tamoxifen (10–30 mg/day)	Antiestrogenic effects. Particularly effective in reducing pain and swelling if used in gynecomastia of recent onset. A 3-month trial before referral for surgery may be of benefit.
Clomifene (50–100 mg/day)	Antiestrogenic. May be effective in reducing breast size in pubertal gynecomastia
Danazol (300–600 mg/day)	Nonaromatizable androgen. May also reduce breast size in adults. Its use is limited by side effects, particularly weight gain and acne.
Testolactone (450 mg/day)	Aromatase inhibitor. May be effective in reducing pubertal gynecomastia. However, tamoxifen appears to be more effective and better tolerated.
Anastrozole (1 mg/day)	Another aromatase inhibitor. Clinical trials have failed to show a beneficial effect on gynecomastia compared with placebo.

Further reading

Khan HN, Blarney RW (2003). Endocrine treatment of physiological gynaecomastia. *BMJ* 327:301–302.

Erectile dysfunction

Definition

Erectile dysfunction (ED) is the consistent inability to achieve or maintain an erect penis sufficient for satisfactory sexual intercourse. ED affects approximately 10% of men and >50% of men >70 years.

Physiology of male sexual function

The erectile response is the result of the coordinated interaction of nerves, smooth muscle of the corpora cavernosa, pelvic muscles, and blood vessels. It is initiated by psychogenic stimuli from the brain or physical stimulation of the genitalia, which are modulated in the limbic system, transmitted down the spinal cord to the sympathetic and parasympathetic outflows of the penile tissue.

Penile erectile tissue consists of paired corpora cavernosa on the dorsum of the penis and the corpus spongiosum. These are surrounded by fibrous tissue known as the tunica albuginea.

In the flaccid state, the corporeal smooth muscle is contracted, minimizing corporeal blood flow and enhancing venous drainage.

Activation of the erectile pathway results in penile smooth muscle relaxation and cavernosal arterial vasodilatation. As the corporeal sinuses fill with blood, the draining venules are compressed against the tunica albuginea so venous outflow is impaired. This results in penile rigidity and an erection.

Corporeal vasodilatation is mediated by parasympathetic neuronal activation, which induces nitric oxide release by the cavernosal nerves. This activates guanyl cyclase, thereby ↑ cGMP, and causing smooth muscle relaxation.

Detumescence occurs after the inactivation of cGMP by the enzyme phosphodiesterase, resulting in smooth muscle contraction and vasoconstriction.

Ejaculation is mediated by the sympathetic nervous system.

Pathophysiology

Erectile dysfunction may occur as a result of several mechanisms:
- Neurological damage
- Arterial insufficiency
- Venous incompetence
- Androgen deficiency
- Penile abnormalities
- Iatrogenic: medications or supplements
- Psychogenic

Evaluation

History

Sexual history
- Extent of the dysfunction, its duration, and progression
- Presence of nocturnal or morning erections
- Abrupt onset of erectile dysfunction that is intermittent is often psychogenic in origin.
- Progressive and persistent dysfunction indicates an organic cause.

Symptoms of hypogonadism
- Reduced libido, muscle strength, and sense of well-being.

Full medical history
- E.g., diabetes mellitus, liver cirrhosis, or neurological, cardiovascular, or endocrine disease
- Intermittent claudication suggests a vascular cause.
- A history of genitourinary trauma or surgery is also important.
- Recent change in bladder or bowel function may indicate neurological cause.
- Psychological history

Drug history
- Onset of impotence in relation to commencing a new medication

Social history
- Stress
- Relationship history
- Smoking history
- Recreational drugs, including alcohol

Physical examination
- Evidence of primary or secondary hypogonadism
- Evidence of endocrine disorders:
  - Hyperprolactinemia, thyroid dysfunction, hypopituitarism.
  - Other complications of diabetes mellitus, if present
- Evidence of neurological disease
  - Autonomic or peripheral neuropathy
  - Spinal cord lesions
- Evidence of systemic disease, e.g.:
  - Chronic liver disease
  - Chronic cardiac disease
  - Peripheral vascular disease

Genital examination
- Assess testicular size—?atrophy
- Penile abnormalities, e.g., Peyronie's disease

📖 See Box 57.1 for causes of erectile dysfunction.

Box 57.1 Causes of erectile dysfunction

Psychological (20%)
- Stress, anxiety
- Psychiatric illness

Drugs (25%)
- Alcohol
- Antihypertensives, e.g., diuretics, β-blockers, methyldopa
- Cimetidine
- Marijuana, heroin, methadone
- Major tranquillizers
- Tricyclic antidepressants, benzodiazepines
- Digoxin
- Glucocorticoids, anabolic steroids
- Estrogens, antiandrogens

Endocrine (20%)
- Hypogonadism (primary or secondary)
- Hyperprolactinemia
- Diabetes mellitus (30–50% of men with DM >6 years)
- Thyroid dysfunction
- Obstructive sleep apnea

Neurological
- Spinal cord disorders
- Peripheral and autonomic neuropathies
- Multiple sclerosis

Vascular
- Peripheral vascular disease
- Trauma
- Diabetes mellitus
- Venous incompetence

Other
- Hemochromatosis
- Debilitating diseases
- Penile abnormalities, e.g., priapism, Peyronie's disease
- Prostatectomy

Investigation of erectile dysfunction

Baseline investigations
- Serum testosterone
- Prolactin, LH, and FSH if serum testosterone is low
- Fasting blood glucose
- Thyroid function tests

- Liver function tests
- Renal function
- Serum lipids
- Serum ferritin (hemachromatosis)

Additional investigations

Evaluate for obstructive sleep apnea

This is rarely required. To assess vascular causes of impotence if corrective surgery is contemplated:

- Intracavernosal injection of a vasodilator, e.g., alprostadil E1 or papaverine. A sustained erection excludes significant vascular insufficiency.
- Penile Doppler ultrasonography: Cavernous arterial flow and venous insufficiency are assessed.

Management

Treat underlying disorder or withdraw offending drugs where possible.

Androgens

This should be first-line therapy in males with hypogonadism (📖 see p. 296). Hyperprolactinemia, when present, should be treated with dopamine agonists and the underlying cause of hypogonadism treated.

Phosphodiesterase (PDE) inhibitors

📖 See Table 57.1 and Box 57.2.

These act by enhancing cGMP activity in erectile tissue by blocking the enzyme PDE-5, thereby amplifying the vasodilatory action of nitric oxide and thus the normal erectile response to sexual stimulation.

Trials indicate a 50–80% success rate.

Alprostadil

Alprostadil results in smooth muscle relaxation and vasodilatation. It is administered intraurethrally and is then absorbed into the erectile bodies.
- 60–66% success rate
- *Side effects:* local pain

Intracavernous injection

This has a 70–100% success rate and is highest in men with non-vasculogenic impotence.

Alprostadil is a potent vasodilator. The dose should be titrated in 1 mcg increments until the desired effect is achieved to minimize side effects.

Papaverine, a PDE inhibitor, induces cavernosal vasodilatation and penile rigidity but causes more side effects.

Side effects
- Priapism in 1–5%. Patients must seek urgent medical advice if an erection lasts >4 hours.

Table 57.1 PDE-5 inhibitors

	Sildenafil	Vardenafil	Tadalafil
Dose (mg/day)	50–100	10–20	10–20
Recommended interval between drug administration and sexual activity	60min	30–60min	>30min
Half life (hours)	3–4	4–5	17
Adverse effects (%)			
Headaches	15–30	7–15	7–20
Facial flushing	10–25	10	1–5
Dyspepsia	2–15	0.5–6	1–15
Nasal congestion	1–10	3–7	4–6
Visual disturbance	1–10	0–2	0.1

Box 57.2 PDE-5 inhibitors—contraindications and cautions

Contraindications
- Recent myocardial infarction or stroke
- Unstable angina
- Current nitrate use, including isosorbide mononitrate/GTN
- Hypotension (<90/50 mmHg)
- Severe heart failure
- Severe hepatic impairment
- Retinitis pigmentosa
- Ketoconazole or HIV protease inhibitors

Cautions (reduce dose)
- Hypertension
- Heart disease
- Peyronies disease
- Sickle cell anemia
- Renal or hepatic impairment
- Elderly
- Leukemia
- Multiple myeloma
- Bleeding disorders e.g., active peptic ulcer disease

Avoid concomitant opiates as they may result in prolonged erections.

- Fibrosis in the injection site in up to 5% of patients. Minimize risk by alternating sides of the penis for injection and injecting a maximum of twice a week.
- Infection at injection site is rare.

Contraindication
- Sickle cell disease

Injection technique
Avoid the midline so as to avoid urethral and neurovascular damage. Clean the injection site, hold the penis under slight tension, and introduce the needle at 90°. Inject after the characteristic "give" of piercing the fibrous capsule. Apply pressure to injection site after removing the needle to prevent bruising.

Vacuum device

Results are good, with 90% of men achieving a satisfactory erection. The flaccid penis is put into the device and air is withdrawn, creating a vacuum that then allows blood to flow into the penis.

A constriction band is then placed on to the base of the penis so that the erection is maintained. This should be removed within 30 minutes.
- *Side effects:* pain, hematoma

Penile prosthesis

This is usually tried in men either reluctant to try other forms of therapy or when other treatments have failed. The prosthesis may be semi-rigid or inflatable.

* *Complications:* infection, mechanical failure

Psychosexual counseling

Consider counseling particularly for men with psychogenic impotence and in men who fail to improve with the above therapies.

Surgical

Surgery is rarely indicated, as results are generally disappointing. Revascularization techniques may be available in some centers.

Ligation of dorsal veins may restore erectile function temporarily in men with venous insufficiency, although rarely permanently.

Further reading

Beckman TJ, Abu-Lebdeh HS, Mynderse LA (2006). Evaluation and medical management of erectile dysfunction. *Mayo Clin Proc* 81:385–390.

Cohan P, Korenman SG (2001). Erectile dysfunction. *J Clin Endocrinol Metab* 86:2391–2394.

Fazio L, Brick G (2004). Erectile dysfunction: management update. *CMAJ* 170(9):1429–1437.

Testicular tumors

Epidemiology

- 6/100 000 men per year
- Incidence is rising, particularly in northwest Europe.

📖 See Table 58.1 for classification.

Risk factors

- Cryptorchidism.
- Gonadal dysgenesis.
- Infertility or reduced spermatogenesis

Table 58.1 Classification of testicular tumors

Tumors		Tumor markers
Germ cell tumors (95%)	Seminoma	None
	Non-seminoma	hCG,
	Mixed	α-fetoprotein, CEA
Stromal tumors (2%)	Leydig cell	
	Sertoli cell	
Gonadoblastoma (2%)		
Other (1%)	Lymphoma	
	Carcinoid	

Prognosis

Seminomas
- 95% cure for early disease. 80% cure for stages II/IV
- ↑ Incidence of second tumors and leukemias 20 years after therapy

Non-seminoma germ cell tumors
- 90% cure in early disease, falling to 60% in metastatic disease
- ↑ Incidence of second tumors and leukemias 20 years after therapy

Stromal tumors
- Excellent prognosis for benign tumors
- Malignant tumors are aggressive and are poorly responsive to treatment.

Further reading
Griffin JE, Wilson JD (1998). Disorders of the testes and male reproductive tract. In Wilson JD, Foster DW, Kronenberg HM, Larson PR (eds.), *William's Textbook of Endocrinology*, 9th ed, Philadelphia: WB Saunders, pp. 819–876.

Infertility

Definition

Infertility, defined as failure of pregnancy after 2 years of unprotected regular (2× week) sexual intercourse, affects approximately 10% of all couples.

Couples who fail to conceive after 1 year of regular unprotected sexual intercourse should be investigated.

If there is a known predisposing factor or the female partner is over 35 years of age, then investigation should be offered earlier.

Causes

📖 See Boxes 59.1 and 59.2.
- Female factors (e.g., PCOS, tubal damage) (35%)
- Male factors (idiopathic gonadal failure in 60%) (25%)
- Combined factors (25%)
- Unexplained infertility (15%)

Box 59.1 Causes of female infertility

Anovulation
- PCOS (80% of anovulatory disorders)
- Secondary hypogonadism
- Hyperprolactinemia
- Thyroid dysfunction
- Hypothalamic disease
- Pituitary disease
- Systemic illness
- Drugs, e.g., anabolic steroids
- POF (5% of anovulatory disorders)

Tubal disorders
- Infective, e.g., *Chlamydia*
- Endometriosis
- Surgery

Cervical mucus defects

Uterine abnormalities
- Congenital
- Intrauterine adhesions
- Uterine fibroids

Box 59.2 Causes of male infertility

Primary gonadal failure
- Genetic, e.g., Klinefelter's syndrome, Y-chromosome microdeletions, immotile cilia/Kartagener syndrome, cystic fibrosis
- Congenital cryptorchidism
- Orchitis
- Torsion or trauma
- Chemotherapy and radiotherapy
- Other toxins, e.g., alcohol, anabolic steroids
- Varicocele
- Idiopathic

Secondary gonadal failure
- Kallman's syndrome (☐ see Secondary hypogonadism, p. 285)
- IHH
- Structural hypothalamic or pituitary disease

Genital tract abnormalities
- Obstructive congenital, infective, postsurgical
- Sperm autoimmunity

Other
- Erectile dysfunction
- Drugs, e.g., spironolactone, corticosteroids, sulfasalazine
- Systemic disease, e.g., cystic fibrosis, Crohn's disease, and other chronic debilitating diseases

Evaluation

Sexual history

- *Frequency of intercourse:* sexual intercourse every 2–3 days should be encouraged.
- *Use of lubricants* should be avoided because of the detrimental effect on semen quality.

Female factors

History

- Age: Fertility declines rapidly after the age of 36 years.

Menstrual history

- Age at menarche
- Length of menstrual cycle and its regularity (e.g., oligo- or amenorrhea)
- Presence or absence of intermenstrual spotting

Other

- Hot flashes may be indicative of estrogen deficiency.
- Spontaneous galactorrhea may be caused by hyperprolactinemia.
- Hypothalamic hypogonadism is suggested by excessive physical exercise (e.g., running >4 miles/day) or weight loss in excess of 10% in 1 year.

Drug history

- Drugs that may cause hyperprolactinemia (□ see Box 16.1, p. 106), including cocaine and marijuana
- Smoking is thought have an adverse effect on fertility.
- The use of anabolic steroids may cause secondary hypogonadism.
- Cytotoxic chemotherapy or radiotherapy may cause ovarian failure.

Medical history

- Diabetes mellitus, thyroid or pituitary dysfunction, and other systemic illnesses

Exclude tubal disease

- Recurrent vaginal or urinary tract infections may predispose to pelvic inflammatory disease (PID).
- Dyspareunia and dysmenorrhea are often present.
- Sexually transmitted disease and previous abdominal or gynecological surgery all predispose to fallopian tube obstruction.

Secondary infertility

- Details of previous pregnancies, including abortions (spontaneous and therapeutic) and ectopic pregnancies, should be ascertained.

Family history

- Suggestive of risk of POI, PCOS, endometriosis

Physical examination

- *BMI:* The ideal BMI for fertility is 20–29.

- *Secondary sexual characteristics:* If absent, look for evidence of Turner's syndrome.
- *Hyperandrogenism:* PCOS
- *Galactorrhea:* hyperprolactinemia
- External genitalia and pelvic examination

Investigations
📖 See Fig. 59.1.

Assess ovulatory function
- In women with regular menstrual cycles, measure midluteal progesterone (day 21 or approximately 7 days before expected onset of menses).
- Check serum FSH and LH. In women who are not amenorrheic this should be measured on days 2–6 of the menstrual cycle (day 1 = first day of menses). Follicular phase FSH >10 is indicative of reduced ovarian reserve. Ovarian failure is diagnosed if FSH is >30.
- Measure TSH, free T$_4$, and serum prolactin in women with irregular menstrual cycles or who are not ovulating.

Other investigations
- *Karyotype:* if primary ovarian failure is present (raised FSH, LH)
- *Serum testosterone, androstenedione, DHEA, sex hormone binding globulin, and 17OH progesterone:* if there is clinical evidence of hyperandrogenism, in the presence of irregular menstrual cycles, or if anovulation is confirmed

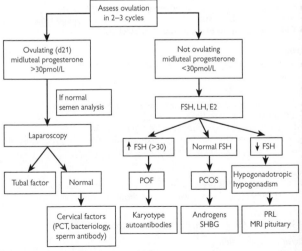

Fig. 59.1 Investigation of female infertility.

- *MRI of the pituitary fossa:* in hyperprolactinemia and hypogonadotropic hypogonadism
- *Exclude cervical infection:* Send vaginal discharge for bacteriology and do *Chlamydia trachomatis* serology
- *Pelvic US:* Assess uterine and ovarian anatomy.

Assess tubal patency (refer to specialist multidisciplinary fertility clinic)
- Hysterosalpingography (HSG) or laparoscopy and dye test (do in the early follicular phase of cycle to avoid doing during pregnancy)
- Give prophylactic antibiotics if *Chlamydia* status is unknown, to avoid postoperative infection.

Postcoital test
- To assess cervical mucus receptivity to sperm penetration and measurement of antisperm antibodies. These tests are rarely performed, as they are unreliable and the results do not alter management.

Male factors

History and physical examination
Symptoms of androgen deficiency
- Reduced libido and potency
- Reduced frequency of shaving
- May be asymptomatic

Drug history
- Drug or alcohol abuse and the use of anabolic steroids may all contribute to hypogonadism.
- Other drugs that may affect spermatogenesis, e.g., sulfasalazine, methotrexate
- Cytotoxic chemotherapy may cause primary testicular failure.

Other factors
- History of infection, e.g., mumps, orchitis, sexually transmitted disease, or epididymitis.
- Bronchiectasis may be associated with epididymal obstruction (Young syndrome) or severe asthenospermia (immotile cilia syndrome).
- Testicular injury or surgery may cause disordered spermatogenesis.
- Secondary sex characteristics may be absent in congenital hypogonadism.
- Anosmia: Kallmann's syndrome
- Eunuchoid habitus (📖 see Box 54.3, p. 293) suggestive of prepubertal hypogonadism
- Gynecomastia may suggest hypogonadism.

Testicular size (using orchidometer)
- Normal: 15–25 mL
- Reduced to <15 mL in hypogonadism
- In Klinefelter's syndrome, they are often <5 mL.
- In patients with normal testicular size, suspect genital tract obstruction, e.g., congenital absence of vas deferens.

Examine the rest of external genitalia, looking for penile and urethral abnormalities and epididymal thickening.

Investigations
📖 See Fig. 59.2.

Semen analysis
This is essential in the diagnostic workup of any infertile couple.
- If normal (📖 see Table 59.1), then a male cause is excluded.
- If abnormal, then repeat semen analysis approximately 6–12 weeks later.
- Semen collection should be performed after 3 days of sexual abstinence. 📖 See Table 59.1 for interpretation of results
- If azoospermia is present, rule out obstruction if FSH and testosterone concentrations are normal.
- Asthenospermia, or immotile sperm, is usually due to immunological infertility or infection, e.g., of the prostate (high semen viscosity and pH, and leukocytospermia).

FSH, LH, and testosterone levels
FSH may be elevated in the presence of normal LH and testosterone levels and oligospermia. This may be seen in men who are normally virilized but infertile as a result of disordered spermatogenesis.

Low FSH, LH, and testosterone concentrations suggest secondary hypogonadism. An MRI of the pituitary gland and hypothalamus is necessary to exclude organic disease.

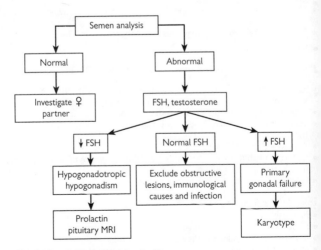

Fig. 59.2 Investigation of male infertility.

Table 59.1 WHO criteria for normal semen analysis*

Test	Normal values (fertile)	Nomenclature for abnormal values
Volume	>2 mL	Aspermia (no ejaculate)
pH	>7.2	
Total sperm number	>40 × 10⁶/ejaculate	Azoospermia (no sperm in ejaculate)
Sperm concentration	>48 × 10⁶/mL	Oligozoospermia
Motility	>63% progressive motilty	Asthenospermia
Morphology	>12% normal forms	Teratospermia
Live sperm	>75%	Necrospermia
Leucocytes	<1 × 10⁶/mL	Leucocytospermia

*Reprinted with permission from Guzick DS, Overstreet JW, Factor-Litvak P, et al. (2001). Sperm morphology, motility, and concentration in fertile and infertile men. *N Engl J Med* 345:1388–1393. Copyright 2001 Massachusetts Medical Society. All rights reserved.

Further investigations

- *Urinary bacteriology* should be performed in men with leukocytospermia.
- *Scrotal US* may help in the diagnosis of chronic epididymitis. Men being investigated for infertility are at ↑ risk of testicular tumors.
- *Karyotyping* may be helpful in men with primary testicular failure. Klinefelter's syndrome (47,XXY) is a cause of infertility, and deletions on the long arm of the Y chromosome have been found in a significant proportion of azoospermic men.
- *Sperm antibodies* in semen should not be measured routinely, as specific treatment is rarely effective.
- *Testicular biopsy* is rarely diagnostic but may be used to retrieve sperm for assisted reproduction techniques in specialist fertility centers.
- *Sperm function tests* are not performed routinely.

Management

Female partner

Anovulation

Hypogonadotropic (WHO class 1)
- If hyperprolactinemic, then dopamine agonists are usually effective
- Lifestyle changes if underweight or excessive exercise
- Otherwise, ovulation induction (📖 see Ovulation induction, p. 328)

Normogonadotropic (WHO class 2)
- Usually PCOS: weight reduction if obese
- Ovulation induction (📖 see Ovulation induction p. 328)

Hypergonadotropic (WHO class 3)
- POF ovum donation followed by IVF is the only option.
- Spontaneous transient remission is possible in early POF.
- If still cycling and FSH is 15–25 IU/L, ovarian hyperstimulation and IVF may be attempted, but with poor results.

Tubal infertility
Surgical tubal reconstruction may be attempted in specialist centers.

There is a 50–60% 2-year cumulative pregnancy rate in patients with mild disease, but only 10% in more severe disease and a high risk of ectopic pregnancy, so IVF may be more appropriate in women with severe disease.

Cumulative pregnancy rate is at least 50% following IVF (20–25% per cycle) unless hydrosalpinx is present. Women with hydrosalpinx should be offered salpingectomy prior to IVF to improve success rates.

Endometriosis

Minimal/mild
- GnRH agonists, danazol, and progestins do not improve fertility.
- Laparoscopic destruction of superficial disease improves pregnancy chances. Resection of ovarian endometriomas may improve ovarian folliculogenesis and thus fertility.
- Assisted reproductive techniques (ART) (Table 59.2) have a pregnancy rate of 25–35% per cycle.

Moderate/severe
- Surgery may improve fertility. However, ART is often necessary.

Vaginal and cervical factors
Each episode of acute PID causes infertility in 10–15% of cases.

Chlamydia trachomatis is responsible for half the cases of PID in the developed countries. Treat both partners with antibiotics.

Uterine factors
Intracavity fibroids, polyps, and uterine septum can be resected hysteroscopically with a high chance of restoring fertility.

Intramural fibroids may also reduce fertility and require myomectomy.
Fibroid embolization is not recommended for women wishing fertility, as safety in pregnancy is not established.

Male partner

Hypogonadotropic hypogonadism

- Gonadotropins: chorionic gonadotropin 1500–2000 IU IM 3×week. Most also require FSH/hMG 75–150 IU IM 3×week. Monitor serum testosterone and testicular size. The main side effect is gynecomastia.

or

- Pulsatile GnRH using an SC infusion pump (📖 see p. 331). Dose varies from 25 to 500 ng/kg every 90–120 minutes. Titrate to normalize LH, FSH, and testosterone. This will not work in pituitary disease.
  - Once testes are >8 mL, get semen analysis every 3–6 months. It takes at least 2 years to maximize spermatogenesis. Normalization of spermatogenesis occurs in 80–90% of men.
  - Once spermatogenesis is induced it may be maintained by hCG alone.

Idiopathic semen abnormalities

There is no evidence to suggest that the use of androgens, gonadotropins, or antiestrogens help improve fertility in men with idiopathic disorders of spermatogenesis.

Obstructive azoospermia

Reversal of vasectomy will result in successful pregnancy in up to 50% of cases within 2 years.

Microsurgery is possible for most other causes, with successful pregnancies in 25–35% of couples within 18 months of treatment. During surgery, sperm is often retrieved and stored for possible future intracytoplasmic sperm injection (ICSI).

Varicocele

There is a controversial association with male subfertility. Surgical correction is currently not recommended for fertility treatment as there is little evidence that surgery improves pregnancy rates.

Unexplained infertility

Definition

This is infertility despite normal sexual intercourse occurring at least twice weekly, normal semen analysis, documentation of ovulation in several cycles, and normal patent tubes (by laparoscopy).

Management

From 30 to 50% will become pregnant within 3 years of expectant management. If not pregnant by then, chances that spontaneous pregnancy will occur are greatly reduced and ART should be considered.

In women >34 years of age, expectant management is not an option and up to 6 cycles of intrauterine insemination (IUI), or IVF should be considered.

Table 59.2 Assisted reproduction techniques (ART)

Technique	Indications	Pregnancy rates	Notes
Intrauterine insemination (IUI) (usually offered up to 6 cycles)	Unexplained infertility mild oligozoospermia (>2 × 10 6 motile sperm)	<15% per cycle 15%.	Washed and prepared motile spermatozoa are injected into the uterine cavity through a catheter just before ovulation Superovulation may improve success rates but is associated with an increased risk of multiple pregnancy
In vitro fertilization (IVF)	Most forms of infertility unless severe male factor	20–30% pregnancy rate per cycle. 80–90% delivery rate after 6 cycles in women under the age of 35 years. Success rates markedly reduced after 40 years of age. Babies conceived by IVF have a 2× increased risk of low birth weight and preterm delivery.	After superovulation, ovarian follicles are aspirated under ultrasonic guidance and are fertilized with prepared sperm in vitro. The embryos are then transferred back into the uterine cavity, usually 48 hours after insemination. Luteal support using progesterone supplementation (pessaries or PO) is then provided until pregnancy is confirmed. May adopt a similar technique in women with premature ovarian failure using donated ova which are then fertilized in vitro with the partner's sperm. Hormonal support will be required following embryo transfer
Gamete intrafallopian transfer (GIFT)	Most forms of infertility unless severe male factor. Do not use in women with tubal disease	Similar to IVF.	Similar to IVF except that retrieved follicles and sperm are injected laparoscopically into a fallopian tube to fertilize naturally. over IVF
Intracytoplasmic sperm injection (ICSI)	Male infertility.	20–30% per cycle if female partner is under 40 years of age. There is a small risk of sex chromosome abnormalities in males (1%) conceived following ICSI	Viable spermatozoa are injected directly into oocytes retrieved following superovulation. Embryos are then implanted into the uterus. Spermatozoa may be concentrated from an ejaculate or be aspirated from the epididymis or testis in men with obstructive azoospermia.

Results

IUI can achieve a pregnancy rate of 15% per cycle, and cumulative delivery rate after several cycles is 50%.

IVF offers a live birth rate per cycle of >25% in younger women and a cumulative delivery rate approaching 80%. ICSI allows IVF to be offered in severe oligospermia, with pregnancy rates equivalent to standard IVF. There is a slight increase in congenital malformations after ICSI.

A significant risk of multiple pregnancy occurs with any form of ART.

Ovulation induction

Indications
- Anovulation due to the following:
  - PCOS
  - Hypopituitarism
  - Hypogonadotropic hypogonadism
- Controlled ovarian hyperstimulation for ART

Pretreatment assessment
- Exclude thyroid dysfunction and hyperprolactinemia.
- Check rubella serology.
- Confirm normal semen analysis.
- Confirm tubal patency (laparoscopy, hysterosalpingogram [HSG], or hysterosalping-contrast sonography [HyCoSy]) prior to gonadotropin use and/or after failed clomifene use.
- Optimize lifestyle: maintain satisfactory BMI, exercise in moderation, reduce alcohol intake, and stop smoking.
- Baseline pelvic US is essential to exclude ovarian masses and uterine abnormalities prior to treatment.

Clomifene citrate

Mode of action
- Binds to estrogen receptors in hypothalamus, blocking normal negative feedback, thereby ↑ pulse frequency of GnRH. This stimulates FSH and LH release, thereby stimulating the production of one or more dominant ovarian follicles.
- Antiestrogen effect on endometrium, cervix, and vagina

Indications
- Eugonadotropic anovulation, e.g., PCOS. May also be used in unexplained infertility. It requires normal hypothalamic–pituitary–ovarian axis to work, thus is ineffective in hypogonadotropic hypogonadism.

Contraindications
- Hepatic dysfunction

Administration
- Start on days 5 of menstrual cycle (may have to induce bleed by giving a progestin for 10 days) and take for a total of 5 days.

Dose
- Start on 50 mg/day and increase by 50 mg every month until midluteal progesterone is >30 nmol/L.
- Spontaneous ovulation should occur 5–10 days after the last day of medication.
- Remain on optimum dose for 6–12 months.
- Most patients require 50–100 mg/day.

- Ideally, follicle growth should be monitored by regular vaginal US to minimize the risk of multiple pregnancies and ovarian hyperstimulation.

Efficacy

- 80–90% ovulate, with conception rates of 50–60% in first 6 ovulatory cycles. Chances of ovulation can be enhanced in nonresponders by administration of 10,000 IU of hCG mid-cycle (use US guidance; administer hCG when leading follicle is at least 20 mm).
- In overweight women with PCOS who remain anovulatory, the addition of metformin (500 mg tid) to clomifene may improve ovulation rates.

Side effects

- Hot flashes in 10%, mood swings, depression and headaches in 1%, pelvic pain in 5%, nausea in 2%, breast tenderness in 5%, hair loss in 0.3%, visual disturbances in 1.5%
- Ovarian hyperstimulation syndrome (OHSS) in 1%
- Multiple pregnancies in 7–10%

Risk of ovarian cancer

This risk is unknown. Infertility is associated with an ↑ risk of ovarian cancer. Additionally, one study suggests a 2-fold ↑ risk of low-grade ovarian cancer following long-term clomifene use. Further studies are necessary, but currently recommended maximum treatment duration is 6–12 months.

Tamoxifen

Tamoxifen is also an antiestrogen that has similar properties to clomifene. It can be used to induce ovulation with results comparable to clomifene. The dose used is 20–40 mg od for 5–7 days starting on days 2–5 of menstrual cycle.

Ovarian drilling

Laparoscopic ovarian drilling by laser or diathermy in 4–10 points on the surface of the ovaries may be used in women with PCOS who have failed to conceive on clomifene.

Its ovulation rate of >80% and pregnancy rate of >60% are comparable to gonadotropin therapy, without the risk of multiple pregnancy or ovarian hyperstimulation syndrome. It is most effective in slim women with PCOS with a high LH. There are few controlled studies, however.

There is a low risk of pelvic adhesions following ovarian diathermy and a theoretical risk of premature ovarian failure.

Gonadotropins

Indications

- Hypogonadotropic hypogonadism
- Women with PCOS who are clomifene resistant
- For superovulation as part of ART

Dose and administration

Several regimens are available, all requiring close monitoring with twice-weekly estradiol (E2) measurements and vaginal US. One suggested regime (low-dose step-up approach) is as follows:

- Start at 50–75 IU/day hMG (or FSH) on days 2–4 of the menstrual cycle. On day 7 (or 14) of treatment measure serum E2 and perform a vaginal US. If E2 <60 pg/mL and there has been no change in follicle development, then increase hMG (or FSH) by 37.5 IU. Continue to monitor and increase hMG (or FSH) by 37.5 IU (maximum dose 225 IU/day) on a weekly basis until there is an ovarian response.
- If >3 mature follicles (>14 mm) develop or E2 >800 pg/mL, then abandon cycle and restart on half-dose hMG/FSH because of risk of OHSS.
- Otherwise, give hCG at a dose of 5000 IU to trigger ovulation when follicle is >18 mm in diameter. The dose may be increased to 10,000 IU in the subsequent cycle if ovulation doesn't occur.
- Gonadotropins may be used for a total of 6 cycles. If unsuccessful, consider ART.

Efficacy

- 80–85% pregnancy rate after 6 cycles

Side effects

- Multiple pregnancy (20%)—OHSS

OHSS

OHSS is a potentially fatal syndrome of ovarian enlargement and ↑ vascular permeability with accumulation of fluid in the peritoneal, pleural, and pericardial cavities. It occurs during the luteal phase of the cycle, i.e., after hCG stimulation, and is more severe if pregnancy occurs, because of endogenous hCG production.

Mild OHSS occurs in up to 25% of stimulated cycles and results in abdominal bloating and nausea. It resolves with bed rest and fluid replacement. Severe OHSS, associated with hypotension, markedly enlarged ovaries, ascites, and pleural and pericardial effusions, occurs in <0.1%.

Women with OHSS need to be hospitalized and resuscitated, as there is ↑ mortality from disseminated intravascular coagulation and pulmonary emboli. Management should be led by an expert reproductive endocrinologist.

OHSS is triggered by hCG, so it is best prevented by withholding hCG during at-risk cycles. Risk factors include the presence of multiple ovarian follicles, PCOS, young age, and a previous history of OHSS.

IVF superovulation

This should be accompanied by use of a GnRH agonist starting from the mid-luteal phase of the preceding cycle (long protocol) or a GnRH antagonist starting in the mid-follicular phase of the stimulation cycle (antagonist protocol). These strategies prevent premature ovulation before eggs can be collected and significantly improve pregnancy rates.

GnRH treatment

Indications

- Hypothalamic hypogonadism with normal pituitary function

Dose and administration
- Pulsatile GnRH using an infusion pump that is worn continuously. This delivers a dose of GnRH every 60–90 minutes. The dose may be administered either intravenously (2.5–10 mcg/90 min) or subcutaneously (20 mcg/90 min).

Monitoring
- Monitor E2 levels because of risk of hypoestrogenemia if GnRH is given too frequently.
- There is little risk of OHSS or multiple pregnancies, so ultrasonic monitoring is not usually necessary.

Side effects
- Allergic reaction

Efficacy
- Cumulative pregnancy rate of 70–90%

Cryopreservation, fertility, and cancer treatment

Chemotherapy and/or radiotherapy for some cancers can adversely affect male and female fertility, resulting in gonadal failure.

Male patients should be offered the chance of sperm cryopreservation and storage prior to starting cancer treatment so that future fertility may be an option.

Cryostorage of oocytes and/or ovarian tissue is less successful. However, it should still be offered to women of reproductive age about to embark on cancer treatment if they are well enough to undergo ovarian stimulation and egg retrieval. They should be counseled about the low chance of a successful pregnancy using such techniques.

Storage of frozen embryos is more successful but requires the young female cancer patient to be in a stable relationship with the potential father of her children. Superovulation/IVF with embryo freezing requires a 3- to 6-week delay in initiation of chemo- or radiotherapy, which must be sanctioned by the lead oncologist.

Further reading

Braude P, Muhammed S (2003).Assisted conception and the law in the United Kingdom. *BMJ* 327:978–981.

Hamilton-Fairley D, Taylor A (2003). Anovulation. *BMJ* 327:546–549.

Hirsh A (2003). Male subfertility. *BMJ* 327:669–672.

Royal College of Obstetrics and Gynaecology (2004). *Fertility assessment and treatment for people with fertility problems.* pp. 1–208.

Disorders of sexual differentiation

Clinical presentation

Infancy
- Ambiguous genitalia (📖 evaluation is discussed in Ambiguous genitalia, p. 456)

Puberty
- Failure to progress through puberty (male or female phenotype)
- Primary amenorrhea in a female phenotype
- Virilization of a female phenotype

Adulthood
- Hypogonadism
- Infertility

Evaluation

- *Karyotype* 46,XX vs. 46, XY male or female

Imaging

Look for presence of testes or ovaries and uterus.

Imaging is most easily performed using pelvic US, but MRI may be more sensitive in identifying internal genitalia and abnormally sited gonads in cryptorchidism.

Hormonal evaluation

- LH/FSH
- Testosterone, androstenedione, SHBG
- 17–hydroxyprogesterone ± ACTH stimulation (📖 see Investigations, p. 499)
- hCG stimulation test (📖 see Clinical assessment, p. 295) to assess the presence of functioning testicular material. Measure testosterone, androstenedione, DHT, and SHBG post-stimulation.
- Others tests, depending on clinical suspicion, e.g., 5-reductase deficiency-check DHT levels before and after hCG stimulation.

For causes, 📖 see Box 60.1.

Box 60.1 Causes of disorders of sexual differentiation

📖 See also Ambiguous genitalia (p. 456).

46,X— undervirilized male
- Gonadal differentiation abnormalities, e.g., gonadal dysgenesis
  - Cause unknown in the majority
  - May result from 45,X/46,XY mosaicism or *SRY* gene mutation
- Leydig cell abnormalities
  - Autosomal recessive
  - Due to inactivating LH receptor gene mutation
- Biochemical defects of androgen synthesis, e.g.:
  - 3β-HSD, 17α-hydroxylase/17,20-desmolase, or 17β-HSD deficiencies
- Androgen receptor defects
  - Androgen insensitivity syndrome (p. 335)
- 5α-reductase deficiency
  - Mutation of 5α-reductase type 2 gene
  - Autosomal recessive inheritance
  - High testosterone but low DHT concentrations
  - Phenotype can range from female external genitalia to males with hypospadias. Patients characteristically become virilized after puberty.
- Persistent Müllerian duct syndrome
  - Müllerian inhibitory substance (MIS), also called anti-Müllerian hormone (AMH), or MIS receptor gene mutation
- True hermaphrodite

46,XX—virilized female
- Excess fetal androgens—CAH
  - 21-OH deficiency (90%)
  - 11B-OH deficiency
- Excess maternal androgens
  - Drugs
  - Virilizing tumors
- Placental aromatase deficiency
- 46,XX male
  - Due to a Y-to-X translocation so that the *SRY* gene is present
  - Phenotype similar to Klinefelter's syndrome
- True hermaphrodite

Androgen insensitivity syndrome

Pathogenesis

This syndrome results from a mutation in the androgen receptor gene located on chromosome Xq11–12. Several mutations may occur, inherited in an X-linked recessive fashion. However, approximately 40% of patients have a negative family history. Major gene deletions result in complete androgen insensitivity, but the more common amino acid substitutions can result in any of the phenotypes.

Incidence is 1:20 000–1:64 000.

Clinical features

Complete androgen insensitivity (testicular feminization) results in normal female external genitalia. However, the vagina is often shorter than normal and may rarely be absent.

No male external sex organs are present, but remnants of Müllerian structures are occasionally present. Testes are usually located in the abdomen or in the inguinal canal. There is no spermatogenesis.

The syndrome often presents during puberty with primary amenorrhea. Height is above the female average and breast development may be normal. Patients have a normal female habitus but little or no pubic and axillary hair. Gender identity and psychological development are female.

Partial androgen insensitivity has a wide phenotypic spectrum, ranging from ambiguous genitalia to a normal male phenotype presenting with infertility.

- Phenotypic female with mild virilization
- Reifenstein's syndrome (undervirilized male with gynecomastia and hypospadias)
- Infertile male

There is a 9% risk of seminoma.

Hormonal evaluation

Testosterone levels are in the normal or often above-normal male range. hCG stimulation results in a further rise in testosterone, with little increase in SHBG.

Estradiol levels are higher than those in normal males, but lower than the female average. Estrogen is produced by the testes and from peripheral aromatization of testosterone.

LH levels are usually markedly elevated, but FSH is normal.

Genetic testing is possible in some centers.

Management

Orchidectomy is performed to prevent malignancy. Exact timing of surgery is controversial but it is usually performed in adolescence after attaining puberty. In phenotypic females with partial androgen insensitivity, gonadectomy may be performed before puberty to avoid virilization.

Estrogen replacement therapy is given in phenotypic females.

High-dose androgen therapy in males with Reifenstein's syndrome may improve virilization.

True hermaphroditism

Pathogenesis

Pathogenesis is unknown. It may be familial.

Affected individuals have both ovarian and testicular tissue, either in the same gonad (ovotestis), or an ovary on one side and a testis on the other. A uterus and a fallopian tube are usually present, the latter on the side of the ovary or ovotestis.

Wolffian structures may be present in a 1/3 of individuals on the side of the testis. The testicular tissue is usually dysgenetic, although the ovarian tissue may be normal.

Clinical features

Most individuals have ambiguous genitalia and are raised as males, but just under 10% have normal female external genitalia.

At puberty, 50% of individuals menstruate, which may present as cyclic hematuria in males, and most develop breasts.

Feminization and virilization vary widely. Most are infertile, but fertility has been reported.

There is a 2% risk of gonadal malignancy, higher in 46,XY individuals.

Evaluation

- 46,XX in 70%, 46,XX/46,XY in 20%, and 46,XY in 10%
- Hypergonadotropic hypogonadism is usual.
- Diagnosis can only be made on gonadal biopsy.

General principles of management

Assignment of gender and reconstructive surgery

Virilized females (female pseudohermaphroditism)
Most individuals are brought up as females.

The timing of feminizing surgery remains controversial but is usually deferred until adolescence. The decision should be made on an individual basis, by a multidisciplinary specialist team, the parents and ideally the patient. It appears that a significant number of children who have surgery performed during infancy will require further surgery in their teens.

The results of feminizing genitoplasty, which involves clitoral reduction and vaginoplasty, with regard to sexual function are unclear.

Undervirilized males (male pseudohermaphroditism)
The decision regarding gender reassignment is more complex and depends on the degree of sexual ambiguity in addition to the cause of the disorder and the potential for normal sexual function and fertility.

Individuals with complete androgen insensitivity are assigned a female sex, as they are resistant to testosterone therapy, develop female sexual characteristics, and have a female gender identity. They may require vaginoplasty in adolescence.

Sex assignment of other forms of male pseudohermaphroditism depends on phallic size. However, the decision should be made by a specialist multidisciplinary team involving parents who should be fully informed.

A trial of 3 months of testosterone may be used to enhance phallic growth.

Penile reconstruction and orchidopexy by an experienced urologist may be considered in some patients. Testicular prostheses may be required if orchidopexy is not possible. The optimal procedure and timing of surgery remain controversial and the decision should ideally be made with the patient when he is old enough to give informed consent. Results of surgery on sexual function are mixed.

Gonadectomy
There is ↑ risk of gonadoblastoma in most individuals with abdominal testes. Risk is highest in those with dysgenetic gonads and Y chromosome material. Bilateral gonadectomy should therefore be performed (usually laparascopically).

Optimal timing of the gonadectomy is unknown. In androgen insensitivity, the risk of gonadoblastoma appears to rise only after the age of 20 years, so orchidectomy is recommended in adolescence after attaining puberty. In most other disorders, gonadectomy prior to puberty is recommended.

Early bilateral orchidectomy should also be performed in 46, XY subjects with 5α-reductase deficiency or 17βHSD deficiency who are being raised as females, to prevent virilization at puberty.

Hormonal therapy
Patients with disorders of adrenal biosynthesis, e.g., CAH, require lifelong glucocorticoid and usually mineralocorticoid replacement therapy.

Most male pseudohermaphrodites and hermaphrodites being raised as males require long-term testosterone replacement therapy.

Individuals with 5α-reductase deficiency usually receive supra-physiological doses of testosterone to achieve satisfactory DHT levels.

Subjects with androgen insensitivity and male pseudohermaphrodites being raised as females should receive estrogen replacement therapy to induce puberty and this should be continued thereafter.

Psychological support

Disorders relating to sexual identity and function require expert counseling.

Patient support groups are often helpful.

Further reading

Creighton S, Minto C (2001). Managing intersex. *BMJ* 323:1264–1265.

MacLaughin DT, Donahoe PK (2004). Sex determination and differentiation. *N Engl J Med* 350:367–378.

Vogiatzi MG, New MI (1998). Differential diagnosis and therapeutic options for ambiguous genitalia. *Curr Opin Endocrinol Diabet* 5:3–10.

Warne GL, Zajac JD (1998). Disorders of sexual differentiation. *Endocrinol Metab Clin North Am* 27(4):945–967.

Transsexualism

Definition

Transsexualism is a condition in which an apparently anatomically and genetically normal person feels that he or she is a member of the opposite sex. There is an irreversible discomfort with the anatomical gender, which may be severe, often developing in childhood.

Epidemiology

• More common in males
• Estimated prevalence of 1:13,000 males and 1:30,000 females

Etiology

Etiology is unknown and controversial.

There is some evidence that it may have a neurobiological basis. There appear to be sex differences in the size and shape of certain nuclei in the hypothalamus. Male-to-female transsexuals have been found to have female differentiation of one of these nuclei, whereas female-to-male transsexuals have been found to have a male pattern of differentiation.

Management

Standards of care

A multidisciplinary approach between psychiatrists, endocrinologists, and surgeons is required. The patient should be counseled about treatment options, risks, and implications and realistic expectations discussed.

Endocrine disorders should be excluded prior to entry into the gender reassignment program—i.e., ensure normal internal and external genitalia, karyotype, gonadotropins, and testosterone/estradiol.

Psychiatric assessment and follow-up is essential before definitive therapy. The transsexual identity should be shown to have been persistently present for at least 2 years to ensure a permanent diagnosis.

Following this period, the patient should dress and live as a member of the desired sex under the supervision of a psychiatrist. This should continue for at least 3–6 months before hormonal treatment and 1 year before surgery.

Psychological follow-up and expert counseling should be available if required throughout the program, including after surgery.

In adolescents, puberty can be reversibly halted by GnRH analog therapy, to prevent irreversible changes in the wrong gender, until a permanent diagnosis is made.

Hormonal manipulation

For contraindications, ☐ see Box 61.1.

Male-to-female transsexuals
- Suppress male secondary sex characteristics: GnRH analog or high-dose sex steroids
- Induce female secondary sex characteristics
  - EE2 100 mcg/day or Premarin 1.25 mg or estradiol patch 100 mcg 2 × /week

Aims
- Breast development—maximum after 2 years of treatment. Add progestin short term after maximal estrogen therapy to differentiate ductules, but not needed long term
- Development of female fat distribution

Box 61.1 Contraindications to hormone manipulation

Feminization

- Prolactinoma
- Family history of breast cancer
- Risk of thromboembolism
- Active liver disease
- Cardiovascular or cerebrovascular disease
- Other contraindication to estrogen therapy (☐ see p. 268).

Masculinization

- Cardiovascular disease
- Active liver disease
- Polycythemia
- Cerebrovascular disease

Table 61.1 Maintenance hormone regimens in treatment of transsexualism

Feminization (post-surgery)	Masculinization (pre- and post- surgery)
< 40 years OCPs Conjugated estrogens 1.25 mg od	Testosterone 200 mg IM every 2 weeks Transdermal testosterone (gel or patch) 5 mg od
> 40 years Conjugated estrogens .625 mg qd Transdermal estradiol .005–0.1 mg	

- ↓ Body hair and smoother skin. However, facial hair is often resistant to treatment.
- Muscle bulk and strength
- Reduction in testicular size
- Hormonal manipulation has little effect on the voice.

Estrogen
- Reduce dose of estrogens following gender reassignment surgery and discontinue if possible. However, some subjects will require an antiandrogen to keep estradiol doses to a minimum (Table 61.1).
- The dose of estrogen may be halved after gender reassignment surgery (Table 61.1).
- Change to transdermal estrogens if >40 years old. Change to HT doses once >50 years old.
- Adjust estrogen dose depending on plasma LH and estradiol levels.

Side effects
Particularly while on high-dose EE2 therapy:
- Venous thromboembolism
- Atherosclerosis
- Abnormal liver enzymes
- Depression
- ?↑ Risk of breast cancer

Female-to-male transsexuals
The aim is to induce male secondary sex characteristics and suppress female secondary sex characteristics: parenteral testosterone (📖 see Table 61.1).

Aims
- Cessation of menstrual bleeding
- Atrophy of uterus and breasts
- Increase muscle bulk and strength
- Deepening of voice (after 6–10 weeks)
- Hirsutism

- Male body fat distribution
- Increase in libido

Once sexual characteristics are stable (after approximately 1 year of treatment) and following surgery, reduce testosterone dose based on serum testosterone and LH levels.

Side effects
- Acne (in 40%)
- Weight gain
- Abnormal liver function
- Adverse lipid profile

Gender reassignment surgery
- Performed at least 6–9 months after starting sex hormone therapy
- A second psychiatric opinion should be sought prior to referral for surgery.
- Usually performed in several stages

Male-to-female transsexuals
- Bilateral orchidectomy and resection of the penis
- Construction of a vagina and labia minora
- Clitoroplasty
- Breast augmentation

Female to male transsexuals
- Bilateral mastectomy
- Hysterectomy and salpingo-oophorectomy
- Phalloplasty and testicular prostheses

Prognosis
- There is significantly ↑ morbidity in male-to-female transsexuals from thromboembolism.
- The risk of osteoporosis is not thought to be ↑ in transsexuals.

Box 61.2 Monitoring of therapy
- Every 3 months for first year then every 6 months
- Hormonal therapy is lifelong and so patients should be followed up indefinitely.

Male to female

- Physical examination
- Liver function tests
- Serum lipids and glucose
- LH, estradiol, prolactin
- PSA (>50 years)
- ?Mammogram (>50 years)
- Bone densitometry

Female to male

- Physical examination
- Liver function tests
- Serum lipids and blood glucose
- LH, testosterone
- FBC (exclude polycythemia)
- Bone densitometry

- There may be a slightly ↑ risk of breast cancer in male-to-female transsexuals.
- Results from reconstructive surgery, particularly in female-to-male transsexuals, remain suboptimal.
- There is an ↑ risk of depressive illness and suicide in transsexual individuals.

Further reading

Gooren LJ, Giltay EJ, Brunck MC (2008). Long-term treatment of transsexuals with cross-sex hormones: extensive personal experience. *J Clin Endocrinol Metab* 93(1):19–25.

Levy A, Crown A, Reid R (2003). Endocrine intervention for transsexuals. *Clin Endocrinol* 59:409–418.

Moore E, Wisniewski A, Dobs A (2003) Endocrine treatment of transsexual people: a review of treatment regimens, outcomes and adverse effects. *J Clin Endocrinol Metab* 88(8):3467–3473.

Schlatterer K, von Werder K, Stalla GK (1996). Multistep treatment concept of transsexual patients. *Exp Clin Endocrinol Diabet* 104:413–419.

Part 5

Endocrine disorders of pregnancy

Boris Draznin

Thyroid disorders

Normal physiology

Effect of pregnancy on thyroid function

- *Iodine stores* fall due to ↑ renal clearance and transplacental transfer to fetus.
- *Thyroid size:* increase in thyroid volume by 10–20% due to hCG stimulation and relative iodine deficiency
- *Thyroglobulin:* rise corresponds to rise in thyroid size.
- *Thyroid-binding globulin (TBG):* 2-fold increase in concentration as a result of reduced hepatic clearance and ↑ synthesis stimulated by estrogen. Concentration plateaus at 20 weeks' gestation and falls again postpartum.
- *Total T4 and T3:* ↑ concentrations, corresponding to rise in TBG
- *Free T4 and T3:* small rise in concentration in first trimester due to hCG stimulation then fall into normal range. During the second and third trimesters, FT_4 concentration is often just below the normal reference range.
- *Thyroid-stimulating hormone (TSH)* is within normal limits in pregnancy. However, it is suppressed in 13.5% in the first trimester, 4.5% in the second trimester, and 1.2% in the third trimester due to hCG thyrotropic effect. There is a positive correlation between free T_4 and hCG levels and a negative correlation between TSH and hCG levels in the first half of pregnancy.
- *Thyrotropin-releasing hormone (TRH)* is normal.
- *TSH receptor antibodies:* When present in high concentrations in maternal serum these may cross the placenta. Antibody titer decreases with progression of the pregnancy.

Fetal thyroid function

TRH and TSH synthesis occurs by 8–10 weeks' gestation, and thyroid hormone synthesis occurs by 10–12 weeks' gestation.

TSH, total and freeT_4 and T_3, and TBG concentrations increase progressively throughout gestation.

Maternal TSH does not cross the placenta, and although TRH crosses the placenta, it does not regulate fetal thyroid function. Iodine crosses the placenta and excessive quantities may induce fetal hypothyroidism. Maternal T_4 and T_3 cross the placenta in small quantities and are important for fetal brain development in the first half of gestation.

Maternal hyperthyroidism

📖 See Thyrotoxicosis in pregnancy (p. 31).

Incidence

This condition affects 0.2% of pregnant women. Most patients are diagnosed before pregnancy or in the first trimester of pregnancy.

In women with Graves' disease in remission, exacerbation may occur in the first trimester of pregnancy.

Graves' disease

The most common scenario is pregnancy in a patient with pre-existing Graves' disease on treatment, as fertility is low in patients with untreated thyrotoxicosis. Newly diagnosed Graves' disease in pregnancy is unusual.

Aggravation of disease occurs in the first trimester with amelioration in second half of pregnancy because of a decrease in maternal immunological activity at that time.

Symptoms of thyrotoxicosis are difficult to differentiate from those of normal pregnancy. The most sensitive symptoms are weight loss and tachycardia. Goiter is found in most patients.

Management

Risks of uncontrolled hyperthyroidism to mother include heart failure and arrhythmias.

Antithyroid drugs (ATDs) are the treatment of choice but cross the placenta. Propylthiouracil is preferred, although the risk of aplasia cutis, a rare fetal scalp defect, with carbimazole is negligible. There is also less transfer to breast milk.

Avoid β-blockers, as they may be associated with fetal growth impairment with prolonged use. They can be used initially for 2–3 weeks while antithyroid drugs take affect.

Most patients will be on a maintenance dose of an ATD. A high dose of ATD may be necessary initially to achieve euthyroidism as quickly as possible (carbimazole 20–40 mg/day or propylthiouracil 200–400 mg/day) in newly diagnosed patients, then the minimal dose of ATD can be used to maintain euthyroidism.

Do not use a block-replace regime, as higher doses of ATDs are required and there is minimal transplacental transfer of T_4, thereby risking fetal hypothyroidism.

Monitor TFTs every 4–6 weeks.

Aim to keep FT_4 at the upper limit of normal and TSH low–normal.

In approximately 30% of women, ATDs may be discontinued at 32–36 weeks' gestation. Consider doing this if the patient is euthyroid for at least 4 weeks on the lowest dose of propylthiouracil, but continue to monitor TFTs frequently. Presence of a large goiter or ophthalmopathy suggests severe disease; the chances of remission are low, so do not stop the ATD.

Risks of neonatal hypothyroidism and goiter are reduced if the woman is on 200 mg propylthiouracil or less (or carbimazole 20 mg) in the last few weeks of gestation.

Propylthiouracil (PTU) is secreted in negligible amounts in breast milk. Carbimazole is secreted in higher amounts. Breast-feeding is not contraindicated if the mother is on <150 mg PTU or 5 mg carbimazole. Give in divided doses after the feeds and monitor neonatal thyroid function.

Surgical management of thyrotoxicosis is rarely necessary in pregnancy. The only indication is serious ATD complication (e.g., agranulocytosis) or drug resistance. There is a possible ↑ risk of spontaneous abortion or premature delivery associated with surgery during pregnancy.

Radioiodine therapy is contraindicated in pregnancy and for 4 months beforehand.

Infants born to mothers with Graves' disease

Risks to fetus of uncontrolled thyrotoxicosis
- ↑ Risk of spontaneous abortion and stillbirth
- Intrauterine growth restriction (IUGR)
- Premature labor
- Fetal or neonatal hyperthyroidism.

Follow-up of babies born to mothers on ATDs shows normal weight, height, and intellectual function.

Fetal hypothyroidism
This may occur following treatment of a mother with high doses of ATDs (>200 mg PTU/day), particularly in the latter half of pregnancy. This condition is rare and may be diagnosed by demonstrating a large fetal goiter on fetal US in the presence of fetal bradycardia.

Fetal hyperthyroidism
This may occur after week 25 of gestation. It results in IUGR, fetal goiter, and tachycardia (fetal heart rate >160 bpm). It may develop if the mother has high titers of TSH-stimulating antibodies (TSAb). Treat by giving the mother an ATD, and monitor fetal heart rate (aim <140 bpm), growth, and goiter size.

Neonatal thyrotoxicosis
This develops in 1% of infants born to thyrotoxic mothers. It is due to placental transfer of TSAb. It is transient, usually subsiding by 6 months, but there is up to 30% mortality if left untreated.

Treat with ATD and β-blockers.

Hyperemesis gravidarum (gestational hyperthyroidism)
- Characterized by severe vomiting and weight loss. Cause unknown
- Begins in early pregnancy (week 6–9 of gestation) and tends to resolve spontaneously by week 20 of gestation
- Biochemical hyperthyroidism in two-thirds of affected women, but T_3 is less commonly elevated. Mechanism: hCG has TSH-like effect, thus stimulating the thyroid gland and suppressing TSH secretion
- Degree of thyroid stimulation correlates with severity of vomiting.
- No other evidence of thyroid disease, i.e., no goiter or history of thyroid disease, no ophthalmopathy, and negative thyroid autoantibodies
- Antithyroid drugs are not required and do not improve symptoms of hyperemesis.

Causes of maternal hyperthyroidism
- Graves' disease (85% of cases)
- Toxic nodule
- Toxic multinodular goiter
- Hydatidiform mole

Maternal hypothyroidism

Prevalence
- 2.5% subclinical hypothyroidism
- 1–2% overt hypothyroidism

Risks of suboptimal treatment during pregnancy
- *Spontaneous abortion:* 2-fold ↑ risk.
- *Pre-eclampsia:* 21% of suboptimally treated mothers have pregnancy-induced hypertension (PIH).
- Also, ↑ risk of anemia during pregnancy and postpartal hemorrhage
- Risk of impaired fetal intellectual and cognitive development
- ↑ Risk of perinatal death
- Other risks to fetus include those associated with PIH (IUGR, premature delivery, etc).
- The risk of congenital malformations is not thought to be ↑.

Management
Spontaneous pregnancy in overtly hypothyroid women is unusual, as hypothyroid women are likely to have anovulatory menstrual cycles.
- *Levothyroxine therapy:* Start on 150 mcg. Measure TSH 4 weeks later.
- If already on T_4 before pregnancy, assess TSH at 6–8 weeks' gestation, then between weeks 16–20, then again between weeks 28–32 of gestation.
- *Aim:* TSH—lower part of normal range; FT4—upper end of normal
- Increase T_4 dose by 30% (an average of 25–50 mcg) when pregnancy is confirmed. After delivery, thyroid requirements decrease to pre-pregnancy levels.Do not give $FeSO_4$ simultaneously with T_4—this reduces its efficacy. Separate times for drug ingestion by at least 2 hours.

Causes of maternal hypothyroidism
- Hashimoto's thyroiditis (most common cause)
- Previous radioiodine therapy or thyroidectomy
- Previous postpartum thyroiditis
- Hypopituitarism

Positive thyroid antibodies but euthyroid
- 2-Fold excess risk of spontaneous abortion
- No other complications
- No risk of neonatal hypothyroidism
- Risk of PIH not ↑
- The occasional mother will develop hypothyroidism toward the end of the pregnancy, so check TSH between weeks 28–32 of gestation.
- ↑ Risk of postpartum thyroiditis, so check TSH at 3 months postpartum

Postpartum thyroid dysfunction

Prevalence
- 5–10% of women within 1 year of delivery or miscarriage
- 3 × more common in women with type 1 diabetes mellitus

Etiology
- Chronic autoimmune thyroiditis (📖 see Other types of thyroiditis, p. 49)

Clinical presentation
Hyperthyroidism (32%)
- Within 4 months of delivery
- The most common symptom is fatigue.
- Usually resolves spontaneously in 2–3 months

Hypothyroidism (43%)
- Develops 4–6 months after delivery
- Symptoms may be mild and nonspecific.
- There may be an ↑ risk of postpartum depression.

Hyperthyroidism followed by hypothyroidism (25%)
- Spontaneous recovery in 80% within 6–12 months of delivery

Differential diagnosis
Graves' disease may relapse in the postpartum period. This is differentiated from postpartum thyroiditis by a high uptake on radioiodine scanning.

Lymphocytic hypophysitis may cause hypothyroidism. However, serum TSH concentrations are inappropriately low.

Investigation
Thyroid peroxidase antibodies are positive in 80%.

Radionuclide uptake scans are rarely necessary. However, there is low uptake during the thyrotoxic phase, differentiating it from Grave's disease where uptake is increased.

Management
- β-blockers if thyrotoxic and symptomatic until TFTs normalize. Antithyroid medication is unnecessary.
- Levothyroxine if TSH>10 or if TSH between 4–10 and symptomatic

There is no consensus on how long to treat with thyroxine. There are two options:
- Halve the dose at about 12 months postnatal and check TFTs 6 weeks later. If normal, then withdraw T$_4$ and check TFTs 6 weeks later.
- Withdraw treatment 1 year after completion of family.

Prognosis
There is recurrence in future pregnancies in 70% of women.

Permanent hypothyroidism develops in up to 50% of women within 10 years. If treatment is withdrawn, then annual TSH measurements are essential.

Thyroid cancer in pregnancy

📖 See Thyroid cancer and pregnancy (p. 77).

Further reading

Abalovich M, Amino N, Barbour LA, et al. (2007).Management of thyroid dysfunction during pregnancy and postpartum: an Endocrine Society Clinical Practice Guideline. *J Clin Endocrinol Metab* 92(8 Suppl):S1–S47.

Alexander EK, Marqusee E, Lawrence J, et al. (2004). Timing and magnitude of increases in levothyroxine requirements during pregnancy in women with hypothyroidism. *N Engl J Med* 351(3):241–249.

Lazarus JH, Kokandi A (2000). Thyroid disease in relation to pregnancy: a decade of change. *Clin Endocrinol* 53:265–278.

LeBeau SO, Mandell SJ (2006). Thyroid disorders during pregnancy. *Endocr Metab Clin North Am* 35:117–136.

Poppe K, Glinoer D (2003). Thyroid autoimmunity and hypothyroidism before and during pregnancy. *Hum Reprod Update* 9(2):149–161.

Stagnaro-Green A (2002). Postpartum thyroiditis. *J Clin Endocrinol Metab* 87(9):4042–4047.

Pituitary disorders

Normal anatomical changes during pregnancy

- *Prolactin (PRL)-secreting cells:* marked lactotrope hyperplasia during pregnancy
- *Gonadotropin-secreting cells:* marked reduction in size and number
- *TSH and ACTH-secreting cells:* no change in size or number
- *Anterior pituitary:* Size increases by up to 70% during pregnancy. It may take 1 year to shrink to near pre-pregnancy size in nonlactating women. Gradual slight increase in size with each pregnancy
- *MRI:* enlarged anterior pituitary gland, but stalk is midline. Posterior pituitary gland may not be seen in late pregnancy.

Normal physiology during pregnancy

Serum PRL

Concentrations increase markedly during pregnancy and fall again to pre-pregnancy levels approximately 2 weeks postpartum in nonlactating women.

Serum LH and FSH

There are undetectable levels in pregnancy and a blunted response to GnRH because of negative feedback inhibition from high levels of sex hormones and PRL.

Serum TSH, T4, and T3

TSH may be suppressed in the first trimester of pregnancy. Free thyroid hormones usually within the normal range.

Growth hormone (GH) and IGF-I

There are low maternal GH levels and a blunted response to hypoglycemia due to placental production of a GH-like substance. IGF-I levels are normal or high in pregnancy.

ACTH and cortisol

CRH, ACTH, and cortisol levels are high in pregnancy, as both CRH and ACTH are produced by the placenta. In addition, estrogen-induced increase in cortisol-binding globulin (CBG) synthesis during pregnancy will further increase maternal plasma cortisol concentrations.

During the latter half of pregnancy there is a progressive increase of ACTH and cortisol levels, peaking during labor. Incomplete suppression of cortisol occurs following dexamethasone suppression test, along with an exaggerated response of cortisol to CRH stimulation. However, normal diurnal variation persists.

Prolactinoma in pregnancy

Effect of pregnancy on tumor size

Risk of significant tumor enlargement (i.e., resulting in visual field disturbances or headaches):
- Microadenoma (1–2%)
- Macroadenoma (15–35%)
- Macroadenoma treated with surgery and/or radiotherapy before pregnancy (4–7%)

Effect of dopamine agonists on the fetus

Bromocriptine

Over 6000 pregnancies have occurred in women receiving bromocriptine in early pregnancy, and the incidence of complications in these pregnancies with regard to fetal outcome is similar to that of the normal population, indicating that bromocriptine is probably safe in early pregnancy.

Data are available on children whose mothers received bromocriptine throughout pregnancy, and again the incidence of congenital abnormalities is negligible.

Cabergoline

This is also probably safe in early pregnancy, with no ↑ risk of fetal loss or congenital abnormalities, although fewer data are available. It is thus recommended that women with prolactinomas seeking fertility receive bromocriptine to induce ovulation, as there are more data on the long-term safety of bromocriptine. Cabergoline is being used increasingly, as it is better tolerated.

Management

Microprolactinoma

Initiate dopamine agonist therapy to induce normal ovulatory cycles and fertility. Stop bromocriptine as soon as pregnancy is confirmed.

Assess for visual symptoms and headache at each trimester, although the risk of complications is low (<5%). Serum PRL levels are difficult to interpret during pregnancy, as they are normally elevated and are thus are not routinely measured.

MRI is indicated in the occasional patient who becomes symptomatic.

In the postpartum period, recheck serum PRL level after cessation of breast-feeding. Reassess size of microprolactinoma by MRI only if the serum PRL level is higher than pre-pregnancy concentrations.

There is a 40–60% chance of remission of microprolactinoma following pregnancy.

Macroprolactinoma

Management is controversial and must therefore be individualized. There are three possible approaches:
- Bromocriptine may be used throughout pregnancy to reduce the risk of tumor growth. The patient is monitored by visual fields at each trimester, or more frequently if symptoms of tumor enlargement develop. This is probably the safest and thus preferred approach.

- Bromocriptine or cabergoline may be used to induce ovulation and then stopped after conception. However, the patient must be monitored very carefully during pregnancy with monthly visual field testing.
- If symptoms of tumor enlargement develop or there is deterioration in visual fields, an MRI should be performed to assess tumor growth. If significant tumor enlargement develops, bromocriptine therapy should be initiated.
- Alternatively, the patient may undergo surgical debulking of the tumor and/or radiotherapy before seeking fertility. This will significantly reduce the risk of complications associated with tumor growth. However, this approach may render them gonadotropin deficient. These patients should again be monitored during pregnancy using regular visual fields.
- There is no contraindication to breast-feeding.
- MRI should be performed in the postpartum period in women with macroprolactinomas to look for tumor growth.

Cushing's syndrome

Pregnancy is rare in women with untreated Cushing's syndrome, as 75% of them will experience oligo- or amenorrhea.

The diagnosis of Cushing's syndrome is difficult to establish during pregnancy. However, the presence of purple striae and proximal myopathy should alert the physician to the diagnosis of Cushing's syndrome.

If suspected, the investigation of Cushing's syndrome should be carried out as in the nonpregnant state. However, high urinary free cortisols and nonsuppression of cortisol production on a low-dose dexamethasone suppression test may be features of a normal pregnancy. The diurnal variation of cortisol secretion is preserved in normal pregnancy.

Diagnosis is important, as pregnancy in Cushing's syndrome is associated with a high risk of maternal and fetal complications (☐ see Table 63.1).

Adrenal disease is the most common cause of Cushing's syndrome developing in pregnancy, responsible for over 50% of reported cases.

Management

First trimester
- Offer termination of pregnancy and instigate treatment, particularly if adrenal carcinoma
- Alternatively, surgical treatment early in the second trimester

Second trimester
- Surgery, e.g., adrenalectomy or pituitary adenomectomy. There is a minimal risk to the fetus.

Third trimester
- ↑ Risk of diabetes mellitus
- Deliver baby as soon as possible (preferably by vaginal delivery to minimize the risk of poor wound healing following a Caesarian section) and instigate treatment.

Table 63.1 Complications of Cushing's syndrome in pregnancy

Maternal complications	Incidence (%)	Fetal complications	Incidence (%)
Hypertension	70	Spontaneous abortion	12
Diabetes mellitus	27	Perinatal death	18
Congestive cardiac failure	7	Prematurity	60
Poor wound healing	6	Congenital malformations	Low risk; no risk of virilization
Death	4		

Metyrapone used in doses of <2g/day appears to be safe in pregnancy. Postoperative glucocorticoid replacement therapy will be required.

Treatment of Cushing's syndrome in pregnancy may reduce maternal and fetal morbidity and mortality.

Acromegaly

Fertility in acromegaly is reduced, partly due to hyperprolactinemia (if present) in addition to secondary hypogonadism. However, there have been several reported cases of pregnancy in acromegaly.

Acromegaly increases the risk of gestational diabetes and hypertension. However, in the absence of diabetes mellitus, there does not appear to be an excess of perinatal morbidity or mortality in babies born to women with acromegaly.

Significant tumor enlargement occasionally occurs together with enlargement of the normal pituitary lactotropes, so monthly visual field testing is recommended. It may be treated with bromocriptine until there are more safety data on other forms of treatment. However, treatment may be deferred until after delivery in the majority of patients.

Few data are available on the use of somatostatin analogs during pregnancy, so their routine use is currently not recommended as they cross the placenta. However, there have been a few reports of uneventful pregnancies in patients treated with octreotide.

Hypopituitarism in pregnancy

Pre-existing hypopituitarism

This is most commonly due to surgical treatment of and/or radiotherapy for a pituitary adenoma. Ovulation and thus conception may be induced by gonadotropin stimulation.

Lymphocytic hypophysitis

📖 See also Lymphocytic hypophysitis (p. 137).

- Rare disorder thought to be autoimmune in origin
- Characterized by pituitary enlargement on imaging and variable loss of pituitary function
- Most commonly seen in women in late pregnancy or in the first year postpartum.
- Symptoms are due to pressure effects, e.g., visual field defects and headaches, or to hormonal deficiency.

The most common hormonal deficiencies are as follows:

- ACTH and vasopressin deficiency
- TSH deficiency may also exist.
- Gonadotropins and GH levels are usually normal.
- PRL levels may be mildly elevated in a third, and low in a third.

Differential diagnosis

- Pituitary adenoma
- Sheehan's syndrome

MRI often reveals diffuse homogenous contrast enhancement of the pituitary gland. However, the diagnosis is often only made definitively by pituitary biopsy.

There is an association with other autoimmune diseases, particularly Hashimoto's thyroiditis.

The course is variable. Pituitary function may deteriorate or improve with time.

Management

- Pituitary hormone replacement therapy as required
- Surgical decompression if pressure symptoms persist
- A course of high-dose steroid therapy is controversial, with mixed results.

Causes of hypopituitarism during pregnancy

- Pre-existing hypopituitarism
- Pituitary adenoma
- Lymphocytic hypophysitis
- Sheehan's syndrome

Management of pre-existing hypopituitarism during pregnancy

Hydrocortisone

The dose may need to be ↑ in the third trimester of pregnancy by 10 mg/day as the increase in CBG will reduce the bioavailability of hydrocortisone. Parenteral hydrocortisone in a dose of 100 mg IM every 6 hours should be given during labor and the dose reduced back to maintenance levels in the postpartum period (24–72 hours).

Thyroxine

Requirements may increase as the pregnancy progresses. Monitor free T$_4$ each trimester and increase T$_4$ dose accordingly.

GH

There are few data on the effects of GH on pregnancy, but case reports do not suggest a detrimental effect on fetal outcome. However, until more data accrue, GH should be stopped prior to pregnancy. Moreover, as the placenta synthesizes a GH variant, GH therapy is unnecessary.

Vasopressin

The placenta synthesizes vasopressinase, which breaks down vasopressin but not desmopressin. Women with partial diabetes insipidus may therefore require desmopressin treatment during pregnancy. Those already receiving desmopressin may require a dose increment during pregnancy. Vasopressinase levels fall rapidly after delivery.

Sheehan's syndrome

Postpartum pituitary infarction or hemorrhage results in hypopituitarism. This syndrome is increasingly uncommon in developed countries with improvements in obstetric care.

Pathogenesis

The enlarged pituitary gland of pregnancy is susceptible to any compromise to its blood supply.

Investigations will confirm hypopituitarism.

Risk factors
- Postpartum hemorrhage
- Type 1 diabetes mellitus
- Sickle cell disease

Clinical features
- Failure of lactation
- Involution of breasts
- Fatigue, lethargy, and dizziness
- Amenorrhea
- Loss of axillary and pubic hair
- Symptoms of hypothyroidism
- Diabetes insipidus is rare.

Management
- Pituitary hormone replacement therapy (☐ see Background, p. 98)

Further reading

Kovacs K (2003). Sheehan syndrome. *Lancet* 361:520–522.

Molitch M (1999). Medical treatment of prolactinomas. *Endocrinol Metab Clin North Am* 28(1):143–169.

Molitch M (2006). Pituitary disorders in pregnancy. *Endocrinol Metab Clin North Am* 35:99–116.

Sam S, Molitch M (2003). Timing and special concerns regarding endocrine surgery during pregnancy. *Endocrinol Metab Clin North Am* 32:337–354.

Adrenal disorders during pregnancy

Normal changes during pregnancy

Changes in maternal adrenocortical function

Markedly ↑concentrations of all adrenal steroids are due to ↑ synthesis and ↓ catabolism.

Fetoplacental unit

Fetal adrenal gland

DHEAS is produced in vast quantities by the fetal adrenal gland. This is the major precursor for estrogen synthesis by the placenta. The fetal adrenal gland has a large capacity for steroidogenesis. Stimulus for fetal adrenal gland is unknown—possibly hCG or PRL.

Placenta

Maternal glucocorticoids are largely inactivated in the placenta by 11βHSD. Maternal androgens are converted to estrogens by placental aromatase, thus protecting the female fetus from virilization.

Addison's disease in pregnancy

There is no associated fetal morbidity in women who have pre-existing primary adrenal insufficiency, as the fetus produces and regulates its own adrenal steroids.

Management of Addison's disease does not differ in pregnancy.

Glucocorticoids metabolized by placental 11βHSD are preferred (i.e., prednisolone or hydrocortisone), to avoid fetal adrenal suppression.

Increase hydrocortisone dose by about 10 mg during the third trimester of pregnancy and at any time in case of intercurrent illness.

High-dose intramuscular hydrocortisone should be given at the time of delivery to cover the stress of labor.

Doses may be tapered to normal maintenance doses in the postpartum period (◻ see Box 64.1).

Addison's disease developing in pregnancy may result in an adrenal crisis, particularly at the time of delivery, because of a delay in diagnosis.

In early pregnancy, vomiting, fatigue, and hyperpigmentation and low BP may be wrongly attributed to pregnancy. However, persisting symptoms should alert the clinician.

If suspected, the diagnosis is confirmed by the presence of low serum cortisol concentrations with failure to rise following ACTH stimulation, and high ACTH levels. However, the normal ranges for serum ACTH and cortisol concentrations have not been established in pregnancy.

Chronic maternal adrenal insufficiency may be associated with intrauterine fetal growth restriction.

There is no ↑ risk of developing Addison's disease in the immediate postpartum period.

Box 64.1 Management of adrenal insufficiency during pregnancy

- Hydrocortisone 20–30 mg PO in divided doses, as per pre-pregnancy dose
- Fludrocortisone 50–200 mcg PO, as per pre-pregnancy dose

During uncomplicated labor
- Hydrocortisone 100 mg IM q6h for 24 hours, then reduce to maintenance dose over 72 hours
- Keep the patient well hydrated.
- Fludrocortisone may be discontinued while on high doses of hydrocortisone.

Congenital adrenal hyperplasia

Fertility is reduced, particularly women with the salt-wasting form of CAH. Reasons for this are as follows:

- Inadequate vaginal introitus despite reconstructive surgery
- Anovulation as a result of hyperandrogenemia
- Adverse effects of elevated progestagen levels on endometrium

From 60 to 80% of women with CAH and an adequate vaginal introitus are fertile. Fertility may be maximized by optimal suppression of hyperandrogenism by glucocorticoid therapy (see Management, p. 244).

No major complications in pregnancy are known in women with CAH, apart from a possibly ↑ incidence of pre-eclampsia. However, women are more likely to require Caesarean section for cephalopelvic disproportion.

Management is the same as in the nonpregnant woman, and steroids are ↑ at the time of delivery as for Addison's disease (p. 203).

Monitor serum testosterone and electrolytes every 6–8 weeks.

Risk to fetus

- There is no risk of virilization from maternal hyperandrogenism, as the placenta will aromatize androgens to estrogens.
- Glucocorticoids do not increase the risk of congenital abnormalities.
- If the partner is a heterozygote or homozygote for CAH, the fetus has a 50% risk of CAH. Prenatal treatment with dexamethasone will then be necessary to avoid virilization of a female fetus (see Management of pregnancy in CAH, p. 245).

Pheochromocytoma

This condition is rare but potentially lethal in pregnancy. Maternal mortality may still be as high as 17%, with 30% fetal mortality if not treated promptly. The highest risk of hypertensive crisis and death is during labor.

Suspect pheochrocytoma in women with hypertension, persistent or intermittent, especially in the absence of proteinuria or edema, hypertension developing before 20 weeks' gestation, or persistent glycosuria.

Suspect it if paroxysmal symptoms are present: palpitations, sweating, and headache.

Prenatal screening is recommended in high-risk women, e.g., those with a history or family history of MEN-2 or von Hippel–Lindau syndrome.

Diagnose by 24-hour urinary catecholamine collection.

Tumor localization is important—MRI is the imaging of choice in pregnancy.

Management

α-blockade

Phenoxybenzamine reduces fetal and maternal morbidity and mortality. It appears to be safe in pregnancy. The starting dose is 10 mg q12h and is built up gradually to a maximum of 20 mg every 8 hours.

β-blockade

Propranolol is given only after adequate α-blockade. It may increase the risk of intrauterine fetal growth restriction if started in the third trimester. Give in a dose of 40 mg q8h.

Surgery

This is controversial. Some clinicians offer surgical removal of pheochromocytoma before 24 weeks' gestation (which is relatively safe following α- and β-blockade). After 24 weeks' gestation, surgery should be deferred until fetal maturity, and then it can be combined with Caesarean section with removal of the tumor.

Ensure adequate adrenergic blockade before surgery. Operate after safe delivery of the fetus.

Further reading

Hadden DR (1995). Adrenal disorders of pregnancy. *Endocrinol Metab Clin North Am* 24(1):139–151.

Sam S, Molitch M (2003). Timing and special concerns regarding endocrine surgery during pregnancy. *Endocrinol Metab Clin North Am* 32:337–354.

Part 6

Calcium and bone metabolism

Sol Epstein

Calcium and bone physiology

Bone turnover

In order to ensure that bone can undertake its mechanical and metabolic functions, it is in a constant state of turnover (see 📖 Fig. 65.1).
- *Osteoclasts*, derived from the hematopoetic stem cell series, resorb bone.
- *Osteoblasts*, derived from the mesenchymal cell precursors, make bone.
- *Osteocytes*, buried osteoblasts, sense mechanical strain and secrete factors important in bone homeostasis.

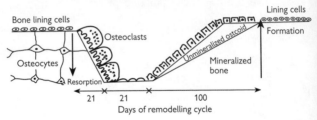

Fig. 65.1 Bone turnover during remodeling cycle.

Bone mass during life

📖 See Fig. 65.2.

Bone is laid down rapidly during skeletal growth at puberty. Following this there is a period of stabilization of bone mass in early adult life. After the age of ~40, there is a gradual loss of bone in both sexes. This occurs at the rate of approximately 0.5% annually.

However, in women after the menopause there is a period of rapid bone loss. The accelerated loss is maximal immediately after the cessation of ovarian function but remains increased throughout life. The excess bone loss associated with the menopause is of the order of 10% of skeletal mass.

This menopause-associated loss coupled with lower peak bone mass largely explains why osteoporosis and its associated fractures are more common in women.

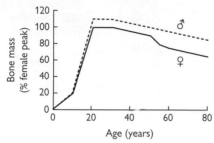

Fig. 65.2 Bone mass and age.

Calcium

Roles of calcium
- Skeletal strength
- Neuromuscular conduction
- Stimulus secretion coupling

Calcium in the circulation
Circulating calcium exists in several forms (📖 see Fig. 65.3).
- Ionized—biologically active
- Complexed to citrate, phosphate etc.—biologically active
- Bound to protein, mainly albumin—inactive

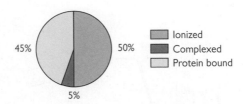

Fig. 65.3 Forms of circulating calcium.

Investigation of bone

Bone turnover markers

These may be useful in
- Assessing overall risk of osteoporotic fracture.
- Judging response to treatments for osteoporosis.

Resorption markers

Collagen cross-links

These make use of the fact that when collagen is laid down in bone, the fibers are held in trimers by covalent links. These links are chemically very stable and are specific to the type of collagen. The excretion of fragments containing these cross-links is a much better indicator of bone turnover.

It can be measured either as the excretion of the linking molecules themselves, known as *deoxypyridinoline cross-links*, or as small fragments of the ends of the collagen molecule including these cross-links, known as *telopeptides*. These latter markers can be derived from either the N- or the C-terminal of the collagen molecule, and separate assays are available for each.

Assays are available for both blood and urine, although the former are subject to less error and are preferred.

Urinary hydroxyproline

This relies on the fact that hydroxyproline is unique to collagen, thus any hydroxyproline in urine must come from collagen breakdown. Unfortunately, this is not specific to bone (type 1) collagen; furthermore, hydroxyproline is variably metabolized before excretion and so its urinary levels are not a true index of collagen destruction. It has accordingly been superseded.

Formation markers

Total alkaline phosphatase is not specific; it is also found in the liver, intestine, and placenta. It is relatively insensitive to small changes in bone turnover and has only found general use in the monitoring of the activity of Paget's disease.

Bone-specific alkaline phosphatase is more specific but its clinical utility is not yet clear.

Osteocalcin is a vitamin K–dependent protein that accounts for about 1% of bone matrix. The serum level of osteocalcin appears to reflect osteoblast activity. However, the results obtained with bone-specific alkaline phosphatase and osteocalcin do not always correlate. This is particularly true in Paget's disease, where the osteocalcin is frequently scarcely elevated despite the marked increase in bone turnover.

P1NP is a procollagen fragment released from the N terminal as type 1 collagen is laid down. When measured in the serum it is the most sensitive and specific marker of bone formation, although its clinical utility is as yet unclear.

Bone imaging

Skeletal radiology

This is useful for the following:
- Diagnosis of fracture
- Diagnosis of specific diseases (e.g., Paget's disease and osteomalacia)
- Identification of bone dysplasia

It is not useful for assessing bone density.

Isotope bone scanning

Bone-seeking isotopes, particularly ^{99m}technetium-labeled bisphosphonates, are concentrated in areas of localized ↑ bone cell activity. They are useful for identifying localized areas of bone disease such as fracture, metastasis, or Paget's disease.

However, isotope uptake is not selective, and so ↑ activity on a scan does not indicate the nature of the underlying bone disease. Hence, subsequent radiology of affected regions is frequently needed to establish the diagnosis.

Isotope bone scans are particularly useful in Paget's disease to establish the extent of skeletal involvement and the underlying disease activity.

Bone mass measurements

📖 See Table 66.1.

Interpretation of results

The differences in normal ranges between the machines of different manufacturers has led to the practice of quoting bone mass measurements in terms of the number of standard deviations (SDs) they lie from an expected mean. This can be done in two ways: T score and Z score; 📖 see Table 66.2.

It is generally accepted that a reduction of 1 SD in bone density will approximately double the risk of fracture.

The WHO has developed guidelines for the diagnosis of osteoporosis in postmenopausal women (📖 see Table 66.3).

No similar criteria have been set in males, but the same thresholds are generally accepted.

For some secondary causes of osteoporosis, particularly corticosteroid use, it has been suggested that the less stringent criterion of T score <–1.5 be used as a treatment intervention threshold.

Table 66.1 Measurement of bone density

Technique	Site	Measures	Radiation	Reproducibility
Dual energy absorptiometry (DXA)	Spine* Femur* Whole body Forearm Calcaneus	Bone mineral per unit area (g/cm²)	~1 Sv per site	<1% at spine <2% at femur
Quantitative computed tomography (QCT)	Spine Forearm	True bone mineral density (BMD) (g/cm³)	~50 Sv at spine	~1%
Quantitative ultrasound (QUS)	Calcaneus Tibia Fingers	Speed of sound or broadband ultrasound attenuation	Nil	Poor

*Accepted as gold-standard measurement.

Table 66.2 T score and Z score

	T score	**Z score**
Definition	Number of SDs bone density lies from peak mean density for that sex	Number of SDs bone density lies from mean density expected for that sex and age
Significance		Age-independent effect on BMD, i.e., secondary osteoporosis
Normal range	Not applicable	−2 to +2

Table 66.3 WHO proposals for diagnosis of postmenopausal osteoporosis

T score	**Fragility fracture**	**Diagnosis**
≥−1		Normal
<−1 but ≥−2.5		Low bone mass (osteopenia)
<−2.5	No	Osteoporosis
<−2.5	Yes	Established (severe) osteoporosis

Bone biopsy

Bone biopsy is occasionally necessary for the diagnosis of difficult patients with metabolic bone disease. This is usually in the context of suspected osteomalacia or a secondary cause of osteoporosis when the diagnosis is uncertain.

Bone biopsy is not indicated for the routine diagnosis of osteoporosis. It is best undertaken in specialist centers and requires fluorescent labeling, e.g., tetracycline.

Investigation of calcium, phosphate, and magnesium

Blood concentration

Calcium

The importance of obtaining blood for calcium measurement in the fasting state with little venous stasis has been overstated. It is, however, important to collect blood for the estimation of parathyroid hormone (PTH) and phosphate levels after an overnight fast.

In most clinical situations, direct measurement of the ionized calcium concentration is not necessary. However, it is important to correct the measured calcium concentration for the prevailing level of albumin (📖 see Box 67.1).

Phosphate and magnesium

Measurements of plasma phosphate and magnesium do not normally require to be corrected for plasma proteins. However, phosphate should be measured after an overnight fast.

Box 67.1 Correction of measured calcium concentration

Corrected Ca = measured Ca + 0.02 × (40 − albumin)

where calcium is in mmol/L and albumin in g/L

Urine excretion

Calcium

A measurement of 24-hour excretion of calcium may be useful for the assessment of the risk of renal stone formation, although the relationship is not that robust to show calcification in states of chronic hypercalcemia.

In other circumstances, particularly the assessment of the cause of hypercalcemia (primary hyperparathyroidism vs. familial hypocalciuric hypercalcemia), an estimate of the renal handling of calcium is more useful. This is most commonly estimated from the ratio of the renal clearance of calcium to that of creatinine in the fasting state (📖 see Box 67.2). If all values are in mmol/L, the ratio is usually >0.02 in primary hyperparathyroidism; values <0.01 are suggestive of hypocalciuric hypercalcemia.

Other causes of hypocalciuria should be excluded, e.g., renal insufficiency, vitamin D deficiency, and some drugs.

Phosphate

A 24-hour measurement of phosphate excretion largely reflects dietary phosphate intake and has little clinical utility.

Box 67.2 Calculation of calcium/creatinine excretion ratio

$$CaE = \frac{\text{urine calcium (micromol)}}{\text{urine creatinine (micromol)}} \times \frac{\text{plasma creatinine}}{\text{plasma calcium}}$$

$$= < 0.01 \text{ in FHH}$$

$$= > 0.02 \text{ in hyperparathyroidism}$$

Calcium-regulating hormones

Parathyroid hormone

Reliable immunoassays for PTH are now available. In general, these are two-site assays aimed at estimating the concentration of the intact PTH molecule. PTH is relatively labile and specimens require careful handling, including early separation from the cells and speedy freezing for storage if the assay is not performed immediately.

Since PTH secretion is suppressed by calcium ingestion, it should be measured in the fasting state. The normal range depends on the precise assay employed, but typical values are 10–60 pg/mL (1–6 pmol/L).

In African Americans, levels are typically higher than in Caucasians.

Vitamin D and its metabolites

25OH vitamin D (25OHD)

This is the main storage form of vitamin D and the best measure of vitamin D status. It is relatively stable, and samples do not require as speedy handling as PTH. In clinical terms, it is the total vitamin D concentration that is important.

The conventionally accepted normal range is 5–30 ng/mL (roughly 12.5–75 nmol/L). However, this normal range was set with the idea of avoiding frank osteomalacia. If the 25OHD is 5–15 ng/mL, there is likely to be a state of vitamin D insufficiency with elevated PTH concentration and ↑ bone turnover. This can be associated with ↑ risk of fracture, particularly in the elderly.

Low levels of 25OHD can result from a variety of causes (⊞ see vitamin D deficiency, p. 399). Likewise, it is unlikely that serious intoxication will occur unless the 25OHD is >100 ng/mL. A more pragmatic reference range might be in the region of 20–80 ng/mL (50–200 nmol/L). (For conversion from ng/mL to nmol/L, multiply by 2.46.)

1,25(OH)₂ vitamin D (1,25(OH)₂D)

Although this is the active form of vitamin D, measurement of its concentration is less often clinically useful than measurement of 25OHD or PTH. It is sometimes useful as a marker of PTH activity and in diseases such as sarcoidosis where there is ↑ extrarenal synthesis of 1,25(OH)₂D.

The normal range is generally accepted as 20–60 pg/mL (50–125 pmol/L), depending on the assay.

Parathyroid hormone–related peptide (PTHrP)

It is possible to measure the level of this oncofetoprotein in serum. Although it is raised in many cases of humoral hypercalcemia of malignancy, the diagnosis is usually readily made from other sources (i.e., Ca with suppressed PTH) and this measurement is noncontributory.

PTHrP is highly labile. Specimens need to be collected into special preservative (Trasylol®), separated, and stored rapidly after venipuncture.

Calcitonin

Calcitonin assays are available but are limited to diagnosis and monitoring of medullary carcinoma of the thyroid. There is no role for calcitonin measurements in routine investigation of calcium and bone metabolism.

Hypercalcemia

Epidemiology

Hypercalcemia is found in 5% of hospital patients but in only 0.5% of the general population.

Causes

Many different disease states can lead to hypercalcemia. These are listed by order of importance in hospital practice in Box 68.1. In asymptomatic community-dwelling subjects, the vast majority of hypercalcemia is the result of hyperparathyroidism.

Box 68.1 Causes of hypercalcemia

Common

Hyperparathyroidism
- Primary
- Tertiary

Malignancy
- Humoral hypercalcemia
- Multiple myeloma
- Bony metastases

Less common
- Vitamin D intoxication.
- Familial hypocalciuric hypercalcemia
- Sarcoidosis and other granulomatous diseases

Uncommon
- Thiazide diuretics
- Lithium
- Immobilization (may be more common with Paget's patients)
- Hyperthyroidism
- Renal failure
- Addison's disease
- Vitamin A intoxication

Clinical features

Notwithstanding the underlying cause of hypercalcemia, the clinical features are similar. With corrected calcium levels <3.0 mmol/L (<12 mg/ml) it is unlikely that any symptoms will be related to the hypercalcemia itself. With progressive increases in calcium concentration the likelihood of symptoms increases.

The clinical features of hypercalcemia are well recognized (listed in Box 68.2). Unfortunately, they are nonspecific and may equally relate to underlying illness.

Clinical signs of hypercalcemia are rare. With the exception of band keratopathy, these are not specific. It is important to seek clinical evidence of underlying causes of hypercalcemia, particularly malignant disease.

In addition to these specific symptoms of hypercalcemia, symptoms of the long-term consequences of hypercalcemia should be sought. These include the presence of bone pain or fracture and renal stones. These tend to indicate the presence of chronic hypercalcemia.

Investigation of hypercalcemia

Confirm the diagnosis
• Plasma calcium (corrected for albumin)

Determine the mechanism
• ↑ *PTH*: parathyroid overactivity (can also occur in familial hypocalciuric hypercalcemia, tertiary hyperparathyroidism, and in lithium therapy due to faulty calcium sensing)

Box 68.2 Clinical features of hypercalcemia

Renal
• Polyuria
• Polydipsia

Gastrointestinal
• Anorexia
• Vomiting
• Constipation
• Abdominal pain

Central nervous system
• Confusion
• Lethargy
• Depression

Other
• Pruritus
• Sore eyes

- ↓ *PTH* : non-parathyroid cause
- *Normal PTH*
  - May imply parathyroid overactivity—incomplete suppression
  - May imply altered calcium sensor—familial hypocalciuric hypercalcemia—calcium/creatine excretion ratio will be low
- Urine calcium to determine calcium/creatinine excretion ratio

Seek underlying illness (where indicated)
- History and examination
- Chest X-ray
- FBC and ESR
- Biochemical profile (renal and liver function)
- Thyroid function tests (exclude thyrotoxicosis)
- 25OHD and 1,25(OH)$_2$D
- Plasma and urine protein electrophoresis (exclude myeloma)
- Serum cortisol (short Synacthen® test [exclude Addison's disease])

To determine end-organ damage
- 24-hour urine calcium (± urine creatinine for reproducibility)
- Renal tract ultrasound (exclude calculi, nephrocalcinosis)
- Skeletal radiographs (lateral thoracolumbar spine, hands, knees)
- BMD
- Bone turnover markers, to confirm increased bone turnover

Hyperparathyroidism

Primary hyperparathyroidism is present in up to 1 in 500 of the general population where it is predominantly a disease of postmenopausal women.

The normal physiological response to hypocalcemia is an increase in PTH secretion. This is termed *secondary hyperparathyroidism* and is not pathological in as much as the PTH secretion remains under feedback control. Continued stimulation of the parathyroid glands can lead to autonomous production of PTH.

This in turn causes hypercalcemia, which is termed *tertiary hyperparathyroidism*. This is usually seen in the context of renal disease but can occur in any state of chronic hypocalcemia, such as vitamin D deficiency or malabsorption.

Pathology: primary hyperparathyroidism

- 85% single adenoma
- 14% hyperplasia
- Often associated with other endocrine abnormalities, particularly multiple endocrine neoplasia (MEN) types I and II (☐ see Chapter 91, MEN type 1, p. 499; Chapter 92, MEN type 2, p. 503).
- <1% carcinoma

Clinical features

- Most patients are asymptomatic.
- Features of hypercalcemia
- End-organ damage—☐ see Box 68.3.

Natural history

In most patients without end-organ damage disease is benign and stable.

A significant minority (2–3% per annum, depending on the series) will develop new indications for surgery.

Excess deaths are due to diabetes and vascular diseases.

Investigation (Box 68.4)

Potential diagnostic pitfalls are as follows:

- Familial hypocalciuric hypercalcemia (FHH)—differentiate with calcium/creatine excretion ratio (☐ see Familial hypocalciuric hypercalcemia, p. 387) (<0.01 in FHH, >0.02 in hyperparathyroidism)
- Long-standing vitamin D deficiency in which the concomitant osteomalacia and calcium malabsorption can mask hypercalcemia, which becomes apparent only after vitamin D repletion. Consider other causes of a raised PTH (Box 68.5.)
- Drugs associated with hypercalcemia (e.g., thiazides and lithium)

Investigation is, therefore, aimed primarily at determining the presence of end-organ damage from the hypercalcemia to determine whether operative intervention is indicated.

Box 68.3 End-organ damage in hyperparathyroidism

Bone

Osteoporosis
- Common
- Affects all sites but predominant loss is in peripheral cortical bone

Radiographic changes
- Uncommon
- Include subperiosteal resorption, abnormal skull vault, eroded lamina dura (around teeth), and bone cysts

Osteitis fibrosa cystica
- Rare
- Usually with tertiary hyperparathyroidism

Kidneys
- Renal calculi
- Nephrocalcinosis
- Renal impairment

Joints
- Chondrocalcinosis
- Pseudogout

Pancreatitis

Box 68.4 Diagnosis of primary hyperparathyroidism

- Ca >2.65 mmol (corrected) repeated; however, this depends on the lab normal values
- Urea and electrolytes normal
- Not on lithium or thiazide diuretic
- PTH >3.0 pmol (depending on the normal lab values)
- Urine Ca >2.5 mmol/day

Box 68.5 Causes of a secondary raised PTH

- GI disorders, e.g., malabsorption
- Renal insufficiency
- Vitamin D deficiency (25 OHD <20 ng/mL)
- Renal hypercalcemia
- Drugs (e.g., lithium, thiazides)

Exclusion of underlying condition

Primary hyperparathyroidism (PHP) can be associated with genetic abnormalities, especially MEN I and II, as well as familial hyperparathyroidism.

These conditions should be sought in patients presenting with PHP and a family history in ≥1 first-degree relative, or at a young age (<40 years).

Localization of abnormal parathyroid glands

This should only form part of a preoperative assessment and is not indicated in the initial diagnosis of hyperparathyroidism.

Localization with two separate techniques (usually US and ^{99m}Tc-sestamibi) is usual before performing minimally invasive parathyroidectomy. Otherwise, bilateral neck exploration by an experienced surgeon is optimal in the first instance.

After failed neck exploration, other techniques may be needed:
- ^{99m}Tc-sestamibi
- −thallium/technetium subtraction scanning (less sensitive)
- CT
- US

Following failed neck exploration, it is often useful to undertake angiography with selective venous sampling. This should be confined to specialist centers.

Treatment

Surgery

This should be done only by an experienced surgeon (>20 procedures per year).
- *Adenoma*: remove affected gland
- *Hyperplasia*: either
  - Partial parathyroidectomy (perhaps with reimplantation of tissue in more accessible site), *or*
  - Total parathyroidectomy with medical treatment for hypoparathyroidism

Observation

This approach is suitable for patients with mild disease with no evidence of end-organ damage. Such patients can continue for many years without deterioration.

They require follow up:
- Annual plasma calcium
- Creatinine annually
- Every 1–2 years BMD

Any significant deterioration is an indication for surgery.

Medical management

This is only indicated if the patient is not suitable for surgery.

Hormone replacement therapy
- Reduces plasma and urine calcium
- Preserves bone mass

Consider the long-term risks (breast cancer, venous thrombosis, heart disease, and stroke).

Bisphosphonates
- Only transient effect on plasma and urine calcium
- Preserve bone mass

Calcium-sensing receptor agonists

Cinacalcet (30 mg tid) will reduce plasma, but not urinary, calcium concentrations. It increases the sensitivity of calcium-sensing receptors decreasing PTH secretion.

It is licensed for use in secondary hyperparathyroidism and parathyroid carcinoma. It is not licensed for use in primary hyperparathyroidism.

Indications for surgery in primary hyperparathyroidism

It is generally accepted that all patients with symptomatic hyperparathyroidism or evidence of end-organ damage should be considered for parathyroidectomy. This would include the following:
- Definite symptoms of hypercalcemia. There is less good evidence that nonspecific symptoms such as abdominal pain, tiredness, or mild cognitive impairment benefit from surgery.
- Impaired renal function

- Renal stones (symptomatic or on radiograph)
- Parathyroid bone disease, especially osteitis fibrosis cystica (low BMD T score <2.5 and/or previous fragility fracture)
- Pancreatitis

Surgery may also be indicated when medical surveillance is neither desired nor required.

Guidelines for the management of asymptomatic hyperparathyroidism have been produced on the basis of a consensus development conference in the United States.[1] Indications for surgery in asymptomatic patients are presented in Table 68.1.

Conservative management

Patients not managed with surgery require regular follow-up (see Table 68.2).

Table 68.1 Indications for parathyroidectomy in asymptomatic patients in the U.S.*

Plasma calcium (>upper limit of normal)	1.0 mg /dL (0.25 mmol/L)
24-hour urine calcium	Not indicated
Creatinine clearance (calculated)	Reduced to less than 60 ml/min
BMD	T score <−2.5 at any site and/or previous fracture fragility
Age	>50 years

*Surgery may also be indicated in patients in whom medical surveillance is neither desired nor possible.

Source: Bilezekeian JP, Kahn AA, Potts JT, et al. (2009). Guidelines for the management of asymptomatic primary hyperparathyroidism: summary statement from the Third International Workshop. *J Clin Endocrinol Metab* 94(2):335–339.

Table 68.2 Management recommendations for patients

Plasma calcium	12 months
Plasma creatinine	12 months
Urine calcium	Not recommended
Creatinine clearance (24-hour collection)	Not recommended
BMD	12 months
Abdominal X-ray/US	Not recommended

1 Bilezikian, JP, Khan AA, Potts JT, et al. (2009). The diagnosis and management of asymptomatic primary hyperparathyroidism revisited. *J Clin Endocrinol Metab* 94(2):335–339.

Complications of parathyroidectomy

Mechanical

Vocal cord paresis
- Usually transient
- May be permanent with extensive exploration, particularly repeated surgery
- May require Teflon® injection of vocal cord

Tracheal compression from hematoma

Metabolic (hypocalcemia)

Transient
- Due to suppression of remaining glands
- Usually causes little problem
- May sometimes require oral therapy with calcium ± vitamin D metabolites

Severe
- Due to hungry bones (calcitriol 1 mcg/day and oral calcium, e.g., calcium citrate 1200 mg daily may be required for several weeks)
- Occurs in patients with pre-existing bone disease
- Prevent postoperative hypocalcemia or hungry bone disease through pretreatment with calcium and vitamin D (1 g and 20 mcg [800 IU], respectively, daily) for several weeks. Vitamin D insufficiency is common in primary hyperparathyroidism. Serum calcium must be monitored while on vitamin D replacement therapy.
- May settle with oral therapy but often requires IV calcium.

Outcome after surgery

Less than 10% fail to become normocalcemic; of these, half will respond to a second operation. Relapse occurs in 1/20 patients with adenoma but in 1/6 with hyperplasia.

All patients with parathyroid hyperplasia (including MEN) need indefinite follow-up.

If the patient is rendered hypoparathyroid by surgery, they will need lifelong supplements of calcium ± active metabolites of vitamin D. This can lead to hypercalciuria, and the risk of stone formation may still be present in these patients.

Other causes of hypercalcemia

Hypercalcemia of malignancy

Mechanism (□ See Table 68.3)

Clinical features

Hypercalcemia is usually a late manifestation of malignant disease and frequently indicates the presence of an untreatable tumor load (50% due within 30 days). One exception to this is in small endocrine tumors such as carcinoids and islet cell tumours, which can produce humoral mediators of hypercalcemia (PTHrP) in the absence of significant spread.

Hypercalcemic symptoms are nonspecific and frequently difficult to distinguish from those of the underlying disease.

Investigation

□ See investigation of hypercalcemia in Clinical features, p. 377.

Factors suggesting hypercalcemia of malignancy include the following:

- ↑ Calcium
- ↓ PTH
- Other features of malignant disease
- ↑ PTHrP—not usually measured in clinical practice

Treatment

Frequently, patients requiring treatment will have severe symptomatic hypercalcemia. Often emergency treatment is necessary to stabilize the patient before confirmation of the diagnosis of the underlying malignant state can be confirmed.

Table 68.3 Types of hypercalcemia associated with cancer

Type	Frequency	Bone metastases	Causing agent	Tumor type
Local osteolytic	20	Common Extensive	Cytokines Chemokines PTHrP	Breast Myeloma Lymphoma
Humoral	80	Minimal	PTHrP	Sqamous carcinoma Renal Ovarian Endometrial Breast HTLV Lymphoma
1,25OH vitamin D	<1	Variable	1,25(OH)$_2$D	Lymphoma, granulomatous diseases
Ectopic PTH	<1	Variable	PTH	Variable

In such circumstances, the principles of management are the same as those for severe hypercalcemia from any cause (see Box 68.6).

Box 68.6 Management of severe hypercalcemia

1. Stabilization

Stabilize the level of hypercalcemia and prevent any further decline in renal function. This requires the IV infusion of large quantities of 0.9% saline, frequently 3–6 L over the first 24 hours.

If there is a danger of salt and water retention, a loop diuretic should be added. This is the only role of diuretics in the management of hypercalcemia. There is no evidence that they lead to sustained reduction in plasma calcium. As they cause intravascular volume depletion, they can worsen the situation and so should otherwise be avoided.

In very severe renal impairment, dialysis might help both stabilize the fluid balance and assist in the removal of calcium from the plasma.

2. Treating hypercalcemia

Once the patient is volume replete, it is necessary to treat the cause of the hypercalcemia. The most effective therapy available for this is IV bisphosphonate. Although these agents are specific inhibitors of bone resorption, they are often beneficial when hypercalcemia is the result of ↑ tubular reabsorption of calcium brought about by PTHrP production.

- Vigorous rehydration 200–500 mL/hr
- Calciuresis with loop diuretics when normovolemia
- Disodium pamidronate 60–90 mg. Zoledronic acid 5 mg IV infusion over 20 minutes, but creatinine clearance should be above 35 mL/min
- Calcium falls within 12 hours nadix 4–7 days
- Remains normal for 1–3 weeks.

IV bisphosphonate therapy is generally well tolerated, but a minority of patient may develop ↑ bone pain or a transient pyrexia and flu-like symptoms. Rarer complications include rashes and iritis.

Bisphosphonates have been associated with deterioration in renal function. For this reason, they should not be given to patients until adequate rehydration has been administered. In addition, dose reduction should be considered for patients with GFR <30 mL/min.

3. Treatment of resistant hypercalcemia

Although most patients will respond to IV bisphosphonates, not all will do so. In such cases, treatment with calcitonin may be helpful. This is usually given as salmon calcitonin and may need to be given as high doses of up to 400 IU by IM injection every 6 hours. In addition to the large volume of injection required, this is frequently poorly tolerated, with side effects such as flushing and nausea.

Some cases of resistant hypercalcemia will respond to corticosteroid therapy, which needs to be given in high doses, such as prednisolone 40 mg daily.

Familial hypocalciuric hypercalcemia (FHH)

FHH is also known as familial benign hypercalcemia.

- 2% of all asymptomatic hypercalcemia
- Autosomal dominant with virtually complete penetrance
- Mutation occurs in the calcium-sensing receptor that reduces its sensitivity such that the body behaves as if it were experiencing normocalcemia, even though the plasma calcium level is elevated.
- Generally benign and is not usually associated with symptoms or adverse effects such as renal stones or bone disease
- Does not usually show any sustained benefit from parathyroidectomy
- A few adults with FHH have had recurrent pancreatitis. In such cases, parathyroidectomy may reduce the frequency of attacks.
- The homozygous state produces severe life-threatening hypercalcemia soon after birth (neonatal severe hyperparathyroidism). In such cases, total parathyroidectomy is life saving.
- Patients have low urine calcium excretion (24 hours <2.5 mmol, fasting calcium/creatine excretion ration <0.01; see Box 68.2, p. 377).

Further Reading

Pallais JC, Kifor O, Chen YB, et al. (2004). Acquired hypocalciuric hypercalcemia due to autoantibodies against the calcium-sensing receptor. *N Engl J Med* 351(4):362–369.

Vitamin D intoxication

The diagnosis is established by the presence of greatly elevated concentrations of 25OHD (>100 ng/mL) and 1,25(OH)$_2$D together with suppressed PTH. If calcitriol or alfacalcidol is the offending compound, then 25OHD levels will not be elevated.

In mild cases, particularly when the active vitamin D metabolites are involved, the only treatment necessary is to withdraw the offending treatment and let the calcium levels settle. If the longer-acting vitamin D metabolites are involved, active treatment may be necessary depending on the level of increased calcium.

Patients should first be stabilized with a saline infusion (see Box 68.4, p. 380).

Following this, the traditional management has been to give high-dose oral corticosteroids such as prednisolone 40 mg daily. This reduces the vitamin D–stimulated calcium absorption and may have beneficial effects on vitamin D metabolism following intoxication.

However, there is now emerging evidence to suggest that bisphosphonates given as for hypercalcemia of malignancy are equally effective.

Sarcoidosis

Together with other granulomatous disorders, sarcoidosis causes hypercalcemia by extrarenal production of $1,25(OH)_2D$ in granulomata. This process is not under feedback inhibition, but is substrate regulated. The hypercalcemia is therefore dependent on vitamin D supply.

Patients frequently present with hypercalcemia in the summer or following foreign holidays when endogenous production of vitamin D is maximal.

The biochemical picture is of normal 25OHD, raised $1,25(OH)_2D$, and suppressed PTH. In addition, other markers of sarcoid activity, such as raised angiotensin-converting enzyme (ACE) activity, are frequently present.

Treatment with high-dose corticosteroids as in vitamin D intoxication is generally recommended to control sarcoid activity and to minimize the GI effects of the excess $1,25(OH)_2D$. The antifungal ketoconazole and the antimalarial chloroquine (or its derivative, hydroxychloroquine) modulate vitamin D metabolism and have been reported to reduce hypercalcemia in patients with sarcoidosis.

If the calcium levels do not respond to these, there is evidence that bisphosphonates might be useful in this situation.

Further reading

Bilezikian JP, Watts JT Jr, Fuleihan Gel-H, et al. (2002). Summary statement from a workshop on asymptomatic primary hyperparathyroidism: a perspective for the 21st century. *J Clinl Endocrinol Metab* 87(12):5353–5361.

Palazzo FF, Sadler GP (2004). Minimally invasive parathyroidectomy. *BMJ* 328(7444):849–850.

Peacock M, Bilezikian JP, Klassen PS, et al. (2005). Cinacalcet hydrochloride maintains long-term normocalcemia in patients with primary hyperthyroidism. *J Clin Endocrinol Metab* 90(1):135–141.

Stewart AE (2005). Clinical practice. Hypercalcemia associated with cancer. *N Engl J Med* 352(4):373–379.

Hypocalcemia

Causes

Although hypocalcemia can result from failure of any of the mechanisms by which plasma calcium concentration is maintained, it is usually the result of either failure of PTH secretion or the inability to release calcium from bone. These causes are summarized in Box 69.1.

Box 69.1 Causes of hypocalcemia

Hypoparathyroidism

Destruction of parathyroid glands
- Autoimmune
- Surgical
- Radiation
- Infiltration

Failure of parathyroid development
- Isolated, e.g., X-linked
- With other abnormalities, e.g., DiGeorge syndrome (with thymic aplasia, immunodeficiency, and cardiac anomalies)

Failure of PTH secretion
- Magnesium deficiency
- Overactivity of calcium sensing receptor

Failure of PTH action
- Pseudohypoparathyroidism—due to G protein abnormality

Failure of 1,25(OH)$_2$D levels
- Drugs, e.g., ketoconazole
- Acute pancreatitis
- Acute systemic illness

Failure of release of calcium from bone
Osteomalacia
- Vitamin D deficiency
- Vitamin D resistance
- Renal failure

Inhibition of bone resorption
- Hypocalcemic drugs, e.g., cisplatin, calcitonin, oral phosphate, bisphosphonates, rankl inhibitors

Box 69.1 (Contd.)

↑ *Uptake of calcium into bone*
- Osteoblastic metastases (e.g., prostate)
- Hungry bone syndrome

Complexing of calcium from the circulation
- ↑ Albumin binding in alkalosis
- Acute pancreatitis
  - Formation of calcium soaps from autodigestion of fat
  - Abnormal PTH and vitamin D metabolism
  - Phosphate infusion
- Multiple blood transfusion—complexing by citrate

Clinical features

The clinical features of hypocalcemia are largely a result of ↑ neuromuscular excitability. In order of ↑ severity, these include the following:

- Tingling—especially of fingers, toes, or lips
- Numbness—especially of fingers, toes, or lips
- Cramps
- Carpopedal spasm
- Stridor due to laryngospam
- Seizures

The symptoms of hypocalcemia tend to reflect the severity and rapidity of onset of the metabolic abnormality.

Clinical signs of hypocalcemia depend on the demonstration of neuromuscular irritability before this necessarily causes symptoms:

- *Chvostek's sign* is elicited by tapping the facial nerve in front of the ear. A positive result is indicated by twitching of the corner of the mouth. Slight twitching is seen in up to 15% of normal women, but more major involvement of the facial muscles is indicative of hypocalcemia or hypomagnesemia.
- *Trousseau's sign* is produced by occlusion of the blood supply to the arm by inflation of a sphygmomanometer cuff above arterial pressure for 3 minutes. If positive, there will be carpopedal spasm, which may be accompanied by painful paraesthesiae.In addition, there may be clinical signs and symptoms associated with the underlying condition:
- *Vitamin D deficiency* may be associated with bone pain, fractures, or proximal myopathy (see p. 399).
- *Hypoparathyroidism* can be accompanied by mental retardation and personality disturbances, as well as extrapyramidal signs, cataracts, and papilloedema, basal ganglia calcification
- If *hypocalcemia* is present during development of the permanent teeth, these may show areas of enamel hypoplasia. This can be a useful physical sign indicating that the hypocalcemia is long-standing.

Pseudohypoparathyroidism

- Resistance to parathyroid hormone action
- Due to defective signaling of PTH action via cell membrane receptor
- Also affects TSH, LH, FSH, and GH signaling
- Most commonly caused by autosomal dominant mutation of *GNAS1* gene
- Significant imprinting:
  - Maternal transmission leads to full-blown syndrome of hormone resistance.
  - Paternal transmission causes only phenotypic features of Albright's hereditary osteodystrophy.

Albright's hereditary osteodystrophy

Patients with the most common type of pseudohypoparathyroidism (type Ia) have a characteristic set of skeletal abnormalities known as Albright's hereditary osteodystrophy. This comprises the following:

- Short stature
- Obesity
- Round face
- Short metacarpals

Some individuals with Albright's hereditary osteodystrophy do not appear to have a disorder of calcium metabolism. In the past, the term *pseudopseudohypoparathyroidism* was used to describe these patients' condition. However, it is now clear that this reflects different manifestations of the same underlying genetic defect as a result of imprinting.

In light of the same underlying cellular abnormality, there has been a tendency to avoid the more cumbersome designations and refer to all such patients as having Albright's hereditary osteodystrophy.

Investigation

- Plasma calcium
- PTH—presence of a low or even normal PTH concentration implies failure of PTH secretion.
- Serum 25 and 1-25 dihydroxy vitamin D
- Magnesium may be needed if the patient fails to respond.
- Ellsworth–Howard test if pseudohypoparathyroidism suspected (📖 see Box 69.2)

In chronic hypocalcemia, skull radiographs will frequently demonstrate calcification of the basal ganglia. As this is of no clinical consequence, it is debatable whether the investigation can be justified.

Box 69.2 Modified Ellsworth–Howard test

Method

1. Fast overnight.
2. Give 200 mL water every 30 minutes from 6 A.M. to 11 A.M.
3. From 8:30 A.M., collect timed 30-minute urine samples for phosphate, creatinine, and cAMP.
4. At 8:45 A.M., 10:15 A.M., and 10:45 A.M., collect blood for creatinine and phosphate.
5. At 10:00 A.M., commence 10-minute infusion of synthetic PTH 1–34, 5 units/kg to a maximum of 200 units.
6. Calculate urinary cAMP excretion as:

   $$cAMPE = [urine\ cAMP] \times [plasma\ creatinine]/[urine\ creatinine]$$

7. Calculate tubular maximum for phosphate reabsorption:

   $$TmP/GFR = ([plasma\ PO_4] - P_E)/(1 - 0.01 \times \log_e([plasma\ PO_4]/P_E)$$

   where $P_E = [urine\ PO_4] \times [plasma\ creatinine]/[urine\ creatinine]$ and all measurements are in mmol/L

   or using the nomogram of Walton and Bijvoet (1975; *Lancet* 2:309).

Interpretation

- Patients with a normal response to PTH will demonstrate a brisk increase in cAMP excretion and a decrease in TmP.
- Patients with pseudohypoparathyroidism type I show neither response.
- There is a rarer condition, pseudohypoparathyroidism type II, in which there is a normal cAMP response but a blunted phosphaturic response.
- A similar pattern can be seen in some patients with profound hypocalcemia due to vitamin D deficiency. It is therefore important to ensure that patients are vitamin D replete before undertaking a PTH infusion test.

Treatment

Acute symptomatic hypocalcemia is a medical emergency and demands urgent treatment, whatever the cause (☐see Box 69.3).

Treatment of *chronic hypocalcemia* is more dependent on the cause.

Chronic hypocalcemia

Hypoparathyroidism

In hypoparathyroidism the aim is not to achieve normalization of the plasma calcium, rather to render the patient asymptomatic with a plasma calcium at or just below the normal lower limit. The reason for this is that the renal retention of calcium brought about by PTH has been lost. Thus, any attempt to raise the plasma calcium well into the normal range is likely to result in unacceptable hypercalciuria, with the risk of nephrocalcinosis and renal stones.

Box 69.3 Treatment of acute hypocalcemia

- Patients with tetany or seizures require urgent IV treatment with calcium gluconate (less irritant than the chloride).
  - This is a 10% w/v solution (10 mL = 2.25 mmol elemental calcium).
  - The solution should always be further diluted to minimize the risk of phlebitis or tissue damage if extravasation occurs.
- Initially, 20 mL of 10% calcium gluconate should be diluted in 100–200 mL of 0.9% saline or 5% glucose and infused over about 10 minutes.
- Repeat if symptoms are not resolved.
- Care must be taken if the patient has heart disease, especially if taking digoxin, as too-rapid elevation of the plasma calcium can cause arrhythmias. In such patients it is advisable to monitor the cardiac rhythm during calcium infusion.
- To maintain the plasma calcium, give a continuous calcium infusion: 40 mL of 10% calcium gluconate should be added to 1 L of saline or glucose solution and infused over 24 hours.
- The plasma calcium should be checked regularly (not less than q6h) and the infusion rate adjusted in response to change in concentration.
- Failure of the plasma calcium to respond to infused calcium should raise the possibility of hypomagnesemia. This can be rapidly ascertained by plasma magnesium estimation and, if appropriate, a magnesium infusion commenced (☐ see Treatment, p. 566).
- In circumstances where hypoparathyroidism could be predicted (such as block dissection of the neck), infusion of calcium gluconate in an initial dose of 50 mL 10% solution (~11 mmol Ca) diluted in normal saline over 24 hours should be given to avoid postoperative hypocalcemia. This dose should be adjusted in light of regular calcium estimations.
- Once oral or NG tube intake is possible, calcium and active vitamin D metabolites should be substituted as above.

In patients with mild parathyroid dysfunction, it may be possible to achieve acceptable calcium concentrations by using calcium supplements alone. If used in this way, these need to be given in large doses, perhaps as much as 1 g elemental calcium 3× daily.

Most patients will not achieve adequate control with such treatment. In those cases it is necessary to use vitamin D or its metabolites in pharmacological doses to maintain plasma calcium. The more potent analogs of vitamin D, such as calcitriol or alfacalcidol, have the advantage over high-dose calciferol that it is easier to make changes in therapy in response to plasma calcium levels.

If hypercalcemia does occur, it settles much more quickly following withdrawal of these compounds than ergocalciferol. The dose of vitamin D is determined by the clinical response but usually lies in the range of 0.5–2 mcg of the potent analogs daily.

Hypercalcemia is the main hazard of such therapy. Plasma calcium levels must be checked frequently after any change in therapy and no less than every 3 months while on maintenance.

It is essential to ensure an adequate intake of calcium as well as vitamin D analogs. In some patients it is necessary to give calcium supplementation, particularly in the young. It is very rarely needed in patients aged >60 years.

Pseudohypoparathyroidism

The principles underlying the treatment of pseudohypoparathyroidism are the same as those underlying hypoparathyroidism.

Patients with the most common form of pseudohypoparathyroidism may have resistance to the action of other hormones that rely on G-protein signaling. They therefore need to be assessed for thyroid and gonadal dysfunction (because of defective TSH or gonadotrophin action). If these deficiencies are present, they need to be treated in the conventional manner.

Vitamin D deficiency

📖 Treatment of osteomalacia and vitamin D deficiency is described on p. 399.

Overactivity of calcium-sensing receptor

This leads to a condition known as autosomal dominant hypocalcemia. It is a benign condition in which the hypocalcemia is usually asymptomatic.

Treatment should be avoided in the absence of symptoms, as elevation of calcium levels even to within the normal range may cause renal impairment.

Further reading

Shoback D (2008). Hypoparathyroidism *N Engl J Med* 359:391–403.

Rickets and osteomalacia

Definitions

Osteomalacia occurs when there is inadequate mineralization of mature bone. *Rickets* is a disorder of the growing skeleton in which there is inadequate mineralization of bone as it is laid down at the epiphysis.

In most instances, osteomalacia leads to build-up of excessive unmineralized osteoid within the skeleton. In rickets there is build-up of unmineralized osteoid in the growth plate. This leads to the characteristic radiological appearance of rickets with widening of the growth plate and loss of definition of the ossification centers.

These two related conditions may coexist.

Clinical features

Osteomalacia
- Bone pain
- Deformity
- Fracture
- Proximal myopathy (depending on the underlying cause)
- Hypocalcemia (in vitamin D deficiency)

Rickets
- Growth retardation.
- Bone pain and fractures often occurring in unusual locations, e.g., scapular, pubic rami
- Skeletal deformity
  - Bowing of the long bones
  - Widening of the growth plates widening of the wrists, "rickety rosary" (costochondral junctions enlarged)

Diagnosis

The diagnosis of osteomalacia is usually based on the appropriate biochemical findings (🕮 see Table 70.1). Most patients with osteomalacia will show no specific radiological abnormalities.

The most characteristic abnormality is the *Looser's zone* or pseudo-fracture. If these are present they are virtually pathognomonic of osteomalacia.

If the diagnosis of osteomalacia remains in doubt, a bone biopsy may be necessary. This is often the only way of establishing the diagnosis in low-turnover conditions such as the toxic osteomalacias.

Bone biopsy shows not only excess osteoid but also prolonged mineralization lag time.

Box 70.1 Vitamin D resistance

Several different kindreds have been shown to have a defective vitamin D receptor. This is inherited as an autosomal recessive condition. It produces hypocalcemia and osteomalacia with elevated serum levels of 1,25(OH)$_2$ D.

Approximately 2/3 of affected individuals have total alopecia. This condition is known as vitamin D–dependent rickets type II. If alopecia is present, it is often termed type IIA, in contrast to type IIB, in which hair growth is normal.

Treatment usually requires administration of large doses of active vitamin D metabolites, sometimes reaching doses of 60 mcg of calcitriol daily.

Box 70.2 Abnormal vitamin D metabolism

Although liver disease could in theory lead to deficient 25-hydroxylation of vitamin D, there is so much functional reserve that this is seldom a clinical problem. Two cases of rickets due to hereditary defects of 25-hydroxylase have been reported.

The most common cause of failure of 1α-hydroxylase is renal failure. Congenital absence of this enzyme leads to a condition known as vitamin D–dependent rickets type I. This is inherited in an autosomal recessive fashion and results in profound rickets with myopathy and enamel hypoplasia.

Very large doses of calciferol are needed to heal the bone lesions, which, in contrast, will respond to physiological doses of alfacalcidol or calcitriol.

Table 70.1 Biochemical findings and causes of rickets and osteomalacia

	Ca	PO4	Alkaline phosphatase	25OHD	1,25(OH)₂D	PTH	Other
Vitamin D deficiency	↓	↓	↑	↓	↓	↑	
Renal failure	↓	↑	↑	N	↓	↑	↓ GFR
VDDR type I (deficient 1 ahydroxylase)	↓	↓	↑	N	↓	↑	
VDDR type II (deficient vitamin D receptor)	↓	↓	↑	N	↑	↑	
X-linked hypo-phosphatemia (vitamin D resistant rickets [VDDR])	N	↓	↑	N	N	N or ↑	
Oncogenic	N or ↓	↓	↑	N	↓	N	May have aminoaciduria, proteinuria
Phosphate depletion	N	↓	↑	N	↑	N	↑ Urine Ca
Fanconi syndrome	↓ or N	↓	↑	N	↓	N	Acidosis, aminoaciduria, glycosuria
Renal tubular acidosis	↓ or N	↓	↑	N	N or ↓	N	Acidosis
Toxic (etidronate, fluoride)	N	N	N	N	N	N	Diagnosed on biopsy

N, normal.

Vitamin D deficiency

Causes
- Poor sunlight exposure
- Elderly and housebound
- Asian women who cover their entire bodies with clothing
- Excess sunscreen application
- Pigmented skin
- Poor diet (especially vegetarians)
  - Malabsorption
  - ↑Catabolism of vitamin D
- Secondary hyperparathyroidism

  - Malabsorption
  - Post-gastrectomy
  - Enzyme-inducing drugs, e.g., phenytoin

Investigation
Diagnosis of vitamin D deficiency is based on the characteristic biochemical abnormalities (📖 see Table 70.1, p. 398). Frank osteomalacia is usually associated with very low levels of 25OHD (<5 ng/mL, but this can occur at <8 ng/ml). The associated secondary hyperparathyroidism often results in normal or even elevated concentrations of $1,25(OH)_2$ D.

Treatment
Treatment is best given in the form of vitamin D_2 or D_3, which will restore the biochemistry to normal and heal the bony abnormalities. Although active metabolites of vitamin D will heal the bony abnormalities, they will not correct underlying biochemical problem and are associated with ↑ risk of hypercalcemia.

In adults, treatment is given as a daily dose of ergocalciferol/cholecalciferol of 20–25 mcg (800–1000 IU), which is often most easily administered in combination with a calcium supplement.

An alternative that is particularly helpful if poor compliance is suspected is to give a single large dose of 3.75–7.5 mg (150,000–300,000 IU). This is most effectively given as a single oral dose (3–6× 1.25 mg tablets of ergocalciferol/cholecalciferol), which can be supervised in the clinic. This can be repeated at 2- to 3-month intervals depending on the dose.

It is possible to give a similar dose by IM injection, but the absorption from this route is variable.

Toxicity is very uncommon and doses of 10,000 IU may be needed for toxicity or above 200 ng/mL serum 25(OH) D.

Following treatment, there usually is a rapid improvement of myopathy and symptoms of hypocalcemia.

Bone pain frequently persists longer, and biochemical abnormalities may not settle for several months. Following the onset of therapy, markers of bone turnover such as alkaline phosphatase might even show a transient increase as the osteoid is mineralized and remodeled.

Watch for hypercalcemia once osteomalacia is healed. Calcium concentrations should be monitored and vitamin D dosage reduced if necessary.

X-linked hypophosphatemia
• X-linked dominant genetic disorder
• Severe rickets and osteomalacia
• Mutation of an endopeptidase gene (*PHEX*)

Clinical features
The abnormal phosphate levels are often detected early in infancy, but skeletal deformities are not apparent until walking commences.

Typically there is severe rickets, with short stature and bony deformity. This continues into adult life with bone pain, deformity, and fracture in the absence of treatment. Proximal myopathy is absent.

Adults suffer from excessive new bone growth affecting particularly entheses and the longitudinal ligaments of the spinal canal. This can cause spinal cord compression, which may need surgical decompression.

Oncogenic osteomalacia
Certain tumors may be able to produce FGF23, which is phosphaturic. This is rare and usually occurs with mesenchymal tumors (such as hemangiopericytomas, hemangiomata, or osteoid tumors) but has also been reported with a variety of adenocarcinomas (particularly prostatic cancer) and hematological malignancies (e.g., myeloma and chronic lymphocytic leukemia).

A similar picture can be seen in some cases of neurofibromatosis. Clinically, such patients usually present with profound myopathy as well as bone pain and fracture.

Biochemically, the major abnormality is hypophosphatemia, but this is usually accompanied by inappropriately low $1,25(OH)_2D$ concentrations. In some patients, other abnormalities of renal tubular function such as glycosuria or aminoaciduria are also present.

FGF_3 levels are elevated and fall with tumor removal. Tumor may be localized by PET or CT.

Complete removal of tumor results in resolution of biochemical and skeletal abnormalities. If this is not possible, or if a causal tumor is not identified, treatment with vitamin D metabolites and phosphate supplements (as for X-linked hypophosphatemia) may help skeletal symptoms.

Fanconi syndrome
The Fanconi syndrome is a combination of renal tubular defects that can result from several different pathologies. In particular, there is renal wasting of phosphate, bicarbonate, glucose, and amino acids.

The combination of hypophosphatemia with renal tubular acidosis means that osteomalacia is a frequent accompaniment. This can be exacerbated by defective 1α-hydroxylation of vitamin D to its active form.

The osteomalacia is treated by correction of the relevant abnormalities. This might involve the administration of phosphate, alkali, or $1,25(OH)_2D$ depending on the precise circumstances.

Further reading
Carpenter TO (2003). Oncogenic osteomalacia—a complex dance of factors. *N Engl J Med* 348:1705–1708.

Hypophosphatemia

Phosphate is important for normal mineralization of bone. In the absence of sufficient phosphate, osteomalacia results. Clinically, the osteomalacia is often indistinguishable from others that are due to other causes, although there may be features that will help distinguish the underlying cause of hypophosphatemia.

In addition, phosphate is important in its own right for neuromuscular function, and profound hypophosphatemia can be accompanied by encephalopathy, muscle weakness, and cardiomyopathy.

Because phosphate is primarily an intracellular anion, a low plasma phosphate does not necessarily represent actual phosphate depletion.

Several different causes of hypophosphatemia are recognized (☐ see Box 70.3).

Treatment

The mainstay is phosphate replacement, usually orally in tablet form. Ideally, patients should receive 2–3 g of phosphate daily between meals, but this is not easy to achieve. All phosphate preparations are unpalatable and act as osmotic purgatives causing diarrhea.

Box 70.3 Causes of hypophosphatemia

↓ *Intestinal absorption*
- Phosphate-binding antacids
- Malabsorption
- Starvation or malnutrition

↑ *Renal losses*
- Hyperparathyroidism
- Primary
- Secondary, e.g., in vitamin D deficiency
- Renal tubular defects
- Fanconi syndrome
- X-linked hypophosphatemia
- Oncogenic osteomalacia
- Alcohol abuse
- Poorly controlled diabetes
- Acidosis
- Drugs
- Diuretics
- Corticosteroids
- Calcitonin

Shift into cells
- Septicemia
- Insulin treatment
- Glucose administration
- Salicylate poisoning

Long-term administration of phosphate supplements stimulates parathyroid activity. This can lead to hypercalcemia, a further fall in phosphate, with worsening of the bone disease due to development of hyperparathyroid bone disease, which may necessitate parathyroidectomy.

To minimize parathyroid stimulation, it is usual to give one of the active metabolites of vitamin D in conjunction with phosphate. Typically, alfacalcidol or calcitriol in a dose of 1–3 mcg daily is used.

Patients receiving such supraphysiological doses of vitamin D metabolites are at continued risk of hypercalcemia and require regular monitoring of plasma calcium, preferably at least every 3 months. The adequacy of calcitriol replacement can be assessed by maintaining 24-hour urinary calcium excretion at >4–6 mmol/day.

In adults, the role of treatment for X-linked hypophosphatemia is probably confined to symptomatic bone disease. There is little evidence that it will improve the long-term outcome. There has even been some evidence that treatment might accelerate new bone formation.

In children, treatment is usually given in the hope of improving final height and minimizing skeletal abnormality. The evidence that it is possible to achieve these goals is conflicting.

Hypomagnesemia

Introduction

Low plasma magnesium levels are common in acutely ill patients. Clinical manifestations of this are less common.

The most common clinical feature of magnesium deficiency is neuromuscular excitability, which is virtually indistinguishable from that associated with hypocalcemia, which frequently coexists. ECG abnormalities include a prolonged P-R interval and Q-T interval.

The diagnosis is made by measurement of serum magnesium, with normal values being 1.5–1.9 mEq/liter (1.8–2.2 mg/day), but it does not reflect the major source, which is intracellular. However, hypomagnesemia must be suspected if low calcium is difficult to correct.

In some circumstances, the magnesium tolerance test is performed but requires a normal renal function. The two major routes of loss are the GI tract and kidney.

With magnesium deficiency, PTH secretion is defective, leading to the presence or worsening of hypocalcemia, which will not respond to treatment unless the magnesium deficiency is corrected. In magnesium depletion there is defective trans-membrane electrolyte transport. This can cause loss of intracellular potassium and of the renal tubule's ability to retain potassium.

See Box 71.1 for various causes of hypomagnesemia.

Treatment with potassium supplementation is often unsuccessful unless magnesium is replaced at the same time.

Box 71.1 Causes of hypomagnesemia

GI losses
- Vomiting
- Diarrhea
- Losses from fistulae
- Malabsorption
- Severe acute pancreatitis
- Defective intestinal transport caused by mutations in the *TRPM6* gene

Renal losses
- Chronic parenteral therapy
- Osmotic diuresis

Box 71.1 (*Contd.*)

Drugs
- Alcohol
- Loop diuretics
- Aminoglycosides
- Cisplatin
- Cyclosporin
- Amphotericin

Other causes
- Diabetes
- Metabolic acidosis
- Hypercalcemia
- Phosphate depletion
- Hungry bone syndrome

Treatment

Symptomatic magnesium deficiency, especially if associated with hypocalcemia or hypokalemia, requires parenteral treatment. The total deficit may be of the order of 200–400 mEq. This should be replaced gradually parenterally.

A dose of 2 g Mg SO4-.7H2O (16.2 mEq Mg) as a 50% solution every 8 hours intramuscularly can be given. However, as these doses are frequently painful, a continuous IV infusion of 48 mEq over 24 hours may be preferred. This should be continued until the clinical and biochemical manifestations (hypocalcemia and hypokalemia) are resolved.

In the presence of renal impairment, plasma magnesium can rise quickly, so particular care must be used if magnesium infusion is contemplated in this situation.

After repletion has been achieved intravenously, or in less severe cases, treatment can be continued orally.

Patients who have chronic Mg loss can be given oral supplementation of 300–600 mg of elemental Mg in divided doses to avoid the purgative effects. In all of these instances the dose is frequently limited by the purgative properties of magnesium salts.

There is some evidence to suggest that the addition of calcitriol or alfacalcidol might improve magnesium absorption.

Further reading

Rude R (2008). Chapter 70. *Primer on the Metabolic Bone Diseases and Disorders of Mineral Metabolism*, 7th ed. American Society for Bone and Mineral Research, pp. 325–328.

Osteoporosis

Introduction

Although the term *osteoporosis* refers to the reduction in the amount of bony tissue within the skeleton, this is generally associated with a loss of structural integrity of the internal architecture of the bone. The combination of both of these changes means that osteoporotic bone is at high risk of fracture, after even trivial injury.

Although most fractures are related to bone mass to some extent, the most common osteoporotic fractures are those of the hip and wrist (Colles) and compression fractures of vertebral bodies. Patients who fracture ribs, the upper humerus, leg, and pelvis also have a higher incidence of osteoporosis.

Pathology

Osteoporosis may arise from a failure of the body to lay down sufficient bone during growth and maturation; an earlier-than-usual onset of bone loss following maturity; or an ↑ rate of that loss. In females, the loss of estrogen at the menopause is the major etiological factor.

Peak bone mass

This is mainly genetically determined:
- Racial effects (bone mass higher in Afro-Caribbean, lower in Caucasians)
- Family influence on the risk of osteoporosis—may account for 60–70% of variation

It is also influenced by environmental factors:
- Exercise—particularly weight-bearing
- Nutrition—especially calcium

Exposure to estrogen is also important. Early menopause or late puberty (in males or females) is associated with ↑ risk of osteoporosis.

Early onset of loss
- Early menopause
- Conditions leading to bone loss, e.g., glucocorticoid therapy

Increased net loss
- Aging
  - Vitamin D insufficiency
  - Declining bone formation
  - Declining renal function
- Underlying disease states (📖 see Box 72.1)

Lifestyle factors affecting bone mass

Increase
- Weight-bearing exercise

Decrease
- Smoking
- Excessive alcohol
- Nulliparity
- Poor calcium nutrition

Box 72.1 Underlying causes of osteoporosis

Gonadal failure
- Premature menopause (age <45)
- Hypogonadism in men, e.g., acquired and Klinefelter's syndrome
- Turner syndrome
- Estrogen receptor defect

Conditions leading to amenorrhea with low estrogen (for >6 months)
- Hyperprolactinemia
- Anorexia nervosa
- Athletic amenorrhea

Endocrine disorders
- Cushing's syndrome
- GH deficiency
- Hyperparathyroidism
- Acromegaly with hypogonadism
- Hyperthyroidism within 3 years
- Diabetes mellitus

GI disorders
- Malabsorption
- Postgastrectomy
- Celiac disease
- Crohn's disease

Liver disease
- Cholestasis
- Cirrhosis

Neoplastic disorders
- Multiple myeloma
- Systemic mastocytosis

Inflammatory conditions
- Rheumatoid arthritis
- Cystic fibrosis

Nutritional disorders
- Parenteral nutrition
- Lactose intolerance
- Immobilization

Drugs
- Systemic corticosteroids (when administered for >3 months)
- Heparin (when given long term, particularly in pregnancy)
- Chemotherapy (primarily by gonadal damage)
- Gonadotrophin-releasing hormone agonists
- Cyclosporin
- Anticonvulsants (long term)
- Aromatase inhibition for breast cancer

Box 72.1 (*Contd.*)

- Androgen deprivation therapy
- Proton pump inhibitors
- Thiaglitizone

Other causes

- Immobilization and chronic bed rest
- Stroke
- Cronic cardiac disease
- Chronic lung disease

Metabolic abnormalities

- Homocystinuria

Hereditary disorders

- Osteogenesis imperfecta
- Marfan syndrome

Epidemiology

The risk of osteoporotic fracture increases with age. Fracture rates in men are approximately one-half those seen in women of the same age. A woman aged 50 has approximately a 1/2 chance of sustaining an osteoporotic fracture during the rest of her life. The corresponding figure for men is 1/5, although this is increasing.

In the United States, 10 million Americans older than 50 years of age have osteoporosis. There are 1.5 million fractures each year, and another 34 million are at risk for the disease.

There are approximately 500,000 hip fractures per year. These are a particular health challenge as they invariably result in hospital admission. One-fifth of hip fracture victims will die within 6 months of the injury and only 50% will return to their previous level of independence.

It has been estimated that the overall cost of osteoporotic fractures in the United States is $22 billion annually.

Presentation

Osteoporosis is usually clinically silent until the onset of fracture. Two-thirds of vertebral fractures do not come to clinical attention.

Typical vertebral fracture has the following features:

- Sudden episode of well-localized pain
- May or may not have been related to injury or exertion
- May be radiation of the pain in a girdle distribution
- Pain may initially require bed rest but gradually subsides over the following 4–8 weeks. Even after this time there may be residual pain at the fracture site.
- Osteoporotic vertebral fractures only rarely lead to neurological impairment.

Any evidence of spinal cord compression should prompt a search for malignancy or other underlying cause.

Following vertebral fracture, a patient may be left with persistent back pain, kyphosis, or height loss.

Although height loss and kyphosis are often thought to be indicative of osteoporosis, they are more frequently the result of degenerative disease. They cannot be the result of osteoporosis in the absence of vertebral fracture.

Peripheral fractures are also more common in osteoporosis.

If a bone breaks from a fall from less than standing height, this represents a low-trauma fracture that might indicate underlying osteoporosis. Osteoporosis does not cause generalized skeletal pain.

Investigation

Establish the diagnosis

Plain radiographs are useful for determining the presence of fracture. Apart from this, they are of little utility in the diagnosis of osteoporosis.

Bone densitometry

In order to identify the presence of osteoporosis, it is important to actually measure the bone mineral density (BMD). This is usually carried out at the hip and/or lumbar spine with dual-energy X-ray absorptiometry (DXA).

The presence of degenerative disease or arterial calcification can elevate the apparent bone density of the spine without adding to skeletal strength. Increased reliance is thus being placed on measurements derived from the hip.

The schema for diagnosis of osteoporosis that was proposed by the WHO has been accepted for general use (🕮 see Table 72.1).

Biochemical markers

Biochemical markers of bone turnover may be helpful in the calculation of fracture risk and in judging the response to antiresorptive therapy, but they have no role in the diagnosis of osteoporosis.

Exclude underlying causes

An underlying cause for osteoporosis is present in approximately 1/3 of women and over 1/2 of men with osteoporosis. Many of the underlying causes (🕮 see Box 72.1, pp. 407–408) should be apparent from a careful history and physical examination.

A few basic investigations are useful to exclude the more common underlying causes. Other investigations may be needed to exclude other specific conditions (see Box 72.2).

It is most helpful to target these investigations at those people who have a lower-than-expected bone mass for their age (Z score < –2).

Monitoring therapy

Repeat bone densitometry is advocated by most, depending on cost and availability. A time interval of 18 months to 2 years is recommended between scans. However, in certain conditions, e.g., glucocorticoid and

Table 72.1 WHO proposals for diagnosis of postmenopausal osteoporosis

T score	Fragility fracture	Diagnosis
–1		Normal
<–1 but ≥ –2.5		Low bone mass (osteopenia)
<–2.5	No	Osteoporosis
<–2.5	Yes	Established (severe) osteoporosis

Box 72.2 Investigations to exclude an underlying cause of osteoporosis

Useful in most patients
- FBC
- ESR
- Biochemical profile
- Renal function
- Liver function
- Calcium
- Thyroid function
- Testosterone and LH (only in men)
- Vitamin D level

Useful in specific instances
- Estradiol and FSH (in women whose menopausal status is not clear)
- Serum and urine electrophoresis (if raised ESR or plasma globulin is elevated)
- Anti-endomysial antibodies (if any suggestion of celiac disease)
- Other investigations for specific diseases
- Bone turnover markers to assess drug efficacy or compliance and response to treatment

Low-trauma fractures associated with osteoporosis
Any fracture other than those affecting the fingers, toes, or face that is caused by less trauma than a fall from standing height is potentially the result of osteoporosis. Patients suffering this kind of fracture should be considered for investigation and/or treatment for osteoporosis.

post-transplantation bone disease, more frequent measurements may be advocated.

Effective treatment leads to increases of 5–8% at the spine. Bone densitometry may be replaced by biochemical markers as assays improve (e.g., P1NP).

Medical management of osteoporosis

Fracture risk assessment and treatment guidelines are essential to management of osteoporosis. One of the tools is FRAX which was developed by the WHO, in collaboration with a number of centers worldwide, t to evaluate an individual's risk of fracture during the ensuing 10 years.

The population-based data incorporate clinical risk factors such as age, low BMI, smoking, oral glucocorticoid use, previous fractures, parental history of fractures, alcohol intake, rheumatoid arthritis, secondary causes of osteoporosis, and femoral neck BMD. On the basis of these risk factors, which are weighted, a score is calculated that determines an individual's 10-year probability of fracture. FRAX can be viewed online.

The National Osteoporosis Foundation (NOF), with consideration of FRAX, has recently revised its guidelines (see Fig. 72.1).

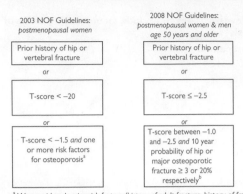

^a We considered major risk factors (history of adult fracture, history of fragility fracture in first degree relative, weight < 127 lbs, current smoking, or oral corticosteroid use for > 3 months) in our application of the 2003 Guidelines. We did not consider additional risk factors (impaired vision, early estrogen deficiency, dementia, frailty, revent falls, low calcium intake, low physical activity, excess alcohol use) in our application of the 2003 Guidelines.

^b Calculated by the FRAX® tool.

Fig. 72.1 NOF guidelines for treatment of osteoporosis: comparison made between old and revised versions. Reprinted with permission from the National Osteoporosis Foundation.

It is recommended that treatment be considered in postmenopausal women or men older than 50 years if they have low bone mass (T score between –1.0 and –2.5) and a 10-year probability of hip fracture ≥3% or a 10-year probability of major osteoporotic-related fracture ≥20%, based on FRAX calculations. These thresholds were determined with heavy emphasis on cost-effectiveness.

These guidelines are not intended to replace clinician judgment and patient preference.

Treatment

Treatments should, whenever possible, be judged by their effect on fracture reduction. Although some treatments are specific to certain clinical situations, there are also general measures that apply to all patients with osteoporosis.

In addition to treatments aimed at improving bone mass, it must be remembered that fractures can be prevented in other ways. Thus it is prudent to try and minimize the risk of falling by adjusting the home environment and reviewing the need for medications such as hypnotics and antihypertensives, antidepressants, proton pump inhibitors, etc.

There is conflicting evidence on the use of wearing hip-protecting pads. These can only be recommended in an institutional setting where compliance can be assured.

Lifestyle measures

- Smoking cessation
- Moderate alcohol consumption. (2 glasses per day)
- Encourage weight-bearing exercise:
  - Impact exercise such as skipping or jumping increases bone mass.
  - Lower-impact exercise, e.g., walking outdoors for 20 minutes 3 × × week may reduce fracture risk.
- Encourage a well-balanced diet.
- Ensure adequate calcium and vitamin D intake: 1000–1200 mg elemental calcium and at least 800 IU vitamin D daily.

Choice of therapy

N-containing bisphosphonates

Either oral or IV agents are the first line of treatment, as they are relatively cheap and are effective in reducing fractures rates by approximately 50% at the spine and hip. They also have a very long history of patient exposure to the drug in clinical practice. Patients who cannot take these drugs orally may benefit from IV preparations.

HRT

The use of estrogen or combined estrogen progesterone preparations has fallen off as a result of the findings of the Women's Health Initiative studies (WHI). The data showed an increased risk of breast cancer and stroke that outweighed the benefits of reduction in hip fracture.

The results are still considered controversial and it is recommended that estrogen be given for the shortest possible time and in the smallest effective dose to control postmenopausal symptoms, e.g., hot flashes, and other therapies, e.g., bisphosphonates, be given as first line for osteoporosis management.

Other agents

Raloxifene is recommended in females who have mainly spinal osteoporosis and who are at risk or have a history of breast cancer. It is not effective in reducing nonvertebral fractures, including hip.

Table 72.2 Drug treatments available

Treatment	Effective dose	Spine BMD	#	Hip BMD	#
HRT					
Oral	2 mg E20 or .625 mg conjugated estrogens	++	?	++	↓
Transdermal	50 mcg daily		↓		
SERMs					
Raloxifene	60 mg daily	+	↓	+	-
Bisphosphonates					
Alendronic acid	10 mg daily/70 mg weekly with or without vitamin D combined	++	↓	++	↓
Risedronate	5 mg daily/70 mg weekly/ 150 mg monthly	++	↓	+	↓
Ibandronic acid	150 mg orally monthly or 3 mg IV every 3 months	++	↓	+	-
Zoledronic acid	5 mg by slow IV infusion once a year for 3 years	++	↓	++	↓
Calcium and vitamin D	1 g + 20 mcg (800 IU)	+	–/↓	+	↓
Calcitonin					
SC or IM		+	?	?	?
Nasal	200 IU daily	+	↓	?	?
Calcitriol	0.25 mcg 2x day	+	↓	?	?
Parathyroid hormone 1-34	20 mcg/daily for median of 19 months	+++	↓	+	-
SC injections					

*No RCT evidence

However, it may be useful in patients in whom bisphosphonates are contraindicated or who are intolerant of the medication.

Calcitonin given as a nasal spray is not a very effective anti-osteoporotic therapy but may reduce spinal fractures in selected patients.

Strontium ranelate, although used elsewhere, is not approved in the United States. *Calcitriol* is also not approved for therapy of osteoporosis in the United States.

Denosumab (Prolia) is a RANK ligand inhibitor indicated for the treatment of postmenopausal women with osteoporosis at high risk of fracture. In a 3-year randomized, double-blind, placebo-controlled trial in 7808 women aged 60–91 years, denosumab decreased new vertebral fractures by a relative risk reduction of 68%, hip fractures by 40%, and nonvertebral fractures by 20%. All fracture reductions were significant.

It must be administered by a health care professional. The dosage is 60 mg every 6 months as an SC injection in the upper arm, upper thigh, and abdomen. Patients should also take 1000 mg calcium and at least 400 IU vitamin D daily.

Physicians should check serum calcium, as it must not be administered in the presence of hypoclacemia. Adverse events include skin infections and osteonecrosis of the jaw. As with other antiosteoporotic drugs, it should not be given to pregnant or lactating women.

Teriparatide is reserved for use in postmenopausal females with severe osteoporosis at high risk of fracture (previous fractures, multiple risk factors, failure or intolerance of previous therapy).

Glucocorticoid-induced osteoporosis

Glucocorticoid treatment is one of the major secondary causes of osteoporosis (Boxes 72.3, 72.4). Not all patients receiving steroid treatment lose bone, and it is not clear what determines this.

There is some suggestion that patients on corticosteroids may have bones that are more fragile than would be suggested by the BMD. It is often suggested that such patients be treated at a higher bone density than would be case for other causes of osteoporosis (Box 72.5).

Box 72.3 Most common form of secondary osteoporosis

- Use in general population between 0.5 and 1.7 % in postmenopausal women >55 years
- Incidence ~ 50% in all patients treated >6 months
- Estimated fracture incidence at spine and ribs in patients on long-term use is 15–40%
- Risk of hip fracture doubled in glucocorticoid users

Box 72.4 Etiological factors for glucocorticoid-induced osteoporosis

- Doses of 5 mg or greater for >3 months
- Underlying disease itself, e.g., rheumatoid arthritis
- Inhibition of sex steroids
- Inhibition of calcium absorption, loss in the urine
- Secondary hyperparathyroidism ???
- Direct effect on bone cells leading to increased apoptosis of osteoblasts and osteocytes

Box 72.5 Management of glucocorticoid osteoporosis

- DXA in patients receiving or will receive glucocorticoids for 3 months or more
- Intervene at T scores of −1 (American College of Rheumatology) or −1.5 (Royal College of Physicians)
- Decrease dose of glucocorticoids as rapidly as possible
- Replace sex hormones if hypogonadal
- Calcium and vitamin D
- Bisphosphonates
- Human PTH with or without HRT

Complications of therapy

HRT

Because of adverse effects (breast cancer, venous thromboembolism, coronary disease, and stroke), HRT is no longer recommended as primary treatment for osteoporosis in normal postmenopausal women.

When a woman is receiving HRT for climacteric symptoms it will provide protection to her skeleton for the duration of treatment. Skeletal protection is rapidly lost on cessation of HRT.

In women with a premature menopause, HRT remains the most appropriate means of preventing bone loss in the absence of other contraindications (e.g., breast cancer) (see Box 72.6).

Women who are unable to take conventional HRT might be able to take progestogens alone (e.g., norethisterone 5 mg daily); several of these agents have been shown to have bone-sparing properties.

Box 72.6 Special considerations in premenopausal women

- Osteoporosis in premenopausal women is rare but well recognized. The Z score should be used.
- It is important to exclude underlying causes of bone loss.
- Osteoporosis can very rarely occur in conjunction with pregnancy or lactation. This is frequently self-limiting and usually requires little treatment other than calcium supplementation.
- In the absence of a pre-existing fracture and continued menses, fracture risk is low. Frequently, all that is needed is calcium and vitamin D supplementation and lifestyle advice until the menopause, when more active therapy is needed to counteract menopausal bone loss.
- In other situations, particularly when fractures are present, most of the therapies that are used in postmenopausal women, with the exception of HRT, can be used (although not approved).
- Some caution needs to be exercised with the use of bisphosphonates in younger people:
  - Teratogenic in animals
  - Long skeletal retention time, making their long-term use cautious

An alternative strategy is to give no treatment unless there is an osteoporotic fracture if the BMD is stable over 2–4 years.

Bisphosphonates

- Difficult dosing schedules to avoid complexing with calcium in GI tract
- GI disturbance, including nausea, gastritis, esophagitis, and diarrhea
- ↑ Bone pain
- Osteonecrosis of jaw
- Atrial fibrillation but no cause and effect found
- Flu-like symptoms following IV administration
- Possible association with atypical subtrochanteric fractures

Calcium and vitamin D
- Constipation
- Hypercalciuria
- Very rarely hypercalcemia

Calcitonin
- Parenteral administration
- Flushing
- Nausea and diarrhea

Side effects are less marked following nasal administration. When given in doses of 50–100 units IM or 200 units nasally daily, it has analgesic properties and can be used in the management of acute fracture pain.

Calcitriol
This has a risk of hypercalcemia and requires regular (ideally every 6 months) plasma calcium measurements.

Raloxifene
- Similar increase in risk of venous thrombosis as HRT
- May induce or worsen climacteric symptoms
- Reduces risk of breast cancer

Strontium ranelate (not approved in the U.S.)
- Diarrhea
- Venous thromboembolism
- Strontium is incorporated into bone making bone densitometry difficult to interpret.
- It may affect measurement of calcium in plasma.

Teriparatide
- Contraindcations include hypercalcemia, renal impairment unexplained elevation of alkaline phosphatase, Paget's disease, prior irradiation.
- Risk of hypercalcemia is not great and no specific monitoring of treatment is needed.
- Vomiting
- Leg cramps
- ↑ Risk of osteosarcoma seen in rats given teriparatide for most of their life. Black box warning in package insert. It should be avoided in patients with ↑ risk of bone tumors (Paget's disease, raised alkaline phosphatase, previous skeletal radiotherapy).

Male osteoporosis
Osteoporosis is less common in men for the following reasons:
- Greater accumulation of bone mass during growth
- Greater bone size and strength
- Absence of a distinct equivalent of menopause
- Shorter life expectancy
- Lesser propensity to fall

Box 72.7 Special considerations in men

- Secondary causes of osteoporosis are more common in men and need to be excluded in all men with osteoporotic fracture.
- Bisphosphonates benefit bone mass in men in a similar way to postmenopausal women.
- Hypogonadal men show an improvement in bone mass on testosterone replacement. This can be used as primary treatment in hypogonadal men. However, hypogonadal men respond to bisphosphonates the same as those with normal testosterone levels.
- Parathyroid hormone SC injections have also been shown to be beneficial in improving BMD.

Box 72.8 BMD testing in males: recommendations

- Men over the age of 50 who have suffered a fracture or with a vertebral deformity
- Men with secondary causes of osteoporosis, e.g., glucocorticoids
- Screening BMD measures recommended for men over 70 years—cost-effectiveness?
- Ideally, male reference range to grade risk is desirable.

Causes of increased bone mineral density

Artifacts
- Excess skeletal calcium (lumbar spondylosis, ankylosing spondylitis)
- Extra skeletal calcium (vascular, gallstones)
- Vertebral fracture
- Radiodense material (surgical implants, strontium)

Focal increase in bone
- Paget's disease
- Tumors (e.g., hemangioma, Hodgkins, plasmacytoma)

Generalized increase in bone
- Acquired osteosclerosis (general osteodystrophy, fluorosis, mastocytosis, hepatitis C, myelofibrosis, acromegaly)

Genetic sclerosing bone dysplasias
- ↓ Absorption (e.g., osteopetrosis)
- ↑ Formation (e.g., sclerosteosis)
- Disturbed balance of formation and resorption

Further reading

Black DM, Delmas, PD, Eastell R, et al. (2007). Once-yearly zoledronic acid for treatment of post-menopausal osteoporosis. *N Engl J Med* 356(18):1809–1822.

Cranney A, Tugwell P, Wells G, et al. (2002). Meta-analyses of therapies for postmenopausal osteoporosis. I. Systematic reviews of randomized trials in osteoporosis: induction and methodology. *Endocr Rev* 23(4):496–507.

Cummings S, San Martin J, McClung M, et al. (2009). Denosumab for prevention of fractures in postmenopausal women with osteoporosis *N Engl J Med* 361:756–765.

Ebeling PR (2008). Osteoporosis in men *N Engl J Med* 358:1474–1482.

Khosla S, et al. (2008). Osteoporosis in men. *Endocr Rev* 29:441–464.

Meunier PJ, Roux C, Seeman E, et al. (2004). The effects of strontium ranelate on the risk of vertebral fracture in women with postmenopausal osteoporosis. *N Engl J Med* 350(5):459–468.

National Osteoporosis Foundation: Clinician's guide to prevention and treatment of osteoporosis. Available at: http://www.nof.org/professionals/Clinicians_Guide.htm. Acessed Jan 2010.

Sambrook P, Cooper C (2006). Osteoporosis. *Lancet* 367(9527);2010–2028.

Paget's disease

Paget's disease is the result of greatly ↑ local bone turnover, which occurs particularly in the middle-aged or elderly.

Pathology

The primary abnormality in Paget's disease is gross overactivity of the osteoclasts, resulting in greatly ↑ bone resorption. This secondarily results in ↑ osteoblastic activity. The new bone is laid down in a highly disorganized manner and leads to the characteristic pagetic abnormality, with irregular packets of woven bone being apparent on biopsy and disorganized internal architecture of the bone on plain radiographs.

Paget's disease can affect any bone in the skeleton but is most frequently found in the pelvis, vertebral column, femur, skull, and tibia. In most patients it affects several sites, but in about 20% of cases a single bone is affected (monostotic disease).

Typically, the disease will start in one end of a long bone and spread along the bone at a rate of about 1 cm per year. Although it can spread within an affected bone, it appears that the pattern of disease is fixed by the time of clinical presentation, and it is exceedingly rare for new bones to become involved during the course of the disease.

Paget's disease alters the mechanical properties of the bone. Thus, pagetic bones are more likely to bend under normal physiological loads and liable to fracture.

This can take the form of complete fractures, which tend to be transverse, rather than the more common spiral fractures of long bones. More frequently, fissure or incremental fractures are seen on the convex surface of bowed pagetic bones. These may be painful in their own right but are also liable to proceed to complete fracture.

Pagetic bones are also larger than their normal counterparts. This can lead to ↑ arthritis at adjacent joints and to pressure on nerves, producing neurological compression syndromes and, when it occurs in the skull base, sensorineural deafness.

Etiology of Paget's disease

The etiology is unclear. There are two major theories.

Familial
• Some genetic associations, especially with sequestomma at 18q.
• These are not invariable.

Viral
• Inclusion bodies similar to those seen in viral infections are present in pagetic osteoclasts.

- Some investigators have found paramyxoviral (measles or canine distemper) protein or nucleic acid in pagetic bone.
- Others are not able to replicate this.

Epidemiology

Paget's disease is present in about 2% of the UK population over the age of 55. Its prevalence increases with age and it is more common in men than women. Only about 10% of affected patients will have symptomatic disease.

It is most common in the UK or in migrants of British descent in North America and Australasia, but is rare in Africa. Recent studies in the UK and New Zealand have suggested that the prevalence may be declining with time.

Clinical features

- 90% asymptomatic
- The most notable feature is pain. This is frequently multifactorial:
  - ↑ Metabolic activity of the bone
  - Changes in bone shape
  - Fissure fractures
  - Nerve compression
  - Arthritis
- Pagetic bones tend to increase in size or to become bowed (16% cases): bowing can be so severe as to interfere with function.
- Fractures (either complete or fissure) are present in 10%.

Investigation

The diagnosis of Paget's disease is primarily radiological (Box 73.1)

Box 73.1 Radiological features of Paget's disease

Early disease—primarily lytic
- V-shaped 'cutting cone ' in long bones
- Osteoporosis circumscripta in skull

Combined phase (mixed lytic and sclerotic)
- Cortical thickening
- Loss of corticomedullary distinction
- Accentuated trabecular markings

Late phase—primarily sclerotic
- Thickening of long bones
- Increase in bone size
- Sclerosis

An isotope bone scan is frequently helpful in assessing the extent of skeletal involvement with Paget's disease. It is particularly important to identify Paget's disease in a weight-bearing bone because of the risk of fracture. The uptake of tracer depends on the disease activity, and isotope bone scans can also be used to assess the response to therapy.

In active disease, plasma alkaline phosphatase activity is usually (85%) elevated. An exception to this is in monostotic disease, when there may be insufficient bone involved to raise the enzyme levels above normal.

Alkaline phosphatase activity responds to successful treatment. There is little advantage in using the more modern markers of bone turnover over the total alkaline phosphatase activity for the monitoring of pagetic activity. A possible exception to this is in patients with liver disease, where changes in bone alkaline phosphatase might be masked by the liver isoenzyme.

Complications

Deafness is present in up to 1/2 of cases of skull base Paget's. Other neurological complications are rare. These can include the following:

- Compression of other cranial nerves with skull base disease
- Spinal cord compression is most common with involvement of the thoracic spine and is thought to result as much from a vascular steal syndrome as from physical compression. It frequently responds to medical therapy without need for surgical decompression.
- Platybasia, which can lead to an obstructive hydrocephalus that may require surgical drainage

Osteogenic sarcoma:

- Very rare complication of Paget's disease
- Rarely amenable to treatment
- Presents with ↑ pain and radiological evidence of tumor, and a mass

Any increase of pain in a patient with Paget's disease should arouse suspicion of sarcomatous degeneration. A more common cause, however, is resumption of activity of disease.

Pagetic sarcomas are most frequently found in the humerus or femur but can affect any bone involved with Paget's disease.

Treatment

Treatment with agents that decrease bone turnover reduces disease activity as indicated by bone turnover markers and isotope bone scans. There is evidence to suggest that such treatment leads to the deposition of histologically normal bone.

Although such treatment has been shown to help pain, there is little evidence that it benefits the other consequences of Paget's disease. In particular, the deafness of Paget's disease does not regress after treatment, although its progression may be halted.

Nonetheless, it has become generally accepted to treat patients in the hope that future complications of the disease will be avoided. Typical indications for treatment of Paget's disease are listed in Box 73.2.

The bisphosphonates have become the mainstay of treatment (Table 73.1). Calcitonin and plicamycin are no longer used.

Patients should also be fully replete in both calcium and vitamin D before and during treatment.

Goals of treatment

- Normalize bone turnover
- Alkaline phosphatase in normal range
- The more aggressive the initial therapy, the longer the disease remission.
- Minimize symptoms
- Prevent long-term complications
- No actual evidence that treatment achieves this

Box 73.2 Indications for treating Paget's disease

- Pain
- Neurological complications (e.g., deafness, spinal cord compression)
- Disease in weight-bearing bones
- Prevention of long-term complications (e.g., bone deformation, osteoarthritis)
- Young patients
- In preparation for surgery
- Hypercalcemia
- Following fracture

Table 73.1 Biophosphonates licensed in the U.S. for Paget's disease

Drug	Dose	Duration of treatment	Side effects
Etidronate	5 mg/kg per day orally in middle of 4-hour fast (max 400 mg)	6 months	Nausea Diarrhea Bone pain ↑ Focal osteomalacia
Pamidronate	3 x 60 mg IV infusion or 6 x 30 mg IV infusion	2-week interval Weekly interval	Influenza-like symptoms ↑ Bone pain\ritis
Risedronate	30 mg orally on rising and wait 30 minutes before breakfast	2 months	Increased bone pain Nausea
Tiludronate	400 mg/day and wait 2 hours before food in the morning	3 months, and 3 months post- treatment observation period	Increased bone pain Nausea
Zoledronic acid	5 mg IV	Single dose	Flu-like symptoms ↑ Bone pain
Alendronate	40 mg orally on rising, wait 30 minutes upright before eating	6 months	Upper GI side effects Bone pain

Monitoring therapy

• Plasma alkaline phosphatase every 6 months
• Clinical assessment

Re-treat if symptoms recur with objective evidence of disease recurrence (alkaline phosphatase or positive isotope scan). If treating for asymptomatic disease, re-treat if alkaline phosphatase increases 25% > nadir.

Further reading

Bilezikian, JP, Watts JT Jr, Fuleihan Gel-H, et al. (2002). Summary statement from a workshop on asymptomatic primary hyperparathyroidism: a perspective for the 21st century. *J Clin Endocrinol Metab* 87(12):5353–5561.

Davies M, Fraser WD, Hosking DJ (2002). The management of primaryhyperparathyroidism. *Clin Endocrinol (Oxf)* 57(2):145–155.

Ralston SH, et al (2008). Pathogenous and management of Paget's disease of Core. 372:155–163.

Selby PL, Davie MW, Ralston SH, et al. (2002). National Association for the Relief of Paget's Disease: guidelines on the management of Paget's disease of the bone. *Bone* 31(3):366–373.

Inherited disorders of bone

Osteogenesis imperfecta

Osteogenesis imperfecta is an inherited form of osteoporosis in which there is a genetic defect in one of the two genes (*COLIA1* and *COLIA2*) encoding the α-chain of collagen type I collagen production.

Several different mutations are recognized, and these produce different clinical pictures. These are generally separated into four and, more recently, seven different types (📖 see Table 74.1).

In addition to the osteoporosis and easy-fracture predisposition, there may also be abnormalities of the teeth (dentigenesis imperfecta), blue sclerae, hearing loss, hypermobility, and cardiac valvular lesions.

Radiological features include the following:
• Generalized osteopenia
• Multiple fractures with deformity
• Abnormal shape of long bones
• Wormian bones in skull

Diagnosis
• Features (as above) and family history
• Analysis of collagen type I genes (detect 90%)
• Differential diagnosis includes Brock syndrome, panostotic fibrous dysplasia, hyper- and hypophatasia, and idiopathic juvenile osteoporosis.

There are three criteria:
• Three fragility fractures aged <20 years
• At least one of the following: blue sclerae, scoliosis, hearing loss, joint laxity, dentinogenesis imperfecta, and affected family member
• Osteoporosis

Recent studies have demonstrated that infusions of pamidronate lead to ↑ bone mass and reduced fracture incidence in affected children. Patients with milder disease might only be recognized in adulthood. It appears that oral bisphosphonates may be helpful in their disease management.

Prenatal diagnosis of severe types is possible from US, and genetic counseling should be offered to at-risk families.

Further reading
Rauch F, Glorieux FH (2004). Osteogenesis imperfecta. *Lancet* 363(9418):1377–1385.

Table 74.1 Classification of osteogenesis imperfecta

Type	Inheritance	Stature	Teeth	Sclerae	Hearing	Genetic defect
I	AD	Normal	Normal	Blue	Variable loss	Substitution for glycine in COL1A1 and COL1A2
II	AD/AR	Lethal deformity				Rearrangement of COL1A1 and COL1A2
III	AD/AR	(Very short severe scaliosis)	Abnormal	Variable (growth)	Loss common	Glycine substitution is COL1A1 and COL1A2
IV	AD	Mild	Abnormal	Normal	Occasional loss	Point mutations in a2(l) or a1(l)

Part 7

Pediatric endocrinology

Kristen Nadeau

Growth and stature

Growth

Regulation of growth
Normal human growth can be divided into three overlapping stages (the Karlberg model), each under the control of different factors.

Infancy
Growth is largely under nutritional regulation, and wide interindividual variation in rates of growth is seen. Many infants show significant "catch-up" or "catch-down" in weight and length, and by 2 years, length is much more predictive of final adult height than at birth.

Childhood
Growth is regulated by growth hormone (GH) and thyroxine. It is characterized by alternating periods of mini-growth spurts with intervening stasis, each phase lasting several weeks. However, over years, a child will tend to maintain their centile position on height charts with a height velocity between the 25th and 75th centiles.

Puberty
The combination of GH and sex hormones promotes bone maturation and a rapid growth acceleration, or growth spurt. In both sexes estrogen eventually causes epiphyseal fusion, resulting in the attainment of final height.

Sex differences
Adult heights differ between men and women by on average 13 cm. During childhood, onset of the pubertal growth spurt is earlier in girls, who are thus on average taller than boys between the ages of 10–13 years.

Tempo
Within each sex there may also be marked interindividual differences in tempo of growth (or rate of attainment of final height) and the timing of puberty. Delay or advance of bone maturation is linked with timing of puberty. Constitutional delay in growth and puberty often runs in families, reflecting probable genetic factors.

Comparison of bone age (estimated from a hand and wrist radiograph) with chronological age is thus an important part of growth assessment.

Final height
Final height is estimated as the height reached when growth velocity slows to <2 cm/year and can be confirmed by finding epiphyseal fusion on hand or wrist radiograph ± knee radiograph.

Final height is largely genetically determined, and a target height can be estimated in each individual from their parent's heights.

Assessment of growth

Measurement

From birth to 2 years old, supine length is measured ideally using a meas- uring board (e.g., Harpenden neonatometer). Two adults are needed to ensure that the child is lying straight with legs extended.

From 2 years old, standing height is measured against a wall-mounted or free-standing stadiometer with the measurer applying moderate upward neck traction and the child looking forward in the horizontal plane.

To minimize error in the calculation of height velocity (cm/year), height measurements should be taken at least 6 months apart using the same equipment and by the same person.

Measurement of sitting height and comparison with leg length (standing height − sitting height) allows an estimate of body proportion.

Growth charts (Figs. 75.1 and 75.2)

Height and weight velocity should be compared to age- and sex-appropri- ate reference data by plotting values on standard growth charts (e.g., US 2000 CDC Growth Charts: http://www.cdc.gov/growthcharts/).

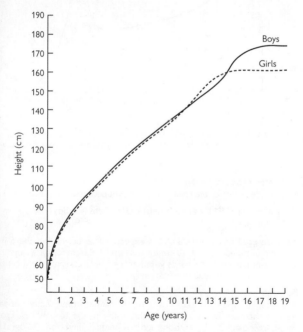

Fig. 75.1 Typical individual height-attained curves for boys and girls (supine length to the ages of 2; integrated curves of Fig. 75.2).

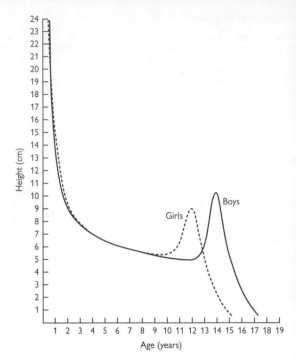

Fig. 75.2 Typical individual velocity curves for supine length or height in boys and girls. These curves represent the velocity of the typical boy and girl at any given instant.

Mid-parental height (MPH)

MPH is an estimate of the child's genetic height potential and is calculated as

[(mother's height + father's height)/2] + 7 cm (for boys) or − 7 cm (for girls).

It can be used to estimate a child's expected final height, but there is a wide target range (MPH ± 10 cm for boys and ± 8.5 cm for girls), and it is more commonly used to assess whether the child's current height centile is consistent with genetic expectation.

Bone age

Skeletal maturation proceeds in an orderly manner from the first appearance of each epiphyseal center to the fusion of the long bones. From chronological age 3–4 years, bone age may be quantified from radiographs of the left hand and wrist by comparison with standard photographs (e.g.,

Greulich and Pyle method) or by an individual bone scoring system (e.g., Tanner–Whitehouse method).

The difference between bone age and chronological age is an estimation of tempo of growth. The initiation of puberty usually coincides with a bone age around 10.5–11 years in girls and 11–11.5 years in boys, although the correlation between bone age and pubertal timing is approximate.

Girls reach skeletal maturity at a bone age of 15 years and boys when bone age is 17 years. Thus, bone age allows an estimation of remaining growth potential and can be used to aid in the prediction of final adult height.

Final height prediction

Predictions of final height can be derived from information on current height, age, pubertal status, and bone age using calculations described by Tanner and Whitehouse, or Bailey and Pinneau, among others (📖 see Further reading, p. 446, De Waal et al., 1996).

Secular trends

Population growth references used should be appropriate to the population studied and may occasionally need to be updated.

Short stature

Definition

Short stature is defined as height at least 2 standard deviations (SD) below the mean for age and sex or at least 2 SD below the predicted MPH. However, abnormalities of growth may be present long before attained height falls below this level and may be detected much earlier by assessing growth velocity and observing height measurements

Assessment

History
- Who is concerned, the child or parents?
- What are the parental heights?
- Has the child always been small, or does the history suggest recent growth failure? Try to obtain previous measurements (e.g., from parents, primary care physician, school).

Ask about maternal illness in pregnancy, drug intake and possible substance abuse in pregnancy, gestation at delivery, size at birth (weight, length, and head circumference), childhood illnesses, medication, and developmental milestones.
- Conduct a systematic inquiry regarding headaches, visual disturbance, asthma and respiratory symptoms, abdominal symptoms, and diet.
- Is there a family history of short stature or pubertal delay?
- What are the psychosocial circumstances of the child and the family?

Examination
- Assess height and height velocity over at least 6 months.
- Measure sitting height and derive subischial leg length (standing height – sitting height [cm] if skeletal disproportion suspected).
- Assess for the presence and severity of chronic disease. Low weight-for-height suggests a nutritional diagnosis, GI cause, or other significant systemic disease.
- Pubertal stage using Tanner's criteria
- Observe for dysmorphic features and signs of endocrinopathy, and presence and severity of chronic disease.
- Measure parents' heights and calculate MPH.

Investigations

Laboratory tests should include CBC, ESR, electrolytes, thyroid function, calcium, phosphate, tissue transglutaminase antibodies, IGF-1 and IGF BP-3 levels, karyotype (of particular importance in girls), and urinalysis.

The following tests may also be clinically indicated: GH provocation testing (e.g., arginine, clonidine, or glucagon) (see Table 75.1) with other anterior pituitary function tests, MRI scan with specific reference to the hypothalamus and pituitary, skeletal survey (for bone dysplasia), and, very rarely, an IGF-1 generation test (📖 for GH resistance, see Growth hormone deficiency, p. 437).

Table 75.1 Comparison of GH provocation tests

	l-arginine (IV)	Clonidine (oral)	Glucagon (IM)
Advantages	Safe	Simple and safe	Safe Also tests ACTH-cortisol axis
Disadvantages	Requires IV infusion	Postural hypotension and somnolence	Nausea may last 3–4 hours Possible late hypoglycemia

Other agents (e.g., L-dopa or Insulin) are less commonly used. Measurement of GH levels after exercise has poor sensitivity and specificity for detecting GH deficiency.

Causes

- Genetic short stature
- Constitutional delay in growth and puberty
  - These first two together account for ~40% of cases.
- Chronic illness (including untreated celiac disease, congenital heart disease, chronic renal failure, inflammatory bowel disease)
- Psychosocial deprivation (which may be associated with reversible GH deficiency)
- Small for gestational age (SGA), including intrauterine growth restriction (IUGR) (7.5%).
- Dysmorphic syndromes (e.g., Turner's, Noonan, or Down syndrome)
- Malnutrition

GH deficiency (8%)

- Undefined etiology (idiopathic, including those with abnormal pituitary morphology on MRI)
- Congenital malformation in the hypothalamus and pituitary (HP) (e.g., septo-optic dysplasia) or acquired HP disorders (e.g., craniopharyngioma, trauma), the GH-1 gene or GH-releasing hormone receptor gene, or rarely, mutations in transcription factors controlling pituitary development
- GH resistance (rare genetic mutations in the GH receptor or GH signaling molecules)
- Endocrine disorders (hypothyroidism, hypoparathyroidism, Cushing's syndrome)

Other

- Skeletal dysplasia (e.g., achondroplasia, hypochondroplasia)
- Metabolic bone disease (e.g., nutritional or hypophosphatemic rickets)

Genetic short stature

Although stature does not follow strict Mendelian laws of inheritance, it does relate to parental height and is probably a polygenic trait. It should be remembered that short parents may themselves have an unidentified dominantly inherited condition (e.g., hypochondroplasia).

Constitutional delay of growth and puberty

Clinical features

This condition often presents in adolescence but may also be recognized in earlier childhood and is more prevalent in boys.

Characteristic features include short stature and delay in pubertal development by >2 SD and/or bone age delay in an otherwise healthy child. In the adolescent years, short sitting height percentile compared to that of leg length is typical. There is often a family history of delayed puberty.

Bone age delay may also develop in a number of other conditions, but in constitutional delay, bone age delay usually remains consistent over time, and height velocity is normal for the bone age. Final height may not reach target height.

GH secretion is usually normal, although provocation tests should be primed by prior administration of exogenous sex hormones if bone age is >10 years.

Management

Often only reassurance is necessary. Treatment is sometimes indicated in adolescent boys who have difficulty coping with their short stature or delayed sexual maturation.

- For the older boy (>14 years) with concerns about puberty: testosterone (50–100 mg IM, monthly for 3–6 months)
- For the older girl (>13 years) with concerns about puberty: estradiol (0.5 mcg qod for 3–6 months) or Premarin 0.3 mg qod.

Growth hormone deficiency

Primary GH deficiency

Primary GH deficiency is usually sporadic, but rarely it may be inherited as autosomal dominant, recessive, or X-linked recessive and may be associated with other pituitary hormone deficiencies. It may represent a defect in homeobox genes (e.g., *Pit1* [leading to GH, TSH, and PRL deficiency], *Prop1* [leading to GH, TSH, PRL, gonadotropin, and later ACTH deficiencies], or *Hesx1*) that control HP development.

Mutation in *Hesx1* has been associated with midline defects, such as optic nerve hypoplasia and corpus callosum defects (i.e., septo-optic dysplasia). GH deficiency usually arises because of failure of release of GHRH from the hypothalamus.

Clinical features

Infancy

GH deficiency may present with hypoglycemia. Coexisting ACTH, TSH, and gonadotropin deficiencies may cause prolonged hyperbilirubinemia and micropenis. Size may be normal, as fetal and infancy growth are more dependent on nutrition and other growth factors than on GH.

Childhood

Typical features include slow growth velocity, short stature, ↓ muscle mass, and ↑ SC fat. Underdevelopment of the mid-facial bones, relative protrusion of the frontal bones because of mid-facial hypoplasia, delayed dental eruption, and delayed closure of the anterior fontanelle may be seen. These children have delayed bone age and delayed puberty.

Secondary GH deficiency

Brain tumors and cranial irradiation

Pituitary or hypothalamic tumors may impair GH secretion, and deficiencies of other pituitary hormones may coexist. Cranial irradiation, used to treat intracranial tumors, facial tumors, and acute leukemia, may also cause GH deficiency.

Risk of HP damage is related to total dose administered, fractionation (single dose more toxic than divided), location of the irradiated tissue, and age (younger children are more sensitive to radiation damage).

GH secretion is most sensitive to radiation damage, followed by gonadotropins, TSH, and ACTH. Central precocious puberty may also occur and may mask GH deficiency by promoting growth but will compromise final height if untreated. At-risk children should therefore be screened regularly by careful examination and multiple pituitary hormone testing.

These survivors of childhood cancer may also have other endocrine problems, including gonadal damage related to concomitant chemotherapy or radiation scatter, hypothyroidism related to spinal radiation, or glucose intolerance related to total body irradiation. It is recommended that all such patients undergo endocrine surveillance.

Psychosocial deprivation

Severe psychosocial deprivation may cause reversible disturbance of GH secretion and growth failure. GH secretion improves within 3 weeks of hospitalization or removal from the adverse environment and catch-up growth is often dramatic (see Fig. 75.3), although these children may continue to exhibit other features of emotional disturbance.

Treatment of GH deficiency (Fig. 75.4)

Recombinant human GH has been available since 1985 and is administered by daily SC injection.

Dose

The replacement dose for childhood GH deficiency is 0.3 mg/kg per week, divided into 7 days/week. Catch-up growth is optimized if GH is commenced early. A higher dose can be used in puberty, reflecting the normal elevation in GH levels at Tanner stage 3–4.

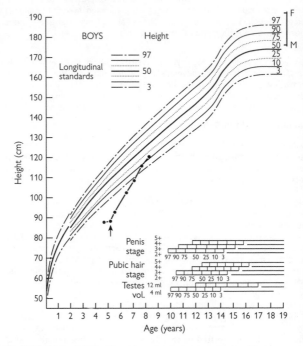

Fig. 75.3 Height of child with psychosocial short stature. Note catch-up on removal, marked by arrow, from parental home. Reprinted with permission from Brook C (2001). *Brook's Clinical Pediatric Endocrinology*. Wiley-Blackwell.

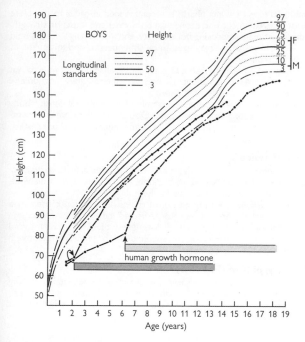

Fig. 75.4 Heights of two brothers with isolated GH deficiency treated with human GH from ages 6 years and 2 years. Catch-up of older brother is partly by high velocity and partly by prolonged growth and is incomplete. Younger brother shows true complete catch-up. F and M, parents' height centiles; vertical thick line, range of expected heights for family. Reprinted with permission from Brook C (2001). *Brook's Clinical Pediatric Endocrinology.* Wiley-Blackwell.

Side effects
Local lipoatrophy and benign intracranial hypertension occur rarely. Slipped upper femoral epiphyses are associated with GH deficiency, but the incidence is similar before or after GH treatment.

Other pituitary hormone deficiencies may be unmasked by GH therapy, and thyroid function should be checked within 4–6 weeks of commencing therapy.

Retesting in adulthood
Once final height is achieved, GH secretion should be retested, as a significant percentage of subjects (25–80%) with GH deficiency in childhood subsequently have normal GH secretion in adulthood.

In those with confirmed GH deficiency, continuation of GH treatment (at a dose of 3–6 mcg/kg/day) through the late adolescent years into early adulthood (the *transition* phase) is recommended in order to complete somatic development (increasing lean body mass and muscular strength, reducing fat mass, improving bone density, and maintaining a healthy lipid profile). GH treatment may need to be continued beyond this phase, as adult GH replacement.

The transition from pediatric to adult care is an important time to not only re-evaluate GH status but also reassess other pituitary function and management of any underlying disorder.

It is also recommended that assessment of bone mineral density, body composition, fasting lipid profile, and QoL by questionnaire be undertaken at this time and repeated at 3- to 5-year intervals for those restarting GH treatment.

GH resistance

GH resistance may arise from primary GH receptor defects or post-receptor defects secondary to malnutrition, liver disease, type 1 diabetes, or, very rarely, circulating GH antibodies.

Laron syndrome is a rare autosomal recessive condition caused by a genetic defect of the GH receptor. Affected individuals have extreme short stature, high levels of GH, low levels of IGF-1, and impaired GH-induced IGF-1 generation (🕮 see Box 75.1, p. 440). Treatment with recombinant IGF-1 is available.

Hypothyroidism (Fig. 75.5)

Congenital primary hypothyroidism is detected by neonatal screening. Hypothyroidism presenting in childhood is usually autoimmune in origin.

Incidence is higher in girls and those with personal or family history of other autoimmune disease.

Box 75.1 GH assessment

GH is normally secreted overnight in regular pulses (pulse frequency 180 minutes). Frequently sampled overnight GH profiles are costly and laborious, thus standardized stimulation tests are more commonly useful.

There can be large variation between different GH assay methods and exact cut-offs must be locally validated.

A number of different agents may be used to stimulate GH secretion (arginine, clonidine, glucagon, or insulin; see Table 75.1, p. 435). All tests should be performed in the morning following an overnight fast, and serial blood samples are collected over 90–180 minutes.

An IGF-1 and IGF BP-3 level should also be measured in the baseline sample, as an additional marker of GH status.

IGF-1 generation test

In those with high basal and stimulated GH levels and low IGF-1 levels, measurement of IGF-1 levels before and following administration of GH 0.1 IU/kg (30 mcg/kg/day) daily SC for 4 days allows an assessment of GH sensitivity and resistance. This test is rarely necessary.

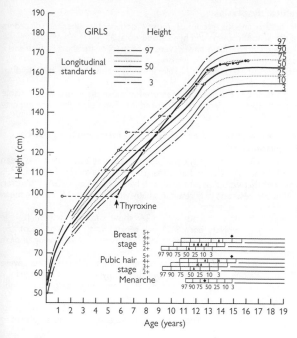

Fig. 75.5 Response of hypothyroid child treated with thyroxine. Solid circles, height for age; open circles, height for bone age. Reprinted with permission from Brook C (2001). *Brook's Clinical Pediatric Endocrinology.* Wiley-Blackwell.

In childhood, hypothyroidism may present with growth failure alone, and bone age is often disproportionately delayed. Very rarely, early puberty may occur.

Investigations show low T_4 and T_3, high TSH, positive anti-thyroglobulin, and antithyroid peroxidase (microsomal) antibodies.

Replacement therapy with oral levothyroxine (100 mcg/m^2 per day titrated with thyroid function) results in catch-up growth unless diagnosis is late.

Celiac disease

This is more common in children with other autoimmune disorders. Although the classical childhood presentation is an irritable toddler with poor weight gain, diarrhea, abdominal pain, and distension, in later childhood poor growth with bone age delay may be the presenting feature.

Measurement of tissue transglutaminase is a valuable screening test, but diagnosis needs to be confirmed by small-bowel biopsy. Catch-up growth usually follows commencement of a gluten-free diet.

Skeletal dysplasias

This heterogeneous group of mostly dominantly inherited disorders includes achondroplasia and hypochondroplasia.

These children usually have severe disproportionate short stature and a positive or suspicious family history.

Radiological assessment by skeletal survey often allows a specific diagnosis to be made.

High-dose GH therapy has been used in these disorders, with variable success. Surgical leg-lengthening procedures before and/or after puberty are also an additional option.

Small for gestational age (SGA) and intrauterine growth restriction (IUGR)

SGA is defined as birth weight and/or length at least 2 SD below the mean for gestational age. *IUGR* is defined as growth failure on serial antenatal US scans, and that would usually lead to a baby being born SGA. However, IUGR in late gestation may result in a baby who is within 2 SD of the mean for birth weight or length.

Ninety percent of infants with SGA show catch-up growth by age 3 years; 8% of subjects born SGA will remain small at 18 years of age. Catch-up growth is more common in infants with relative sparing of birth length and head circumference (>10th centile).

In severe IUGR, length and head circumference are also reduced. Severe IUGR may be due to maternal factors such as hypertension in pregnancy, placental dysfunction, or a wide range of chromosomal or genetic conditions in the fetus.

Russell-Silver syndrome is characterized by severe IUGR, lateral asymmetry, triangular facies, clinodactyly, and extremely poor infancy feeding and postnatal weight gain.

Children with severe IUGR who do not undergo catch-up growth may have early-onset puberty despite bone age delay and therefore achieve a very poor final height.

Numerous epidemiological studies have shown a relationship between low birth weight and an ↑ risk of a number of disorders in later life, including hypertension, ischemic heart disease, cerebrovascular disease, metabolic syndrome, and type 2 diabetes. The risk is ↑ with rapid postnatal weight gain. These associations relate to relatively low birth weight and not exclusively to those born SGA.

Management

GH therapy is used in the SGA/IUGR child who has failed to show catch-up growth by age 3 years. GH (at doses of 0.48 mg/kg/week) can increase growth velocity and final height. The effect of GH on later risk of insulin resistance as type 2 diabetes is not known.

Turner's syndrome

📖 Also see Box 50.1 (p. 258).

Turner's syndrome should always be considered in a girl who is short for her parental target. The classical dysmorphic features may be difficult to identify at younger ages. Karyotype usually confirms the diagnosis.

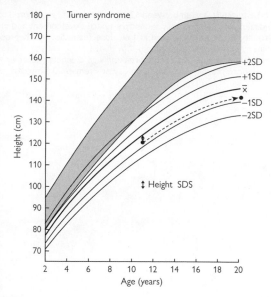

Fig. 75.6 Height SDs for chronological age extrapolated to final height. Reprinted with permission from Brook C (2001). *Brook's Clinical Pediatric Endocrinology*. Wiley-Blackwell.

although sufficient cells (>30) should be examined to exclude the possibility of mosaicism.

Clinical features

There may be a history of lymphedema in the newborn period. Typically, growth velocity starts to decline from 3 to 5 years old (Fig. 75.6) and gonadal failure combined with a degree of skeletal dysplasia results in loss of the pubertal growth spurt.

Mean final height is consistently 7.9 inches below the normal average within each population (4 ft 8 inches in the U.S).

GH secretion is normal, although IGF-1 levels may be low. Ten percent progress through puberty spontaneously but only 1% develop ovulatory cycles.

Management

High-dose *GH therapy* (0.375 mg/kg/week) increases final height, although individual responses are variable. The height gained is related to time on GH treatment, and thus GH therapy should be started early. If the diagnosis has been made in early life, treatment is usually started at 3 to 5 years of age.

Oral *estrogen* is started between 12 and 14 years of age, tailored to the individual patient, to promote secondary sexual development and pubertal growth. It should be started in low dose (estradiol 0.5 mcg qod or Premarin 0.6 mg qod), and gradually ↑ with age.

Progesterone should be added if breakthrough bleeding occurs or when estrogen dose reaches estradiol 1 mg/day or Premarin 0.6 mg/day.

Tall stature and rapid growth

Definition

Although statistically as many children have heights >2 SD above the mean as have heights >2 SD below the mean, referral for evaluation of tall stature is much less common than for short stature.

Socially, for boys heights up to 6 ft 9 in are typically considered acceptable, whereas for girls heights >6 ft may be problematic. Tall stature and particularly accelerated growth rates in early childhood can indicate an underlying hormonal disorder, such as precocious puberty.

For causes, see Box 75.2.

Assessment

History

- Is tall stature long-standing, or does the history suggest recent growth acceleration? Try to obtain previous measurements.
- Inquire about size at birth, infancy weight gain, intellectual development, and neurological development.
- Inquire about headaches, visual disturbance, and evidence of puberty.
- Is there a family history of tall stature or early puberty?

Box 75.2 Causes of tall stature in childhood

Normal variants
- Familial tall stature
- Early maturation (largely familial but also promoted by early-childhood nutrition and obesity. Height is not excessive for bone age, which is advanced)

Hormonal
- See Precocious puberty (p. 449)
- GH or GHRH excess (pituitary gigantism) resulting from pituitary adenoma or ectopic adenomas is a very rare cause of tall stature (📖 p. 110).
- Other hormonal excess, e.g., hyperthyroidism, congenital adrenal hyperplasia (associated with signs of virilization), familial glucocorticoid deficiency
- Rarely, estrogen receptor or aromatase deficiencies delay puberty and epiphyseal fusion, resulting in tall adult height.

Chromosomal abnormalities
- XXY (Klinefelter's syndrome)
- XYY, XYYY (each extra Y confers on average 13 cm additional height)

Other rare syndromes
Overgrowth and dysmorphic features are seen in Marfan syndrome, homocystinuria, Sotos syndrome, Beckwith–Wiedemann syndrome, and Weaver syndrome.

Examination
- Assess height and height velocity over at least 4–6 months.
- Measure sitting height and arm span.
- Pubertal stage?
- Dysmorphic features?
- Measure parents' heights and calculate MPH (📖 see Assessment of growth, p. 445).

Investigations
The following investigations may be clinically indicated:
- Left hand and wrist radiograph for bone age
- Sex hormone levels (testosterone, estrogen, androstenedione, DHEAS), baseline and stimulated LH and FSH levels
- Karyotype
- Serum IGF-1 and IGFBP-3 levels
- Oral glucose tolerance test—GH levels normally suppress to low or undetectable levels (<1 mU/L)
- Specific molecular tests for overgrowth syndromes

Management of tall stature

After excluding abnormal pathology, often only reassurance and information on predicted final height are necessary. In younger children, early induction of puberty using low-dose sex steroids advances the pubertal growth spurt and promotes earlier epiphyseal fusion.

In older children already in puberty, high-dose estrogen therapy in girls, or testosterone in boys, has been used to induce rapid skeletal maturation. However, theoretical side effects of high-dose estrogen therapy include thromboembolic disease and oncogenic risk.

Further reading

Carel JC, Léger J (2008). Precocious puberty *N Engl J Med* 358:2366–2377.

Clayton PE, Cianfarani S, Czernichow P, et al. (2007). Management of the child born small for gestational age child (SGA) through to adulthood: a consensus statement of the International Societies of Paediatric Endocrinology and the Growth Hormone Research Society. *J Clin Endocrinol Metab* 92(3):804–810.

Clayton PE, Cuneo RC, Juul A, et al. (2005). Consensus statement on the management of the GH-treated adolescent in the transition to adult care. *Eur J Endocrinol* 152:165–170.

Dattani M, Preece M (2004). Growth hormone deficiency and related disorders: insights into causation, diagnosis, and treatment. *Lancet* 363:1977–1987.

De Waal WJ, Greyn-Fokker MH, Stijnen T, et al. (1996). Accuracy of final height prediction and effect of growth-reductive therapy in 362 constitutionally tall children. *J Clin Endocrinol Metab* 81:1206–1216.

Growth Hormone Research Society (2000). Consensus guidelines for the diagnosis and treatment of growth (GH) deficiency in childhood and adolescence: summary statement of the GH Research Society. *J Clin Endocrinol Metab* 85:3990–3993.

Saenger P, Wikland KA, Conway GS, et al. (2000). Recommendations for the diagnosis and management of Turner's syndrome. *J Clin Endocrinol Metab* 86:3061–3069.

Puberty

Normal puberty

Puberty is the sequence of physical and physiological changes occurring at adolescence culminating in full sexual maturity.

Age at onset

Average age at onset of puberty is earlier in girls (~11 years) than in boys (~12 years) but varies widely (~±2 years from the mean age of onset) and is influenced by a number of factors:
- *Historical:* Age of menarche has ↓ this century from 17 years in 1900 to 12.8 years today, presumably as a result of improved childhood nutrition and growth.
- *Genetic:* Age at onset of puberty is partly familial.
- *Ethnicity:* Afro-Caribbean girls tend to have earlier puberty than whites.
- *Weight gain:* Earlier puberty is seen in girls who are overweight, whereas girls who engage in strenuous activity and are thin often have delayed puberty.

Hormonal changes prior to and during puberty

Adrenal androgens (DHEAS and androstenedione) rise 2 years before puberty starts (adrenarche). This usually causes no physical changes but occasionally results in early pubic hair and acne (premature adrenarche).

Pulsatile secretion of LHRH from the hypothalamus at night is the first step in the initiation of puberty and occurs well before physical signs of puberty. This results in pulsatile secretion of LH and FSH from the pituitary, and the gonadotropin response to LHRH administration reverses from the prepubertal FSH predominance to a higher response in LH levels.

Physical changes

The first indication of puberty is typically breast development in girls and increase in testicular size in boys. In each sex, puberty then typically progresses in an orderly manner through distinct stages (see Table 76.1).

Puberty rating by an experienced observer involves identification of pubertal stage, particularly breast development in girls and testicular volume (by comparison with an orchidometer) in boys.

Pubertal growth spurt

Increased estrogen levels in both boys and girls lead to ↑ GH secretion. Peak height velocity occurs at puberty stage 2–3 in girls and is later in boys, at stage 3–4 (testicular volume 10–12 mL).

Table 76.1 The normal stages of puberty (Tanner stages)

Boys

Stage	Genitalia	Pubic hair	Other events
I	Prepubertal	Vellus, not thicker than on abdomen	TV* <4 mL
II	Enlargement of testes and scrotum	Sparse long, pigmented strands at base of penis	TV 4–8 mL Voice starts to change
III	Lengthening of penis	Darker, curlier, and spreads over pubis	TV 8–10 mL Axillary hair
IV	Increase in penis length and breadth	Adult-type hair but covering a smaller area	TV 10–15 mL Upper lip hair Peak height velocity
V	Adult shape and size	Spread to medial thighs (Stage 6: spread up linea alba)	TV 15–25 mL Facial hair spreads to cheeks Adult voice

Girls

Stage	Genitalia	Pubic hair	Other events
I	Elevation of papilla only	Vellus, not thicker than on abdomen	
II	Breast bud stage: elevation of breast and papilla	Sparse long, pigmented strands along labia	Peak height velocity
III	Further elevation of breast and areola together	Darker, curlier, and spreads over pubis	
IV	Areola forms a second mound on top of breast	Adult-type hair but covering a smaller area	Menarche
V	Mature stage: areola recedes and only papilla projects	Spread to medial thighs (Stage 6: spread up linea alba)	

*TV, testicular volume: measured by size-comparison with a Prader orchidometer.

Reprinted with permission from Tanner JM (1978). *Growth at Adolescence*, 2nd ed. Wiley-Blackwell.

Precocious puberty

Definition

Early onset of puberty is defined as <8 years in girls and <9 years in boys.

Gonadotropin-dependent ("central" or "true") precocious puberty is characterized by early breast development in girls or testicular enlargement in boys.

Gonadotropin-independent puberty occurs from abnormal peripheral sex hormone secretion, resulting in isolated development of certain secondary sexual characteristics. This may involve autonomous testosterone production in a boy or autonomous estrogen production in a girl. In addition, testosterone production from the adrenal or an ovarian tumor can induce virilization in a girl.

Assessment of precocious puberty

History

- Age when secondary sexual development first noted
- What features are present and in what order did they appear? E.g., virilization (pubic, axillary, or facial hair, acne, body odor), genital or breast enlargement, galactorrhea (very rare), menarche, or cyclical mood changes?
- Is there evidence of recent growth acceleration?
- Family history of early puberty?
- Past history of adoption or early weight gain or prior CNS abnormality or insult (e.g., radiation)?

Examination

- Breast or genital and testicular size; degree of virilization (clitoromegaly in girls indicates abnormal androgen levels)
- Neurological examination, particularly visual field assessment and fundoscopy
- Abdominal or testicular masses
- Skin (?café-au-lait patches —McCune–Albright [see Chapter 85, McCune–Albright syndrome, p. 486], or NF1)
- Assess height and height velocity over 4–6 months.

Investigations

The following investigations may be clinically indicated:

- Radiograph of left wrist and hand for bone age
- Thyroid function
- Sex hormone levels (testosterone, estrogen, androstenedione, DHEAS)
- LH, FSH, and estradiol levels (baseline and after SQ leuprolide)
- 17αOH progesterone levels (baseline and 60 minutes post IV cortrosyn) if congenital adrenal hyperplasia is suspected
- Tumor markers (αFP, βhCG)
- Midnight salivary cortisol
- Abdominal US scan (adrenal glands; ovaries)
- MRI scan (cranial; adrenal glands)

Central precocious puberty

This is due to premature activation of pulsatile LHRH secretion from the hypothalamus, and the normal progression in physical changes is maintained. As precocious puberty is defined as occurring younger than 2 SD before the average age, in a normal distribution, 2.5% of children will have early-onset puberty.

In practice, in girls, central precocious puberty is more likely to be idiopathic or familial, whereas boys have a greater risk of intracranial or other pathology.

Causes

- Idiopathic or familial
- Intracranial tumors, hydrocephalus, or other lesions
- Post–cranial irradiation or trauma
- Intracranial tumors (in particular, optic nerve glioma and hypothalamic germinoma), harmatoma, hydrocephalus, and nonspecific brain injury (e.g., cerebral palsy)
- May also be triggered by long-standing elevation in sex hormones resulting from any peripheral source or adrenal enzyme defect (e.g., late-presenting simple virilizing CAH or inadequately treated CAH)
- Hypothyroidism (elevated TRH stimulates FSH release)—rare
- Gonadotropin-secreting tumors (e.g., pituitary adenoma or hepatoblastoma) are rare.

Treatment

The aims of treatment are as follows:

- Avoid psychosocial problems for the child or family
- Prevent reduced final height due to premature bone maturation and early epiphyseal fusion. A final height prediction is often necessary when considering the need for inhibition of puberty

Pituitary LH and FSH secretion can be inhibited by the use of LHRH analogs, e.g., Lupron 0.3 mg/kg IM monthly (comes as 7.5, 11.25, or 15 mg doses).

Treatment efficacy should be monitored regularly by clinical observation. The dose may need to be increased if there is evidence of inadequate suppression of pubertal development.

Gonadotropin-independent precocious puberty

At least two genetic syndromes have been identified, both resulting in abnormal activation of gonadotropin receptors independent of normal ligand binding. Thus, in these conditions, the gonads autonomously secrete sex hormones and levels of LH and FSH are suppressed by feedback inhibition.

McCune–Albright syndrome

📖 Also see Chapter 85, McCune–Albright syndrome (p. 486). This is a sporadic condition due to a somatic activating mutation of the GSα protein subunit that affects bones (polyostotic fibrous dysplasia) and skin (café-au-lait spots) and potentially contributes to multiple endocrinopathies.

A number of different hormone receptors share the same G protein–coupled cyclic AMP second messenger system, and hyperthyroidism or hyperparathyroidism may also be present.

All cells descended from the mutated embryonic cell-line are affected, while cells descended from nonmutated cells develop into normal tissues. Thus, the phenotype is highly variable in physical distribution and severity. Treatment is with an aromatase inhibitor (letrozole).

Testotoxicosis

This is a rare familial condition resulting in precocious puberty only in boys, due to an activating LH receptor mutation. Testes show only little increase in size and on biopsy Leydig cell hyperplasia is characteristic. Treatment is with a combination of androgen receptor–blocking agents (cyproterone acetate) and aromatase inhibitors or with ketoconazole.

Peripheral sex hormone secretion

Excessive peripheral androgen secretion may occur due to CAH or androgen-secreting adrenal or gonadal tumors. These children usually have rapid growth, advanced bone age, and moderate to severe virilization in the absence of testicular or breast development. (Note: a testicular tumor may cause asymmetrical enlargement).

Peripheral estrogen production from ovarian tumors is a rare cause of precocious breast development in girls.

Premature thelarche

Premature breast development in the absence of other signs of puberty may present at any age from infancy. Breast size may fluctuate and is often asymmetrical.

The cause is unknown, although typically FSH levels (but not LH) are elevated and ovarian US may reveal a single large cyst. Bone maturation, growth rate, and final height are unaffected.

Thelarche variant

This is an intermediate condition between premature thelarche and central precocious puberty. The etiology is unknown.

These girls demonstrate ↑ height velocity and rate of bone maturation and ovarian US reveals a more multicystic appearance, as seen in true puberty. There is probably a whole spectrum of presentations between premature thelarche and true precocious puberty.

The decision to treat should take into account height velocity and final height prediction as well as the rate of physical maturation and the severity of accompanying pubertal features (e.g., mood swings and difficult behavior).

Premature adrenarche and pubarche

The normal onset of adrenal androgen secretion (adrenarche) occurs 1–2 years before the onset of puberty. Premature or exaggerated adrenarche is thought to be due to ↑ androgen production or sensitivity and presents with mild features of virilization, such as onset of pubic hair (pubarche) or acne, in the absence of other features of puberty.

Clitoromegaly in girls suggests a more severe pathology with excessive androgen production (e.g., CAH or androgen-secreting tumor).

The diagnosis is made in the presence of pubic hair and/or axillary hair; the absence of breast or testicular development in children aged <8 years. It is more common in girls.

Management

The management of premature adrenarche usually only requires reassurance after exclusion of other causes, as there is no significant impact on final height and onset or progression of puberty.

Some of these girls may subsequently develop features of polycystic ovary disease. In these cases, treatment should be directed at the presenting feature (e.g., hirsutism, menstrual irregularities).

Delayed or absent puberty

Definition

Delayed puberty is defined as failure to progress into puberty by >2 SD later than the average, i.e., >13 years in girls and >14 years in boys. Clinically, boys are more likely to present with delayed puberty than girls. In addition, some children present with delay in progression from one pubertal stage to the next for >2 years.

Psychological distress may be exacerbated by declining growth velocity relative to that of peers. In the long term, severe delay may be a risk factor for ↓ bone mineral density and osteoporosis.

Causes

General

- Constitutional delay of growth and puberty (this is the most common cause; 📖 see Constitutional delay of growth and puberty, p. 436).
- Chronic childhood disease, malabsorption (e.g., celiac disease, inflammatory bowel disease), or undernutrition

Hypergonadotropic hypogonadism

Gonadal failure may be either of the following:

- Congenital (e.g., Turner's syndrome in girls, Klinefelter's syndrome in boys)
- Acquired (e.g., following chemotherapy, local radiotherapy, infection, torsion)

In these conditions, basal and stimulated gonadotropin levels are raised.

Gonadotropin deficiency

- Kallman syndrome (including anosmia)
- HP lesions (tumors, post-radiotherapy, dysplasia)
- Rare inactivating mutations of genes encoding LH, FSH (or their receptors)

These conditions may also present in the newborn period with micropenis and undescended testes in boys.

Investigation

The following investigations may be clinically indicated:

- LH and FSH levels
- Plasma estrogen or testosterone levels
- Measurement of androgen levels before and after hCG therapy may be used to indicate presence of functional testicular tissue in boys.
- Karyotype
- Pelvic US in girls to determine ovarian morphology
- US or MRI imaging in boys to detect an intra-abdominal testes

It may be difficult to distinguish between constitutional delay and gonado-tropin deficiency, as gonadotropin levels are low in both conditions. In these cases, pharmacological induction of puberty may be indicated with regular assessment of testicular growth in boys (which is independent of testosterone therapy) followed by withdrawal of treatment and reassessment when final height is reached.

Management

Depending on the age and concern of the child and parents, short-course exogenous sex steroids can be used to induce pubertal changes. If gonadotropin deficiency is permanent or the gonads are dysfunctional or absent, then exogenous sex steroids are required to induce and maintain pubertal development (📖 see Constitutional delay of growth and puberty, p. 436).

Long-term treatment

See Table 76.2.

Boys

Testosterone (by IM injection): 50 mg q4–6 weeks, gradually ↑ to 250 mg q4 weeks.

- Monitor penile enlargement, pubic hair, height velocity, and adult body habitus.
- Side effects include severe acne and rarely priapism.

Girls

Estrogen (oral): Start at low dose (estradiol 0.5 mcg qod or Premarin 0.3 mg qod) and gradually increase.

- Promotes breast development and adult body habitus
- *Progesterone* (oral) should be added if breakthrough bleeding occurs or when estrogen dose reaches 1 mcg/day.

Table 76.2 Suggested schema for pubertal induction and maintenance in boys and girls

Testosterone dose	Testosterone Interval	Duration	Estradiol dose (daily)	Duration
50 mg	4 weeks	6 months	0.5 mcg	qod 6 months
100 mg	4 weeks	6 months	0.5 mcg	qd 6 months
125 mg	4 weeks	6 months	1 mcg (+ a progesterone when bleed)	6 months
250 mg	3–4 weeks	Onwards	2 mcg	Onwards

Treatment could be started at age 12–13 years in boys and 11–12 years in girls. Duration for each stage of treatment is determined by individual responses.

Sexual differentiation

Normal sexual differentiation

Gonadal development

In the male or female embryo, the bipotential gonad develops as a thickening of mesenchymal cells and coelomic epithelium around the primitive kidney. This *genital ridge* is then colonized by primordial germ cells that migrate from the yolk sac to form the *gonadal ridge*. In the absence of a Y chromosome, the gonad will develop into an ovary.

In the presence of a normal Y chromosome, immature Sertoli cells, germs cells, and seminiferous tubules can be recognized by 7 weeks, and testis differentiation is complete by 9 weeks. The *SRY* gene is an essential sex-determining region on the Y chromosome that signals for testis differentiation.

Internal genitalia

Embryonic Müllerian structures form the uterus, fallopian tubes, and upper 1/3 of the vagina.

In males, by 6 weeks, anti-Müllerian hormone is secreted by immature Sertoli cells in the testis, and this causes regression of the Müllerian structures. Leydig cells appear in the testis around day 60 and produce testosterone under placental hCG stimulation.

Testosterone promotes growth and differentiation of the Wolffian ducts to form the epididymis, vas deferens, and seminal vesicles.

External genitalia

In the absence of any androgen secretion, the labia majora, labia minora, and clitoris develop from the embryonic genital swelling, genital fold, and genital tubercle, respectively.

Development of normal male external genitalia requires testosterone production from the testis and its conversion to dihydrotestosterone by the enzyme 5α-reductase. In the presence of dihydrotestosterone, the genital tubercle elongates to form the corpora cavernosa and glans penis, the urethral fold forms the penile shaft, and the labioscrotal swelling forms the scrotum.

This process commences at around 9 weeks and is completed by 13 weeks. Testicular descent in males occurs in the later two-thirds of gestation under control of fetal LH and testosterone.

Assessment of ambiguous genitalia

Most cases of ambiguous genitalia present at birth. Involvement of an experienced pediatric endocrinologist and surgeon should be sought as early as possible.

History
- Any maternal medications during pregnancy?
- Are parents consanguineous, or is there a family history of ambiguous genitalia?
- Is there a neonatal history of hypoglycemia or prolonged jaundice?

Examination
- Assess clitoris or phallus size, degree of labial fusion, and position of urethra and urogenital sinus (anterior or posterior).
- Are gonads palpable? Check along line of descent.
- Are there any signs indicating panhypopituitarism (e.g., midline defects, hypoglycemia, hypocortisolemia, prolonged jaundice)?
- Dysmorphic features of Turner's syndrome may be seen in XO/XY mosaicism.

Investigations
- Blood for karyotype, electrolytes, glucose, 17αOH progesterone
- US of pelvis and labial folds (for Müllerian structures and gonads)
- After the infant is 48 hours old, when the neonatal hormonal surge has decreased, repeat blood tests for 17αOH progesterone, cortisol, LH, FSH, and androgen levels.
- Examination under anesthesia (EUA) and cystogram may be required.

Specific tests
- ACTH stimulation test may be required when CAH is suspected, to assess cortisol secretion and aid in diagnosis.
- 3-day HCG test in an undervirilized "male" (testes present or 46, XY) assesses stimulated gonadal production of androgens and may be diagnostic of androgen biosynthesis defects or androgen insensitivity.
- Glucagon test is an alternative test to examine cortisol and GH secretion.
- Androgen receptor function can be tested on cultured fibroblasts from a genital skin biopsy.
- DNA analysis for androgen receptor mutation, CAH mutations, and androgen biosynthesis mutations

Disorders of sex development (DSD)

Male and female internal and external genitalia develop from common embryonic structures. In the absence of male-differentiating signals, normal female genitalia develop.

Genital ambiguity may therefore occur as a result of chromosomal abnormality, gonadal dysgenesis, biochemical defects of androgen synthesis, inappropriate exposure to external androgens, or androgen receptor insensitivity.

46XX DSD

Disorders of ovarian development

Normal male differentiation can occur if the *SRY* gene has been translocated onto an autosome.

Biochemical defects leading to androgen oversecretion

Congenital adrenal hyperplasia (CAH, 21-hydroxylase deficiency most commonly) is the most common cause of ambiguous genitalia in 46, XX.

Maternal hyperandrogenism

The female fetus may be virilized if maternal androgen levels exceed the capacity of placental aromatase to convert these to estrogen.

This may occur from maternal disease (e.g., CAH, adrenal and ovarian tumors) or use of androgenic medication in pregnancy or, rarely, placental aromatase deficiency.

46XY DSD

Disorders of testis development

XY gonadal dysgenesis can be caused by mutations in a number of genes controlling male sexual differentiation, including *SRY, SF-1, WT-1*, and *SOX*, and can present with normal external genitalia.

There is early testicular failure resulting from torsion or infarction.

Biochemical defects of androgen synthesis

Rare deficiencies of the enzymes 5α-reductase, 17β-hydroxysteroid dehydrogenase, or 3β-hydroxysteroid dehydrogenase, which are also associated with glucocorticoid and mineralocorticoid deficiencies, are autosomal recessively inherited and may result in variable degrees of undervirilization.

Androgen receptor insensitivity syndrome

📖 Also see Androgen insensitivity syndrome (p. 335).

Defects of the androgen receptor gene on the X chromosome, or autosomal post-receptor signaling genes, may result in complete or partial androgen insensitivity.

Complete androgen insensitivity results in normal female external genitalia and usually only presents with testicular prolapse in childhood or primary amenorrhea in adolescence.

In partial androgen insensitivity, presentation may vary from mild virilization to micropenis, hypospadias, undescended testes, or only ↓ spermatogenesis.

Gonadotropin defects

Gonadotropin deficiency may occur in hypopituitarism or may be associated with anosmia (Kallmann syndrome). It usually presents with delayed puberty but is an occasional cause of micropenis and undescended testes.

LH receptor gene defects are rare and result in complete absence of virilization, as the testes are unable to respond to placental hCG.

Anti-Müllerian hormone deficiency or insensitivity

Testes are usually undescended and uterus and fallopian tubes are present.

Management of ambiguous genitalia

In the newborn period, the infant should be monitored in the hospital for the following:

- Hypoglycemia (until hypopituitarism is excluded)
- Salt-wasting (until CAH is excluded)

Explain to the parents that the infant appears to be healthy but has a defect that interferes with determining sex. It is helpful to show the parents the physical findings as you explain this. Advise them to postpone the registration of the birth until after further investigations, and discuss what they will say to relatives and friends.

Sex assignment

Decision on the sex of rearing should be based on the optimal expected outcome in terms of psychosexual and reproductive function. Parents should be allowed discussion with an endocrinologist, a surgeon specializing in urogenital reconstruction, a psychologist, and a social worker.

Following the necessary investigations and discussions, early gender assignment is thought to optimize the psychosexual outcome, but further research into this area is still required.

Further management

- If female sex is assigned, any testicular tissue should be removed.
- Reconstructive surgery may include clitoral reduction, gonadectomy, and vaginoplasty in girls, and phallus enlargement, hypospadias repair, and orchidopexy in boys. In both sexes, multiple-stage procedures may be required.
- Testosterone may enhance phallus size in male infants and a trial of therapy is sometimes useful before sex assignment.
- Hormone replacement therapy may also be required from puberty into adulthood.
- Continuing psychological support for the parents and child is very important.

Congenital adrenal hyperplasia

📖 Also see Chapter 47, Congenital adrenal hyperplasia in adults (p. 239).

A number of autosomally inherited enzyme deficiencies result in cortisol deficiency, excess pituitary ACTH secretion, and adrenal gland hyperplasia.

21-hydroxylase deficiency (>90%)

The most common cause of CAH results in cortisol and mineralocorticoid deficiency, while the build-up of precursor steroids is channeled toward excess adrenal androgen synthesis. Different gene defects in the 21-hydroxylase gene (e.g., deletion, splice site, or point mutation) result in different degrees of enzyme dysfunction and thus wide variation in phenotypes.

Clinical features

Virilization of female fetuses may result in clitoromegaly and labial fusion at birth. 75% have sufficient mineralocorticoid deficiency to cause renal salt-wasting.

Because males have normal genitalia at birth, they may present acutely ill in the neonatal period with vomiting, dehydration, collapse, hyponatremia, and hyperkalemia. Non-salt-wasting boys present with early genital enlargement, pubarche, and rapid growth.

If untreated or poorly treated, both sexes may develop pubic hair, acne, rapid height velocity, advanced bone maturation, and precocious puberty that may result in very short final height.

Nonclassic CAH is due to milder 21-hydroxylase deficiency, and affected girls present in later childhood or adulthood with hirsutism, acne, premature or exaggerated adrenarche, menstrual irregularities, and infertility.

11β-hydroxylase deficiency (~5%)

This enzyme, which converts 11-deoxycortisol to cortisol, is the final step in cortisol synthesis. In addition to excess adrenal androgens, the overproduced precursor corticosterone has mineralocorticoid activity. Thus, in contrast to salt-wasting in 21-hydroxylase deficiency, these subjects may have hypernatremia and hypokalemia.

Hypertension is rarely seen in infancy but may develop during childhood and affects 50–60% of adults.

Specific investigations for CAH

📖 See also Assessment of ambiguous genitalia (p. 456).

- *Plasma 17αOH progesterone:* An elevated level indicates 21-hydroxylase deficiency. It may be difficult to distinguish this from the physiological hormonal surge that occurs in the first 2 days of life. This test should therefore be repeated (together with 11-deoxycortisol) after 48 hours of age.
- An ACTH stimulation test may be required to discriminate between the different enzyme deficiencies.
- Plasma electrolytes may need to be monitored over the first 2 weeks.
- Plasma renin level is also useful to confirm salt-wasting in those with normal serum sodium and relatively mild 21-hydroxylase deficiency.

Other rare enzyme deficiencies

17α-Hydrolxylase deficiency
This impairs cortisol, androgen, and estrogen synthesis, but overproduction of mineralocorticoids leads to hypokalemia and hypertension.

3β-Hydroxysteroid dehydrogenase deficiency
This impairs cortisol, mineralocorticoid, and androgen biosynthesis. Males have hypospadias and undescended testes. However, excess DHEA, a weak androgen, may cause mild virilization in females.

Steroid acute regulatory protein

- *STAR mutation:* 46XY sex reversal and severe adrenal failure. Heterozygous defect. Extremely rare
- *CYPIIAI* (P450: side-chain cleavage cytochrome enzyme): 46XY sex reversal and severe adrenal failure. Heterozygous defect. Extremely rare
- *P450 oxidoreductase deficiency:* Biochemical picture of combined 21-hydroxylase/17α-hydrolxylase/17, 20 Lyase deficiencies. Spectrum of presentation from children with ambiguous genitalia, adrenal failure, and the Antley–Bixler skeletal dysplasia through to mildly affected individuals with polycystic ovarian syndrome

Management

- *Hydrocortisone* (10–20 mg/m^2 per day orally in 3 divided doses). In older patients, prednisone or dexamethasone can also be employed. In addition to treating cortisol deficiency, this therapy suppresses ACTH and thereby limits excessive production of adrenal androgens. Occasionally, higher doses are required to achieve adequate androgen suppression, however overtreatment may suppress growth.

Box 77.1 Definitions

Disorders of chromosomes
These include the following:
- 45X Turner and variants
- 47XXY and variants
- 45X/46XY mixed gonadal dysgenesis
- 46XX/46XY gonadal chimera

46XX DSD
These include the following:
- Disorders of gonadal (ovarian) development
- Androgen excess
- Structural disorders, e.g., cloacal extrophy, vaginal atresia

46XY DSD
These include the following:
- Disorders of gonadal (testicular) development
- Disorders in androgen synthesis and action
- Structural disorders, e.g., severe hypospadias, cloacal extrophy

- In salt losers, initial *IV fluid resuscitation* (10–20 mL/kg normal saline) may be required to treat circulatory collapse. Long-term mineralocorticoid replacement (fludrocortisone 0.05–0.3 mg/day) may have incomplete efficacy, particularly in infancy, and sodium chloride supplements are also needed. Up to 4–5 meq/kg/day split qid may be needed in infancy.
- *Reconstructive surgery* (clitoral reduction, vaginoplasty) is often performed in infancy and further procedures may be required during puberty. This requires an experienced surgeon.
- Warn of the need for extra steroid during stress.

Monitoring of hormonal therapy

Height velocity and bone age
If hydrocortisone therapy is insufficient, the growth rate will be above normal and bone age will be advanced. Conversely, if hydrocortisone therapy is excessive, growth is suppressed.

17AOHP
Blood levels should be assessed periodically, especially when clinical signs of rapid growth or bone age advancement occur. Complete normalization of 17αOHP levels should be avoided, as this often leads to overtreatment.

In girls and prepubertal boys, androgen levels (testosterone and androstendione) can be measured if there is concern about poor control and/or virilization.

Mineralocorticoid and sodium replacement
This should be monitored by measuring plasma electrolytes and renin levels and by regular blood pressure assessments.

Genetic advice
The inheritance of CAH is autosomal recessive, and parents should be informed of a 25% risk of recurrence in future offspring.

If the mutation is identifiable on DNA analysis in the child and parents, chorionic villus sampling may allow prenatal diagnosis.

Maternal dexamethasone therapy from around 5 -6 weeks of pregnancy can be used to prevent virilization of the female fetus.

Further reading

Brook CGD (Ed.) (1995). *Clinical Paediatric Endocrinology*, 3rd ed. Oxford: Blackwell Science.

Fluck CE, Miller WL (2006). P450 oxidoreductase deficiency: a new form of congenital adrenal hyperplasia. *Curr Opin Paediatr* 18:435–441.

Hochberg Z (Ed.) (1998). *Practical Algorithms in Pediatric Endocrinology*. Basel: Karger

Hughes IA (1989). *Handbook of Endocrine Investigations in Children*. Bristol, UK: John Wright & Sons.

Hughes IA, Houk C, Ahmed SF, et al. (2006). Consensus statement on management of intersex disorders. *Arch Dis Child* 91:554–563.

Joint LWPES/ESPE Working Group (2002). Consensus statement on 21 hydroxylene deficiency. *J Clin Endocrinol Metab* 87:4048–4053.

Wilkins L (1994). In Kappy MS, Blizzard RM, Migeon CJ (Eds.), *The Diagnosis and Treatment of Endocrine Disorders in Childhood and Adolescence*, 4th ed. Springfield, IL: Charles C Thomas.

Part 8

Neuroendocrine disorders

Emily Jane Gallagher and Dina Green

The neuroendocrine system

Introduction

Neuroendocrine cells are found in many sites throughout the body. They are particularly prominent in the GI tract and pancreas and share a common embryological origin. These cells have the ability to synthesize, store, and release peptide hormones.

Given the prevalence of neuroendocrine cells, most neuroendocrine tumors occur within the gastroenteropancreatic axis. Of these tumors, >50% are traditionally termed *carcinoid* tumors and have been usually sub-classified into foregut, midgut, and hindgut lesions, with the remainder largely comprising pancreatic islet cell tumors.

Carcinoid and islet cell tumors are generally slow growing.

Further reading

Barakat MT, Meeran K, Bloom SR (2004). Neuroendocrine tumours. *Endocr Relat Cancer* 11(1):1–18.

Carcinoid tumors

Definition and classification

Historically, these tumors have been divided into those arising in the foregut, midgut, or hindgut.

Strictly speaking, carcinoid tumors are serotonin secreting and argentaffin positive (take up silver stain), so the term should be reserved for those tumors that fulfill these criteria. Increasingly, the remainder are being classified as neuroendocrine tumors together with their tissue of origin.

About 85% of carcinoid tumors develop in the GI tract, 10% in the lung, and the rest in various organs such as the thymus or ovary.

In 30% of patients, carcinoid tumors are multiple, and associations with other malignancies such as adenocarcinomas of the GI tract and prostate are recognized.

Incidence

The annual incidence of carcinoid tumors is approximately 2.5 per 100,000 population, although postmortem studies suggest that this may be a significant underestimate.

Carcinoid syndrome

This syndrome only occurs in a subset of patients with carcinoid tumors (<10%). It occurs when sufficient vasoactive substances (e.g., serotonin, histamine, tachykinins, kallikrein, and prostaglandins) are released into the systemic circulation. For this reason, almost all patients with the carcinoid syndrome due to GI tumors have hepatic metastases.

In contrast, some bronchial carcinoids may present with classical features of the syndrome without metastatic disease.

The original description of the syndrome includes flushing, diarrhea, asthma, right heart valvular lesions, and pellagra-like skin lesions.

In a published series of patients from Sweden with known GI carcinoids, 84% presented with diarrhea, 75% with flushing, and 44% with intestinal obstruction. During the course of the illness, it was noted that 33% of the patients had carcinoid heart disease and 15% complained of symptoms of wheezing.[1]

The carcinoid flush may be precipitated by spicy food, hot drinks, alcohol, exercise, and postural changes. The cause of flushing is heterogeneous and results from the release of a variety of vasoactive substances. Acute attacks typically cause a diffuse erythematous flush affecting the face and upper thorax, whereas long-standing carcinoid may be associated with a violacious flush and facial telangiectasia.

A life-threatening carcinoid crisis (flushing, BP fluctuations, bronchoconstriction, arrhythmias, altered mental status) can be provoked in these patients as a result of anesthesia or surgical manipulation of the tumor.

Box 79.1 Carcinoid heart disease

- Occurs in up to two-thirds of patients with the carcinoid syndrome
- The mechanism is poorly understood although is thought to be related to serotonin.
- Pathologically, the lesions are characterized by fibrous thickening of the endocardium in plaques.
- The right side of the heart is typically involved. Thickening and retraction of the tricuspid and pulmonary valve leaflets lead to tricuspid regurgitation in nearly all cases and, less commonly, to pulmonary regurgitation, tricuspid stenosis, and pulmonary stenosis. The left side of the heart is involved in <10% of cases.
- Valve replacement can be beneficial, but surgery may be associated with significant morbidity and mortality.

---

1 Norheim I, berg K, Theodorsson–Norheim E, et al. (1987). Malignant carcinoid tumors: an analysis of 103 patients with regard to tumor localization, hormone production, and survival. *Ann Surg* 206(2):115–125.

Diagnostic investigations

Pathology

Historically, carcinoid tumors have been identified by their reaction to silver stains (argentaffin positive).

Characterizing the tumor histpathologically is very important and currently includes the use of specific immunohistochemical stains such as chromogranin A, synaptophysin, serotonin, and gastrin.

Ki67, a marker of cell proliferation, is also used by some centers to guide treatment.

Biochemical investigations

A 24-hour urinary 5HIAA (serotonin metabolite) assessment has traditionally been the mainstay of both diagnosis and monitoring. The test offers a specificity of nearly 100% and a sensitivity of 70%.

Elevated levels are usually only associated with midgut tumors and only once they have metastasized. Elevated levels correlate well with symptoms of the carcinoid syndrome and are useful in monitoring response to treatment.

False-positive tests may result from dietary sources of serotonin (e.g., bananas, avocados, tomatoes, walnuts, pecan nuts, caffeine, pineapples, and chocolate) and interference from drugs (e.g., acetaminophen, nicotine, phenobarbital, phenacetin).

Plasma or platelet serotonin are alternatives to urine testing, although the specificity is uncertain.

The most sensitive biochemical marker for neuroendocrine tumors is plasma chromogranin A (false positive—renal/liver failure, proton pump inhibitors [PPIs], gastritis, inflammatory bowel disease; false negative—L-dopa, phenothiazines). For carcinoid tumors the sensitivity of the test is nearly 100%, but the specificity is lower than for urinary 5HIAA as raised levels are found in most neuroendocrine tumors.

A plasma gut hormone profile may also be useful for identification of tumor markers such as gastrin, pancreatic polypeptide, and somatostatin.

Liver biochemistry is an unreliable marker of hepatic involvement as the alkaline phosphatase may remain in the normal range despite extensive metastatic disease.

Exclude associated inherited syndromes

Carcinoid tumors may rarely be associated with multiple endocrine neoplasia syndrome type 1 (MEN1), von Hippel–Lindau syndrome (VHL), type 1 neurofibromatosis (NF1), and tuberous sclerosis.

Tumor localization and staging

The aim of imaging with abdominal US, CT, and MRI is to both localize the primary tumor and assess the extent of metastatic spread.

On CT, hepatic carcinoid metastases are usually multifocal, showing enhancement after IV contrast and frequently with low-attenuation areas of necrosis. MRI is at least as sensitive as CT, with lesions being iso-intense on T1-weighted images but of high signal on T2-weighted images.

More than 80% of carcinoid tumors have somatostatin receptors, and scanning with radiolabeled octreotide can provide very useful information about the localization and extent of metastatic disease. It frequently reveals previously unidentified extrahepatic sites of disease.

PET scanning, where available, can be useful for tumor localization and staging in difficult cases.

Box 79.2 Monitoring treatment

- Urinary 5HIAA or serum chromogranin A can be useful to monitor response to therapy if these markers were elevated at diagnosis.
- Imaging modalities are also essential to monitor tumor bulk.

Treatment

A multidisciplinary approach to the treatment of these tumors is essential.

Surgical treatment

In patients with local disease, surgery can be curative, but most patients have metastatic disease by the time they seek treatment.

Even in patients with widespread local disease or distant metastases, surgery may still be of benefit by reducing overall tumor bulk and thereby affording a more favorable response to subsequent nonsurgical therapies. Surgery may be required to alleviate obstructive intestinal disease.

Liver transplantation may be considered in a very few selected patients in whom extrahepatic tumor spread and primary tumor recurrence has been excluded.

Box 79.3 Perioperative management of carcinoid tumors

It may be useful to give IV octreotide in the perioperative period, as anesthesia, surgery, and embolization may be associated with the release of various vasoactive peptides that can result in hypotension and bronchospasm, leading to a potentially fatal carcinoid crisis.

Medical treatment

Certain symptom specific medical agents can be useful, such as loperamide or codeine for diarrhea.

Somatostatin analogs

Octreotide and its longer-acting analogs reduce the level of biochemical tumor markers in the majority of patients and control symptoms in around 70% of cases. However, radiological evidence of tumor regression with these agents is rare.

Patient resistance to somatostatin analogs is common after a few years. This potential for tachyphylaxis makes the early use of somatostatin analogs in asymptomatic patients controversial.

Patients are usually given a test dose of SC octreotide and then generally started on the more convenient longer-acting analogs. Short-acting SC octreotide tid may be continued until cover with the longer-acting analog is complete.

A continuous IV infusion of octreotide is the most effective treatment for a carcinoid crisis and is generally given at a rate of 50–100 mcg/h.

A new somatostatin analog (SOM230—pasireotide) with high affinity for receptor subtypes 1, 2, 3, and 5 is currently under evaluation in phase III trials.

Hepatic embolization

This can be performed by surgeons or, increasingly, by interventional radiologists. It is a palliative procedure offering symptom relief by decreasing tumor bulk.

The duration of improvement may be short-lived, and occasionally significant side effects such as the hepatorenal syndrome may occur.

External beam radiotherapy

This may provide palliation in those with symptomatic bone metastases or spinal cord compression.

Chemotherapy

Cytotoxic chemotherapy may be considered in patients with advanced, progressive, or uncontrolled symptomatic disease. The benefit is debatable.

The most promising combination of streptozotocin and 5-fluorouracil (5-FU) produces only short-lasting responses in 10–30% of patients with carcinoid tumors, in contrast to the 50–60% response rate of pancreatic neuroendocrine tumors. Capecitabine (prodrug of 5-FU) can be administered orally, and it may offer a more specific antitumor effect.

Side effects (e.g., flu-like symptoms, fatigue, weight loss, bone marrow suppression) are generally less severe than with conventional chemotherapy but are still the main limitation to its use.

Alpha2b-Interferon

There is a good biochemical response rate (about 45%), with clinical improvement of the symptoms of carcinoid syndrome in 70% of patients. Tumor shrinkage has rarely been described.

A combination of octreotide and α2b-interferon has been shown to produce biochemical and symptomatic improvement in some patients previously resistant to either drug alone. However, there is limited effect on tumor size.

Radioactive isotope therapy

These are relatively new modalities with few long-term data.

There is increasing evidence to suggest that if a positive diagnostic uptake scan is obtained, therapeutic treatment with the relevant radionuclide can offer at least significant symptomatic improvement. A few studies have suggested tumor stabilization or regression may be achieved in some cases.

Radiolabeled somatostatin analogs

Radiolabeled somatostatin analogs, such as ^{111}InDTPA octreotide, the newer ^{90}YDOTA octreotide, and ^{177}Lu octreotate, which have high affinity for type 2 somatostatin receptors, have been used as therapy. Because ^{111}InDTPA octreotide has low tissue penetration, and a stable coupling of alpha- or beta-emitting isotopes to DTPA octreotide could not be achieved, newer compounds (^{90}YDOTA octreotide, ^{177}Lu octreotate) were developed.

^{90}YDOTA octreotide may result in partial remission in 10–25% of patients, while ^{177}Lu octreotate has proved very successful in achieving tumor regression in animal models with encouraging preliminary human studies (remission in 38% and stable disease in 4% at 3 months).

Radiolabeled MIBG

MIBG is structurally related to norepinephrine. After IV injection, up to 70% of carcinoid tumors concentrate significant amounts of the compound.

Limited published data suggest 65–80% of these patients treated with MIBG have palliation of symptoms for varying lengths of time (6–24 months).

Future treatments

Antiangiogenic agents such as inhibitors of vascular endothelial growth factor are currently being evaluated and may be of benefit in preventing tumor progression.

Pellagra

Rarely, pellagra may develop due to nicotinamide deficiency secondary to excessive tryptophan metabolism.

Nicotinamide supplementation is therapeutic.

Prognosis

The site of origin and the size of the primary tumor, together with the extent of metastatic disease, largely determine the prognosis.

Many carcinoid tumors are indolent and are frequently a postmortem finding having caused no significant symptoms during life.

When the disease is confined locally to the region of the primary tumor, the 5-year survival is >90%.

Individual patients have been reported to live 20–30 years after the diagnosis of metastatic carcinoid tumor, but this should not be considered a benign disease. The 5-year survival rate when hepatic metastases are present is approximately 20–40% with a median survival time being about 2 years.

Increasingly, evidence is suggesting that both survival time and quality of life for patients are improved by the use of more active and aggressive therapy.

The prognosis is greatly influenced by the development of carcinoid heart disease and whether it is then amenable to treatment by heart valve replacement.

Further reading

Kaltsas G, Rockall A, Papadogias D, et al. (2004). Recent advances in radiological and radionuclide imaging and therapy of neuroendocrine tumors. *Eur J Endocrinol* 151(1):15–27.

Oberg K (2002). Carcinoid tumors: molecular genetics, tumor biology, and update of diagnosis and treatment. *Curr Opin Oncol* 14(1):38–45.

Insulinomas

Definition

An *insulinoma* is a tumor of the endocrine pancreas that causes hypoglycemia through its inappropriate secretion of insulin. Unlike other endocrine tumors of the pancreas, where malignancy is common, >90% of insulinomas are benign.

More than 80% of insulinomas are solitary, 10% are multiple and 10% are malignant. 50% of patients with multiple insulinomas have MEN1.

Insulinomas are found with equal frequency throughout the head, body and tail of the pancreas.

Incidence

The annual incidence of insulinoma is of the order of 1–2 per million population.

Clinical presentation

Symptoms of hypoglycemia may include both adrenergic (e.g., pallor, sweating, tremor, and tachycardia) and neuroglycopenic (e.g., irritability, confusion, aggression, seizures, and coma) symptoms.

Patients typically give a history of relief of symptoms with food. Weight gain occurs in at least 30% of patients.

Biochemical investigations

The gold standard test remains the supervised 72 hour fast. More than 95% of cases can by diagnosed by the 72 hour fast. While fasting, the patient may consume only caffeine-free beverages, must remain active and exercise normally. A laboratory glucose measurement of <40 mg/dL should be found during symptoms in association with an inappropriately normal or elevated insulin and C-peptide level. An insulin/glucose ratio of >0.3 is abnormal and consistent with organic hyperinsulinism.

The presence of sulfonylurea metabolites in the urine or plasma should be excluded, and the abuse of exogenous insulin considered.

Tumor localization

See Table 80.1.

Islet cell tumors are often small and may not be detected by any imaging technique. The available radiological modalities have a wide reported range of sensitivity that is frequently dependent on the equipment and the operator.

MRI or spiral CT correctly detects >60% of tumors, but preoperative localization can be difficult in tumors <1 cm in diameter.

Arterial stimulation (with calcium or secretin) followed by venous sampling can localize approximately 90% of insulinomas but carries the risks of a more invasive technique.

Endoscopic US, which requires specialized equipment and expertise, may identify tumors as small as 5 mm. The head of the pancreas is visualized with the probe in the duodenum and the body and tail with it in the stomach.

Intraoperative US using a transducer applied directly to the pancreas improves the sensitivity of US to over 90%.

Experienced surgeons can frequently identify the lesions intraoperatively by palpation alone. The risk of multiple tumors makes a thorough examination of the whole pancreas essential at operation.

Somatostatin receptor scintigraphy has been shown to be useful in detecting insulinomas but it is dependent on somatostatin receptor subtype expression by the tumor.

Table 80.1 Radiological localization of pancreatic insulinomas

Localization technique	Reported sensitivity (%)
Transabdominal US	30–61
Endoscopic US	80
Intraoperative US	90
CT	42–78
MRI	20–100
Octreotide scanning	68–86
Pancreatic arteriography	29–90
Venous sampling	84

Treatment

The treatment of choice in all but very elderly or debilitated patients is surgical removal. The perioperative mortality rates are <1% in the hands of an experienced surgeon. The mortality is largely influenced by the incidence of acute pancreatitis and peritonitis.

Postoperative hyperglycemia may occur even following partial pancreatectomy.

Medical treatment to control symptoms may be achieved using a combination of diazoxide and octreotide.

Radiolabeled somatostatin analog therapy may induce a biochemical and symptomatic response in patients with malignant insulinomas, and some small-scale studies report tumor regression.

Prognosis

Following removal of a solitary insulinoma, life expectancy is restored to normal.

Malignant insulinomas, with metastases usually to the liver, have a natural history of years rather than months and symptoms may be controlled with medical therapy or specific antitumor therapy using streptozotocin and 5-FU.

Average 5-year survival estimated to be approximately 35%.

Gastrinomas

Definition

Gastrin, synthesized by the G cells situated predominantly in the gastric antrum, is the principal gut hormone stimulating gastric acid secretion.

The Zollinger–Ellison (gastrinoma) syndrome is due to the excessive release of gastrin by neuroendocrine tumors of the GI tract and pancreas. Gastrinomas most commonly arise in the duodenum (70%), with the remainder arising from the pancreas or adjacent lymph nodes.

About 60% of patients have metastatic disease at the time of diagnosis.

Prevalence

The estimated prevalence is of the order of 1 per million population.

Clinical presentation

Patients typically present with peptic and/or esophageal ulcers that are multiple and refractory to standard medical treatment.

Complications of peptic ulcer disease, such as perforation, hemorrhage, and pyloric stenosis, are frequently seen.

Malabsorption and diarrhea may be the main presenting complaint in 10–20% of patients and is due to acid-related inactivation of enzymes and mucosal damage in the upper small bowel.

Up to 25% of gastrinoma patients may have MEN1. In this context, the prevalence of multiple gastrinomas is higher than for sporadic tumors.

Biochemical investigations

The diagnosis rests on finding an inappropriately elevated fasting plasma gastrin in the presence of increased gastric acid secretion.

Patients should have antisecretory treatment stopped prior to the test (3 days for H_2 blockers and 2 weeks for PPIs), since these drugs are associated with hypergastrinemia. However, gastrin levels above 1000 pg/mL in the presence of elevated gastric acid production, are virtually diagnostic of a gastrinoma.

The secretin stimulation test is the most sensitive and specific stimulation test. A dose of 2 mcg/kg of secretin is given intravenously and blood samples are drawn for gastrin at 2, 5, 10, 20, and 30 minutes. A rise of >150 pg/mL is highly suggestive of gastrinoma.

A gut hormone profile may identify elevated plasma levels of pancreatic polypeptide or other gut hormones.

The tumor localization techniques described for insulinomas are also relevant for gastrinomas (Tumor localization, p. 473). Very small tumors or duodenal tumors can be very hard to localize and even small tumors are frequently associated with local lymph node disease.

Selective arterial angiography may be combined with a provocative test for gastrin release using a bolus of calcium gluconate or secretin for elusive small tumors.

For causes of hypergastrinemia, see Box 81.1.

Box 81.1 Causes of hypergastrinemia

Low or normal gastric acid production
- H_2 blockers
- PPIs
- Vagotomy
- Hypochlorhydria
- Short gut syndrome
- Renal failure
- Hypercalcemia

Elevated gastric acid production
- Gastrinoma
- G-cell hyperplasia

Treatment

The treatment of choice is complete surgical tumor removal, although this is usually only considered after the tumor has been identified preoperatively. Surgery is rarely justified in patients with known hepatic metastases, but some small studies have raised the possibility of benefit from tumor debulking.

Where preoperative imaging has failed to identify a tumor, the patient is often best maintained on medical therapy with regular imaging to reassess (PPIs need to be given less frequently than H_2 antagonists). Check B_{12} annually.

Somatostatin analogs do not appear to be more effective at controlling gastric acid hypersecretion and relieving symptoms than PPIs or H_2 blockers.

The data are currently limited, but as for insulinomas, radiolabeled somatostatin analogs may be a future treatment option for gastrinomas.

In patients with MEN1, management is more controversial. The usual policy is to operate when a well-defined tumor can be identified.

Table 81.1 Treatment options for gastrinomas

Medical treatment	Surgery	Palliation
• H_2 blockers	• Tumor resection	• Chemotherapy
• PPIs	• Tumor debulking	• Hepatic artery embolization
• Octreotide	• Liver transplant	

Glucagonomas

Definition

Glucagonomas are neuroendocrine tumors that usually arise from the alpha cells of the pancreas and produce the glucagonoma syndrome through the secretion of glucagon and other peptides derived from the preproglucagon gene.

The large majority of glucagonomas are malignant, but they are also very indolent tumors, and the diagnosis may be overlooked for many years.

Up to 90% of patients will have lymph node or liver metastases at the time of presentation.

They are classically associated with the rash of necrolytic migratory erythema.

Incidence

The annual incidence is estimated at 1 per 20 million population.

Clinical presentation

See Table 82.1.

The characteristic rash—necrolytic migratory erythema—occurs in >70% of cases and usually manifests initially as a well-demarcated area of erythema in the groin before migrating to the limbs, buttocks, and perineum.

Mucous membrane involvement is common, with stomatitis, glossitis, vaginitis, and urethritis being frequent features.

Glucagon antagonizes the effects of insulin, particularly on hepatic glucose metabolism, and glucose intolerance is a frequent association (>90%). Sustained gluconeogenesis also causes amino acid deficiencies and results in protein catabolism, which can be associated with unrelenting weight loss in >60% of patients.

Glucagon has a direct suppressive effect on the bone marrow, resulting in a normochromic normocytic anemia in almost all patients.

Up to 20% of glucagonoma patients will have associated MEN1.

Table 82.1 Clinical features of the glucagonoma syndrome

Site	Clinical features
Skin	Necrolytic migratory erythema
Mucous membranes	Angular stomatitis
	Atrophic glossitis
	Vulvovaginitis
	Urethritis
Nails	Onycholysis
Scalp	Alopecia
Metabolism	Glucose intolerance
	Protein catabolism and weight loss
Hematological	Anemia
	Venous thromboses
Psychiatric	Depression
	Psychosis

Biochemical investigations

The diagnosis is confirmed on finding raised plasma glucagon levels.

A gut hormone profile may also show elevated neuroendocrine markers such as pancreatic polypeptide.

Impaired glucose intolerance and hypoaminoacidemia may be present.

Tumor localization

At the time of diagnosis >60% of glucagonomas will have metastasized to the liver and most primary tumors will be >3 cm in diameter.

These tumors rarely present problems of radiological localization. Transabdominal US and CT scanning are usually adequate.

Small tumors may require more sophisticated imaging techniques (📖 see Tumor localization, p. 473). Octreotide scanning probably offers the best means of evaluating the extent of metastatic disease.

Treatment

Surgery is the only curative therapeutic option, but the potential for a complete cure may be as low as 5%.

In malignant disease, a surgical cure may still be achieved in those rare cases where the metastases are confined to the liver and the patient is deemed suitable for a liver transplant.

Somatostatin analogs are the treatment of choice with excellent response rates in treating the necrolytic migratory erythema. They are less effective at reversing the weight loss and have an inconsistent effect on glycemic control such that diabetes mellitus may need to be managed with insulin therapy.

If octreotide fails, the rash may be improved using IV amino acids and fatty acids.

Palliative chemotherapy using streptozotocin and 5-FU has been shown to produce a 50% reduction in glucagon levels in 75% of patients, but the benefit is frequently only temporary.

Hepatic artery embolization may result in a dramatic relief of symptoms with remissions of several months recorded.

As for the other pancreatic islet cell tumors, there are preliminary data to suggest that radiolabeled somatostatin analogs may be therapeutic in the glucagonoma syndrome.

VIPomas

Definition

In 1958, Verner and Morrison[1] first described a syndrome consisting of refractory watery diarrhea and hypokalemia associated with a neuroendocrine tumor of the pancreas.

The syndrome of watery diarrhea, hypokalemia, and acidosis (WDHA) is due to secretion of vasoactive intestinal polypeptide (VIP).

Tumors that secrete VIP are known as *VIPomas*. VIPomas account for <10% of islet cell tumors and mainly occur as solitary tumors. More than 60% are malignant and metastasize to the lymph nodes, liver, kidneys, and bone.

Clinical presentation

The most prominent symptom in most patients is profuse watery diarrhea that is secretory in nature and therefore rich in electrolytes (Box 83.1). Other causes of secretory diarrhea should be considered in the differential diagnosis (see Box 83.2).

VIPomas are rare in MEN1 patients, occurring in <1% of cases.

Box 83.1 Clinical features of the VIPoma syndrome

- Watery diarrhea
- Hypokalemia
- Achlorhydria
- Metabolic acidosis
- Hypercalcemia
- Hyperglycemia
- Hypomagnesemia
- Facial flushing

Box 83.2 Differential diagnosis of secretory diarrhea

- Infection, e.g., *Escherichia coli* or cholera toxins
- Laxative abuse
- Villous adenoma
- Other gut neuroendocrine tumors, e.g., carcinoid tumors or gastrinomas
- Carcinoma of the lung
- Medullary carcinoma of the thyroid
- Systemic mastocytosis
- Immunoglobulin A deficiency

---

1 Verner JV, Morrison AB (1958). Islet cell tumor and a syndrome of refractory watery diarrhea and hypokalemia. *Am J Med* 25(3):374–380.

Biochemical investigations

Elevated levels of plasma VIP are found in all patients with the VIPoma syndrome, although false positives may occur in dehydrated patients due to diarrhea from other causes.

A gut hormone profile may identify other raised tumor markers such as pancreatic polypeptide and aid detection of some other causes of watery diarrhea, e.g., gastrinomas.

Urinary catecholamine excretion should be assessed, especially in children, in whom it is common to find the tumors residing in the adrenal medulla.

Tumor localization

The majority of tumors secreting VIP originate in the pancreas, whereas others arise from the sympathetic chain.

Primary VIPomas have very rarely been reported to arise from a variety of other sites, such as the lung, esophagus, small bowel, colon, and kidney.

Most patients present with large tumors that can be easily identified by transabdominal US or CT, although small tumors may require additional methods of tumor localization as previously discussed (📖 p. 473).

Treatment

Severe cases require IV fluid replacement and careful correction of electrolye disturbances.

Surgery to remove the tumor is the treatment of first choice if technically possible and may be curative in around 40% of patients. Surgical debulking may also be of palliative benefit.

Somatostatin analogs produce effective symptomatic relief from the diarrhea in most patients. Long-term use does not result in tumor regression.

Glucocorticoids in high dosage have also been shown to provide good relief of symptoms. A trial of lithium may be warranted in resistant cases and this therapy may be combined with octreotide.

Chemotherapy using streptozotocin in combination with 5-FU has resulted in response rates of >30%.

Hepatic artery embolization can offer temporary respite from severe diarrhea.

Somatostatinomas

Definition

Somatostatinomas are very rare neuroendocrine tumors occurring both in the pancreas and in the duodenum. More than 60% are large tumors located in the head or body of the pancreas.

The clinical syndrome may be diagnosed late in the course of the disease when metastatic spread to local lymph nodes and the liver has already occurred.

Clinical features

See Box 84.1.

Glucose intolerance or frank diabetes mellitus may have been observed for many years prior to the diagnosis and retrospectively often represents the first clinical sign. It is probably due to the inhibitory effect of somatostatin on insulin secretion.

A high incidence of gallstones has been described similar to that seen as a side effect with long-term somatostatin analog therapy.

Diarrhea, steatorrhea, and weight loss appear to be consistent clinical features and may be associated with inhibition of the exocrine pancreas by somatostatin.

Small duodenal somatostatinomas may occur in association with NF1 (43%). Although these rarely cause the inhibitory clinical syndrome, they present with obstructive biliary disease through local spread of the tumor. Somatostatinomas are infrequently associated with MEN1 (7%).

Box 84.1 Clinical features of the somatostatin syndrome

- Glucose intolerance/diabetes mellitus (95%)
- Gallstones (68%)
- Diarrhea and steatorrhea
- Weight loss (25%)
- Anemia (14%)
- Hypochlorhydria

Biochemical investigations

Plasma somatostatin levels will be raised and may also be associated with raised levels of other neuroendocrine tumor markers, including ACTH and calcitonin.

Multisecretory activity is more common with pancreatic (33%) than with duodenal (16%) somatostatinomas.

Tumor localization

Transabdominal US and CT scanning may demonstrate the tumor, since metastatic disease is often apparent at presentation.

Additional methods of tumor localization as previously described may also be required (☐ see p. 473)

Treatment

Surgery should be considered first-line treatment. Although a cure is rare, even debulking surgery may result in significant palliation.

Hepatic embolization can be considered and chemotherapy with streptozotocin and 5-FU may be used to control malignant disease.

Part 9

Inherited endocrine syndromes and multiple endocrine neoplasia (MEN)

Boris Draznin

McCune–Albright syndrome

Definition

The syndrome is characterized by the following:
- Polyostotic fibrous dysplasia
- Café-au-lait pigmented skin lesions
- Autonomous function of multiple endocrine glands

A clinical diagnosis requires two of these pathologies.

Genetics

This syndrome is a genetic but not an inherited condition due to a postzygotic somatic mutation in the gene (*GNAS1*) that encodes the α-chain of the stimulating G protein of adenyl cyclase (GSα mutation). This results in activation of adenyl cyclase.

The somatic mutation results in mosaicism. Consequently, the proportion and distribution of affected cells in a tissue will be determined by the precise stage in development at which the mutation occurred.

Mutational analysis of the *GNAS1* gene from affected tissues or blood may be available.

Clinical features

Polyostotic fibrous dysplasia

Solitary or multiple expansile bony lesions that can cause fracture deformities and nerve entrapment typically develop before the age of 10 years.

The femoral and the pelvic bones are most frequently affected. Radiographs of these bones are useful for screening. Osteosarcomas are a rare complication.

For treatment, 📖 see Box 85.1.

Box 85.1 Treatment of polyostotic fibrous dysplasia

- Surgery may be complicated by bleeding, and radiotherapy has a limited effect.
- There is recent evidence to support the use of bisphosphonates, particularly pamidronate, for both symptomatic pain relief and the radiological healing of bone.

Café-au-lait pigmentation

The lesions are characterized by an irregular border (in neurofibromatosis the border is smooth), do not cross the midline, and tend to be ipsilateral to the bone lesions.

Endocrinopathies

See Table 85.1.

Involvement of other organs

Hepatobiliary complications such as neonatal jaundice, elevated transaminases, and cholestasis are relatively common.

Cardiomegaly, tachyarrythmias, and sudden cardiac death may occur. Gastrointestinal polyps, splenic hyperplasia, and pancreatitis are reported complications. Recognized CNS associations include microcephaly, failure to thrive, and developmental delay.

Table 85.1 Endocrinopathies in McCune-Albright syndrome

Condition	Presentaion	Treatment
Precocious puberty	Frequent initial presentation Typically aged 1–9 years Low gonadotrophins Adults fertile Less frequent in boys	Cyproterone acetate
Thyroid nodules	Present in almost 100% of patients 50% become toxic due to autonomous nodule function	Antithyroid drugs, radioiodine, surgery
GH-secreting pituitary tumors and prolactinomas	Present with features of acromegaly or hyperprolactinemia	Somatostatin analogs, dopamine agonists, surgery
Cushing's syndrome	Adrenal hyperplasia or adenoma	Adrenalectomy
Hypophosphatemic rickets	↓ Phosphate ↓ 1,25 vitamin D ↑ ALP Normal calcium, 25 OH vitamin D, and PTH	Calcitriol, phosphate supplements

Prognosis

Most patients live well beyond reproductive age. Bone deformities may reduce life expectancy.

Sudden cardiac death is uncommon.

Further reading

Lumbroso S, Paris F, Sultan C (2002). McCune–Albright syndrome: molecular genetics. *J Paediatr Endocrinol Metab* 15(3):875–882.

Spiegel AM, Weinstein LS (2004). Inherited diseases involving G proteins and G protein–coupled receptors. *Annu Rev Med* 55:27–39.

Neurofibromatosis

Definition

Neurofibromatosis type 1 (NF1) is also known as *von Recklinghausen disease* and refers to the occurrence of multiple neurofibromas, café-au-lait spots, and Lisch nodules affecting the iris.

Endocrinopathies are sometimes associated with NF1. The prevalence of NF1 is estimated to be 1 in 3500 of the population.

NF type 2 (NF2) is characterized by the presence of bilateral acoustic neuromas typically resulting in deafness. Other features of NF2 include posterior subcapsular cataracts, retinal gliomas, pigmented retinopathy, and gaze palsies.

NF2 has no common associated endocrinopathies. NF2 is rare with an estimated frequency of 1 in 40,000 live births.

NF1

Genetics

NF1 is a highly penetrant, autosomal dominant condition.

The NF1 gene is located on chromosome 17 and encodes a GTPase-activating protein (neurofibromin).

Neurofibromin promotes cleavage of GTP to GDP.

Epidemiology

The incidence of NF1 is 1 per 3000 of the population. NF1 is nearly 100% penetrant but shows variable clinical expression.

Approximately 50% of cases are sporadic.

Clinical features

Diagnosis is generally apparent by the age of 1 year. The café-au-lait spots become visible shortly after birth (95%), and 70% have axillary or grain freckling.

The multiple cutaneous and subcutaneous neurofibromas appear around puberty (95%). Lisch nodules affecting the iris start to appear typically after the age of 5 years (95%).

The endocrine features are detailed in Box 86.1.

Learning disabilities occur in 60% of patients with NF1.

Box 86.1 Endocrine features of NF1

Puberty and pregnancy
- Both are associated with a change in size of neurofibromas.

Hypothalamus and pituitary
- Optic gliomas impinge on adjacent tissues and may affect hypothalamic and/or pituitary function.

Pheochromocytoma 0.1–5.0%
- Serious complication of NF1
- Uncommon before age 20 years
- Most commonly adrenal (20% bilateral) but extra adrenal lesions are reported

Gut neuroendocrine tumors
- Found in around 1% of NF1 patients—carcinoid

Gliomas may be found in around 15% of patients, most commonly affecting the optic pathways. Neurofibrosarcomas complicate around 6% of cases.

Skeletal dysplasias (e.g. sphenoid wing dysplasia, scoliosis, tibial pseudoarthrosis, pectus excavatum) may be found in up to 5% of cases.

Vascuar dysplasia may occur, the most common region affected being the renal vasculature, resulting in renovascular hypertension in up to 3% of cases.

Macrocephaly (16%), seizures (5%), and short stature (6%) are all reported features of NF1.

Associated pheochromocytomas are seen in <5% of NF1 patients.

Further reading

Arun D, Gutmann DH (2004). Recent advances in neurofibromatosis type 1. *Curr Opin Neurol* 17(2):101–105.

Rose VM (2004). Neurocutaneous syndromes. *Mol Med* 101(2):112–116.

Von Hippel–Lindau disease

Definition

Characterized by
- CNS hemangioblastomas
- Retinal angiomas
- Renal cysts and carcinomas
- Pheochromocytomas
- Pancreatic neuroendocrine tumors (less common) and pancreatic cysts
- Occasional endolymphatic sac tumors

See Box 87.1.

Box 87.1 Less common manifestations of von Hippel–Lindau disease

Pancreas	Cysts
	Adenomas
Epididymis	Cystadenoma
CNS	Syringomyelia
	Meningioma
Liver	Adenoma Hemangioblastoma
	Cysts
Lung	Angioma
	Cysts
Spleen	Angioma

Clinical diagnosis established by
- Two or more hemangioblastomas
- A hemangioblastoma and a visual manifestation
- One hemangioblastoma or visual manifestation and a family history of hemangioblastoma

The condition occurs in approximately 1 in 36,000 live births. The average age of presentation is 27 years, and the condition is nearly 100% penetrant by the age of 65 years.

VHL may be subdivided into type 1 and type 2 disease.

- Type 1 VHL is the commonest form of the disease and is characterized by a tendency to develop tumors in the eyes, brain, spinal cord, kidney, and pancreas
- Affected family members with VHL type 2 are also susceptible to developing pheochromocytomas. This may be further subdivided into VHL type 2A (develop phecochromocytomas and renal cell carcinomas).

Genetics

VHL is a highly penetrant, autosomal dominant condition. The VHL gene is on chromosome 3 and is a tumor suppressor gene.

Genetic testing in affected families is recommended from the age of 5 years.

Clinical features

Retinal angiomas are the initial manifestation of VHL in 40% of patients. They are uncommon before the age of 10 years but continue to develop throughout life. They tend to be peripheral in the retina, appearing as red, oval lesions. Bleeding and retinal detachment may occur, and treatment is with laser therapy.

Seventy-five percent of hemangioblastomas occur in the cerebellum. They are the initial presenting feature in 40% of VHL patients. Treatment is with surgery or radiotherapy.

Renal carcinoma is the most common cause of death in VHL patients. By the age of 60 years, 70% of VHL patients will be affected, with a mean age of presentation of 44 years. The lesions tend to be multifocal. The management of choice is surgical resection.

Pheochromocytomas occur in up to 20% of VHL families and are bilateral in 40% of cases. The frequency of this condition varies widely among families, as certain mutations are particularly associated with a high risk of pheochromocytoma. Regular biochemical screening is essential in these high-risk families. Treatment is with α- and β-blockade followed by surgical resection.

Most pancreatic tumors associated with VHL are nonfunctioning, but they may secrete VIP, insulin, glucagons, or calcitonin. They occur in 10–20% of VHL patients and should be treated expectantly unless symptomatic, enlarging, or >2–3 cm.

Table 87.1 lists the recommended ages to start tests for VHL.

Table 87.1 Testing for VHL

Test	Recommended age to start (years)
Palpation (renal and epididymal lesions)	5
Urinalysis	5
24-hour urinary catecholamines	5
Fundoscopy and fluorescein angiography	5
Cerebral MRI	10
Abdominal MRI for renal, adrenal, and pancreatic lesions	5

Prognosis

Until recently, the median survival for a VHL patient was 40–50 years of age with the majority of deaths attributable to renal cell carcinoma.

Currently, the prognosis for individual patients depends on the location and complications of the tumors but overall is improving as a result of the institution of screening programs and consequent earlier therapeutic interventions.

For surveillance in VHL, 📖 see Table 87.2.

Table 87.2 Surveillance in VHL

	Affected	**At risk**
Annual	Clinical examination	Clinical examination
	Urinalysis	Urinalysis
	24-hour urinary catecholamines	24h urinary catecholamines
	Fundoscopy	Fundoscopy (aged 5–60 years)
Triennial	Cerebral MRI (to age 50, then every 5 years)	Cerebral MRI (aged 5–40 years, then every 5 years to age 60)
	Abdominal MRI	Abdominal MRI (aged 25–65 years)

Further reading

Kaelin WG Jr (2003). The von Hippel–Lindau gene, kidney cancer and oxygen sensing. *Am Soc Nephrol* 14(11):2703–2711.

Lonser RR, et al. (2003). Von Hippel-Lindau disease. *Lancet* 361:2059–2067.

Richard S, Graff J, Lindau J, et al. (2005). Von Hippel–Lindau disease. *Lancet* 363:1231–1234.

Carney complex

Definition

A clinical diagnosis is made by finding two of the clinical features listed in Clinical presentation (below) or one of these features *plus* either an affected first-degree relative or an inactivating mutation in the relevant gene (*PRKARIα*).

Genetics

- Autosomal dominant
- An inactivating mutation of the *PRKARIα* gene on the long arm of chromosome 17q2 can be identified in approximately 50% of families.

Clinical presentation

- Spotty skin pigmentation
- Cardiac, skin, or mucosal myxomas
- Endocrine tumors (📖 see Box 88.1).
- Psammomatous melanotic schwannoma

Box 88.1 Endocrine tumors associated with Carney complex

- The most common endocrine manifestation is primary pigmented nodular adrenocortical disease (PPNAD) causing Cushing's syndrome.
- Large-cell calcifying Sertoli cell tumor (LCCSCT)
- GH/PRL-secreting pituitary adenoma (also somatotrope/mammotrope hyperplasia)
- Thyroid adenoma
- Ovarian cysts

Further reading

Sandrini F, Stratakis C (2003). Clinical and molecular genetics of Carney complex. *Mol Genet Metab* 78(2):83–92.

Stergiopolous SG, Abu-Asab MS, Tsokos M, et al. (2004). Pituitary pathology in Carney complex patients. *Pituitary* 7:73–82.

Stratakis CA, Kirschner LS, Carney JA (2001). Clinical and molecular features of the Carney complex. *J Clin Endocrinol Metab* 86(9):4041–4046.

Cowden syndrome

Incidence

This syndrome is estimated to affect 1 in 200,000 individuals.

Genetics

- Autosomal dominant condition
- Inactivating mutations in the *PTEN* tumor suppressor gene can be identified in approximately 80% of affected probands.

Clinical presentation

Also 📖 see Box 89.1.

The condition is characterized by multiple hamartomas involving organ systems derived from all three germ cell layers. Patients are also at risk for breast, thyroid, and endometrial carcinomas.

Thyroid pathology occurs in >2/3 of patients, and the lesions may be multifocal.

> **Box 89.1 Endocrine features of Cowden syndrome**
>
> - Nonmedullary thyroid carcinomas, especially follicular thyroid carcinoma
> - Multinodular goiter
> - Thyroid adenomas
> - Parathyroid adenomas are extremely rare.

Further reading

Pilarski R, Eng C (2004). Will the real Cowden syndrome please stand up (again)? Expanding mutational and clinical spectra of the PTEN hamartoma tumour syndrome. *J Med Genet* 41(5):323–326.

POEMS syndrome

Definition

Progressive polyneuropathy, organomegaly, endocrinopathy, monoclonal gammopathy, and skin changes (POEMS) is a rare disorder of unclear pathogenesis that is probably mediated by ↑ production of λ light chains from abnormal plasma cells.

Clinical presentation

- Progressive polyneuropathy
- Organomegaly, especially hepatosplenomegaly and lymphadenopathy
- Common endocrinopathies (84%) (multiple in 65%) include hypogonadotrophic hypogonadism (70%—2/3 central, 1/3 primary), hypothyroidism (60%), hypoadrenalism (60%), and diabetes mellitus (50%) hyperprolactinemia (20%).
- Monoclonal gammopathy
- Skin changes

Treatment

Treatments include chemotherapy, irradiation, and surgery.

Further reading

Dispenzieri A, Gertz MA (2004). Treatment of POEMS syndrome. *Curr Treat Options Oncol* 5(3):249–257.

MEN type 1

Definition

Characterized by
- Parathyroid tumors/hyperplasia
- Anterior pituitary adenomas
- Pancreatic neuroendocrine tumors

A clinical diagnosis of MEN1 is reached in the presence of two out of three of these tumors or one of these tumors in the context of a family history of MEN1.

The prevalence of MEN1 has been estimated at 1 in 10,000 of the population.

Genetics

MEN1 is an autosomal dominant condition with an estimated penetrance of 98% by the age of 40 years.

The *MEN1* gene is located on the long arm of chromosome 11 (11q13) and is a tumor suppressor gene, although the function of the encoded protein, MENIN, is unknown.

The mutations causing MFN1 are inactivating mutations. Many mutations in the *MEN1* gene have been described in affected families. There is no clear genotype–phenotype correlation.

Mutational analysis is available in the US, although it is important to note that up to 10% of MEN1 patients will not have mutations identifiable within the coding region of the *MEN1* gene.

Clinical features

Primary hyperparathyroidism is the most common presenting feature in MEN1 and occurs in up to 95% of patients with MEN1.

Pituitary adenomas are found in approximately 30% of MEN1 patients (📖 see Table 91.1).

The incidence of pancreatic endocrine tumors varies between 30% and 80% in different series (📖 see Table 91.2).

Other lesions are also associated with MEN1 (📖 see Table 91.3).

Table 91.1 Pituitary tumors in MEN1

Tumor	Frequency
Prolactinoma	60%
Acromegaly	25%
Nonfunctioning tumor	1%
Cushing's disease	<1%

Table 91.2 Pancreatic tumors in MEN1

Tumor	Frequency
Gastrinoma	60%
Insulinoma	30%
Glucagonoma	2%
VIPoma	<1%
PPoma	<1%
Nonfunctioning tumor	1%

Table 91.3 Other lesions in MEN1

Tumor	Frequency
Adrenal cortical tumors	5%
Carcinoid tumors	4%
Lipomas	1%
Pheochromocytoma	0.5%
Malignant melanoma	0.5%
Testicular teratoma	0.5%
Multiple (>3) angiofibromas	75%

Management

Primary hyperparathyroidism

The hypercalcemia is frequently mild with an early age of onset and is the first manifestation of the disease in 90% of patients.

Multiple gland disease (adenomas or hyperplasia) is common, in contrast with sporadic primary hyperparathyroidism, where usually a single adenoma is found.

No effective medical treatments are currently available and surgical management is the gold standard. In view of the potential for multigland disease, total parathyroidectomy with lifelong oral calcitriol replacement should always be considered.

The timing of surgery in asymptomatic patients with borderline hypercalcemia is still controversial.

Pituitary adenomas

These are managed with surgery, medical therapies, or radiotherapy as per sporadic pituitary tumors (see p. 87).

Pancreatic tumors

An experienced surgeon is essential to resection of these tumors.

For patients with aggressive disease, the pancreas and duodenum together with surrounding lymph nodes may be removed, whereas simple enucleation may be sufficient for some lesions.

Gastrinomas are the major cause of morbidity and mortality in MEN1 patients and these may respond to medical therapy with proton pump inhibitors.

Mutational analysis

The criteria for performing mutational analysis are controversial. One approach is to recommend assessing the following categories of patient:

- Patients with 2 MEN1 tumors
- First- and second-degree relatives of patients with MEN1
- Consider screening in patients with primary hyperparathyroidism <40 years of age, particularly in the presence of multigland disease.
- Consider screening in patients with isolated pancreatic neuroendocrine tumors, especially gastrinomas or insulinomas.

Screening

Screening is relevant for affected patients, asymptomatic mutation carriers, and first- and second-degree relatives in families with a clinical diagnosis of MEN1 but where a mutation has not been identified.

Manifestations of MEN1 are very rare before the teenage years but have been described in patients as young as 5 years. Careful parental counseling can encourage some childhood monitoring, which should include a careful history for symptoms (e.g., hypoglycaemia) and height and weight assessment in addition to calcium and prolactin measurements.

Screening involves a careful clinical history and examination as well as biochemical assessment and imaging modalities (🕮 see Table 91.4).

Age-related penetrance is as follows: age 10–7%, age 20–52%, age 30–87%, age 40–98%, age 60–100%.

Table 91.4 Screening adults in MEN1

Tumor	Frequency
Calcium, phosphate, and PTH	Annual
Basal anterior pituitary function (particularly prolactin and IGF-1)	Annual
Fasting gut hormones	Annual
Fasting glucose	Annual
24-hour urinary 5HIAA and chromogranin A	Annual
MRI abdomen	Annual–every 3 years
MRI pituitary	Baseline

Box 91.1 Prognosis

Malignant pancreatic tumors, especially gastrinomas, are the major cause of mortality in MEN1, but outcomes have been improving with the introduction of appropriate screening programs for affected and at-risk individuals.

Further reading

Asgharian B, Turner ML, Gibril F, et al. (2004). Cutaneous tumours in patients with multiple endocrine neoplasm type 1 (MEN1) and gastrinomas: prospective study of frequency and development of criteria with high sensitivity and specificity for MEN1. *J Clin Endocrinol Metab* 89:5328–5336.

Brandi ML Gagel AF, Angeli A, et al. (2001). Guidelines for diagnosis and therapy of MEN type 1 and 2. *J Clin Endocrinol Metab*, 86(12):5658–5671.

MEN type 2

Definition

MEN2 may be divided into three forms (see Table 92.1):
- MEN2a comprises familial medullary thyroid carcinoma (FMTC) in combination with pheochromocytoma and parathyroid tumors.
- MEN2b is defined as the occurrence of familial MTC in association with pheochromocytoma, mucosal neuromas, and a marfanoid habitus.
- FMTC may also occur in isolation.

MEN2a accounts for >75% of all MEN2 cases.

Table 92.1 Classification and presentation of MEN2

Pathology	MEN2a	MEN2b	FMTC
MTC	95%	~100%	~100%
Pheochromocytoma	50%	50%	Not present
Parathyroid neoplasia	20–30%	Not present	Not present
Marfanoid habitus	Not present	75%	Not present
Mucosal neuromas	Not present	10–20%	Not present
Intestinal ganglioneuromatosis	Not present	~40%	Not present

Genetics

MEN2 is an autosomal dominant condition. The C-RET protooncogene, mutations in which cause MEN2, is located on the long arm of chromosome 10 (10q11.2).

This gene encodes RET, which is a transmembrane receptor with an extracellular cysteine-rich domain and an intracellular tyrosine kinase domain.

The mutations causing MEN2 are activating mutations.

Different germline mutations cause different clinical syndromes, so in contrast to MEN1, MEN2 shows a strong genotype–phenotype correlation.

The C-RET proto-oncogene is also involved, via inactivating mutations, in the etiology of Hirschsprung's disease.

Clinical features—MEN2a

Medulllary thyroid cancer (MTC)

MTC is often the initial manifestation and is generally multifocal. Pheochromocytoma and parathyroid disease typically develop later.

Diagnosis of MTC requires histological analysis that reveals C-cell hyperplasia and stromal amyloid. Circulating calcitonin levels are generally elevated (see Box 92.1), but hypocalcemia is not seen.

With metastatic disease, diarrhea is common (30%).

Rarely, these tumors secrete ACTH, resulting in Cushing's syndrome due to ectopic ACTH secretion.

Box 92.1 Pentagastrin test

- Indication borderline basal calcitonin and screening of families with medullary carcinoma (calcitonin slightly raised with thyroiditis)
- Patient fasting
- 0.5 mcg/kg pentagastrin IV over 5 seconds and flush cannula
- Calcitonin measured at 0, 2, and 10 minutes
- Elevated basal levels of calcitonin, which do not rise with pentagastrin stimulation, are seen in children, pregnancy, with some tumors (e.g., carcinoids), pernicious anemia, thyroiditis, and chronic renal failure.
- Side effects of the test include nausea, flushing, and substernal tightness, which typically resolves in <5 minutes.

Stimulated calcitonin	30–100 ng/L	Follow-up screening recommended
Stimulated calcitonin	100–200 ng/L	Probable C-cell hyperplasia or early medullary thyroid carcinoma
Stimulated calcitonin	200 ng/L	Medullary thyroid carcinoma very likely

---

Pheochromocytoma

- Tend to present later than MTC
- 50% will be bilateral but malignancy is rare (<10%).
- These lesions must be excluded prior to surgery for any other indication.

Primary hyperparathyroidism

- Generally results from hyperplasia of the glands
- Hypercalcemia is typically mild.

Clinical features—MEN2b

Mucosal neuromas can be found on the distal tongue, conjunctiva, and throughout the gastrointestinal tract.

A marfanoid habitus is typically evident.

MTC tends to present earlier than in MEN2a and frequently follows a more aggressive course.

Management

MTC

The definitive treatment is adequate surgery by total thyroidectomy and careful lymph node dissection. Postoperative levothyroxine is administered to all patients.

Tumor spread is usually local but distant metastases do occur.

Regular postoperative calcitonin assessment (first 3 months, then every 6–12 months) is used to monitor for disease recurrence.

MRI, octreotide scanning, and venous catheterization may all be helpful in staging disease recurrence.

Treatment of recurrent disease responds poorly to radiotherapy or chemotherapy and consequently is generally surgical if appropriate.

Somatostatin analogs may help symptom control, e.g., diarrhea, but do not appear to have an antitumor effect.

Few data are available to date, but therapy with radiolabeled MIBG or somatostatin analogs appears to offer significant symptomatic improvement, although tumor stabilization and/or regression was observed only rarely.

Children with MEN2 should be considered for early prophylactic surgery. This should generally be performed before the age of 5 years, and before the age of 1 year in patients with the highest risk mutations.

Pheochromocytoma

These tumors are best treated medically with α- and β-blockade followed by surgical removal.

The risk of multifocal and/or recurrent disease must be considered.

Screening has resulted in earlier detection of these lesions.

Primary hyperparathyroidism

The criteria for diagnosis and the indications for surgery are broadly similar to those for sporadic primary hyperparathyroidism.

Mutational analysis

Mutational analysis is indicated for first- and second-degree relatives of patients with MEN2 and genetic analysis should be performed as early as possible in at-risk children.

Consider screening in patients with sporadic MTC or sporadic pheochromocytoma or in patients with mucosal neuromas or other phenotypic features compatible with MEN2b.

Somatic RET oncogene mutations confer a worse prognosis in sporadic medullary carcinoma.

Screening

Biochemical and radiological screening is relevant for affected patients, asymptomatic mutation carriers, and first- and second-degree relatives in families with a clinical diagnosis of MEN2 but where a mutation has not been identified (📖 see Table 92.2).

Table 92.2 Screening in MEN2

Test	Frequency
Calcitonin ± pentagastrin stimulation test	Annual
24h urinary catecholamines	Annual
Calcium	Annual
CT/MRI adrenals	Annual–every 3 years

Box 92.2 Prognosis

- Variable
- Overall 10-year survival rate for MEN2b is 65% and for MEN2a is 80%.
- The prognosis for these patients is improving with earlier screening and intervention.

Further reading

Brandi ML, Gagel AF, Angeli A, et al. (2001). Guidelines for diagnosis and therapy of MEN type 1 and 2. *J Clin Endocrinol Metab* 86(12):5658–5671.

Carling T. (2005). Multiple endocrine neoplasia syndrome: genetic basis for clinical management. *J Curr Opin Oncol* 17:7–12.

Constante G, Meringolo D, Durante C, et al. (2007). Predictive value of serum calcitonin levels for preoperative diagnosis of medullary thyroid carcinoma in a cohort of 5817 consecutive patients with thyroid nodules. *J Clin Endocrinol Metab* 92(2):450–455.

Karges W, Dralle H, Raue F, et al. (2004). Calcitonin measurement to detect medullary thyroid carcinoma in nodular goitre: German evidence-based consensus recommendations. *Exp Clin Endocrinol Diabetes* 112(1):52–58.

Marx SJ (2005). Molecular genetics of multiple endocrine neoplasia types 1 and 2. *J Nat Rev Cancer* 5:67–75.

Inherited primary hyperparathyroidism

Epidemiology

Parathyroid tumors affect 1 per 1000 population. Primary hyperparathyroidism is inherited in up to 10% of patients.

Causes

- MEN1
- MEN2a
- Hyperparathyroidism–jaw tumor syndrome (HPT-JT)
- Familial isolated hyperparathyroidism (FIHP)

HPT-JT

This is an autosomal dominant condition. It is characterized by pathology in three main tissues:

- Parathyroid tumors, which show a high penetrance in these patients and in up to 15% of cases will be parathyroid carcinomas
- Ossifying fibromas, which affect the maxilla and/or mandible in around 30% of HPT-JT patients

Renal manifestations may also occur, the most common being bilateral renal cysts (19% of patients) but also including hamartomas and Wilms' tumors.

Benign and malignant uterine pathology is seen in up to 75% of women with HPT-JT and reduces reproductive fitness.

Other tumors have also been reported in these patients, including pancreatic adenocarcinomas, testicular mixed germ-cell tumors, Hürthle cell thyroid adenomas, and benign and malignant uterine tumors.

The gene (HRPT2) in activating mutations that are responsible for HPT-JT has been identified on the long arm of chromosome 1. Mutational analysis is available in the US.

The function of the protein product (parafibromin) encoded by this tumor suppressor gene is unknown.

FIHP

Affected individuals within a kindred suffer only from primary hyperparathyroidism as an isolated endocrinopathy.

In some kindreds, mutations in the *MEN1* or *HRPT2* genes have been identified, but in the majority the cause is still unknown.

Further reading

Carpten JD, Robbins CM, Villablanca A, et al. (2002). HRPT2, encoding parafibromin, is mutated in hyperparathyroidism-jaw tumor syndrome. *Nat Genet* 32(4):676–680.

Marx SJ (2002). Hyperparathyroidism in hereditary syndromes: special expressions and special managements. *J Bone Miner Res* 17(2):N37–N43.

Inherited renal calculi

Definitions

Renal calculi affect 12% of men and 5% of women by the seventh decade of life. Renal calculi arise due to a reduced urine volume or ↑ excretion of stone-forming components such as calcium, oxalate, urate, cystine, xanthine, and phosphate.

A variety of causes for renal stones are established (☐ see Box 94.1 for general causes of nephrolithiasis), but the most common etiology is hypercalciuria.

Calcium stones account for >80% of all renal calculi. Uric acid stones comprise 5–10% of all renal calculi.

The most common cause of hypercalciuria is hypercalcemia. This in turn is most frequently secondary to primary hyperparathyroidism.

Nephrolithiasis is frequently a recurrent condition with a relapse rate of 75% in 20 years.

Features associated with recurrence include early age of onset, positive family history, and lithiasis related to infection or underlying medical conditions.

Box 94.1 Causes of renal calculi

- Hypercalciuria
- Hyperoxaluria
- Hyperuricosuria
- Hypocitraturia
- Urinary tract infection, e.g., *Proteus*, *Pseudomonas*, *Klebsiella*.
- Primary renal disease, e.g., polycystic kidney disease
- Drugs, e.g., indinavir, diuretics, salicylates, allopurinol, some chemotherapeutic agents

Genetics

Renal calculi generally arise from complex multifactorial disease resulting from an interaction between genetic and environmental factors. The disorder may be familial in up to 45% of patients.

The majority of causative genes are probably as yet unidentified and account for much of "idiopathic" calcium nephrolithiasis.

Many cases of hypercalciuria are likely to be polygenic, but two examples of monogenic causes are Dent's disease and autosomal dominant hypocalcemic hypercalciuria (ADHH).

Box 94.2 Mutational analysis

- Currently largely a research tool
- Mutations in a variety of genes have been reported to result in renal calculi due to hypercalciuria, hyperoxaluria, cystinuria, or hyperuricosuria.
- As these research tests move into the clinical domain, family screening will become increasingly relevant.

Dent's disease

- X-linked condition
- Due to inactivating mutations in a chloride channel (*CLC5*) gene
- Characterized by hypercalciuria, nephrocalcinosis, β2 microglobinuria, progressive glomerular disease, and mild rickets due to renal phosphate loss in affected males

ADHH

- Autosomal dominant condition
- Due to activating mutations in the calcium-sensing receptor gene
- May be asymptomatic or present early with neonatal or childhood seizures

Investigation of renal calculi

- 24-hour urine volume and urine osmolarity (low urine volume raises production of solutes)
- 24-hour urinary calcium excretion
- Urine pH
- Stone composition, if possible
- Exclude causes of hypercalcemia (hyperparathyroidism, immobilization, or renal tubular acidosis)
- Exclude hypercalciuria (excess chloride, excess sodium, malignancy, sarcoidosis, renal calcium leak, and drugs, e.g., levothyroxine or loop diuretics)
- Exclude causes of hyperoxaluria (primary hyperoxaluria, vitamin B$_6$ deficiency, short bowel syndrome, and excess dietary oxalates)
- Exclude urinary tract infection
- Exclude causes of hyperuricosuria (gout, dietary, uricosuric drugs, binge drinking, or myeloproliferative disorders)

- Exclude causes of hypocitraturia—citrate is the primary agent for removal of excess calcium (renal tubular acidosis, potassium or magnesium deficiency, urinary tract infection, renal failure, and chronic diarrhea)
- Exclude cysteine (usually genetic in origin) or xanthine (usually secondary to allopurinol treatment) stones

Management

- Increase fluid intake.
- Appropriate dietary modifications
- Treat underlying cause.

Further reading

Langman CB (2004). The molecular basis of kidney stones. *Curr Opin Paediatr* 16(2):188–193

Thakker RV (2004). Diseases associated with the extracellular calcium-sensing receptor. *Cell Calcium* 35(3):275–282.

Part 10

Miscellaneous endocrinology

Marc-Andre Cornier

Hypoglycemia

Definition (Whipple's triad)

- Plasma glucose of <50 mg/dL *associated with*
- Symptoms of neuro-glycopenia *and*
- Reversal of symptoms with correction of glucose levels.

For causes, see Box 95.1.

Box 95.1 Causes of hypoglycemia

- Spontaneous hypoglycemia
- Drug induced (the most common cause; both accidental and non-accidental)
  - Antidiabetic agents used either alone (e.g., insulin, sulfonylureas, prandial glucose regulators) or in combination (e.g., insulin and thiazolidinediones)
  - Alcohol (impairs hepatic gluconeogenesis and is often associated with poor glycogen stores)
  - Quinine can promote hyperinsulinemia.
  - Salicylates can act by inhibiting hepatic glucose release and increase insulin secretion.
- Organ failure and critical illness
  - Acute liver failure
  - Chronic renal failure
- Hormone deficiency
  - Addison's disease
  - Isolated ACTH deficiency
  - GH deficiency
  - Hypopituitarism
- Insulinoma
  - Benign 85%, malignant 15%
  - Occasionally part of MEN1 (~10%)
- Other tumors
  - Excessive IGF-2 secretion from large mesenchymal tumors (non–islet cell tumor hypoglycemia [NICH]), e.g., fibrosarcoma, mesothelioma (~ 1/3 are retroperitoneal, 1/3 intra-abdominal, and 1/3 intra-thoracic)
  - Hepatocellular carcinoma
  - Adrenal carcinoma, pheochromocytoma
  - Lymphoma, myeloma, leukemia
  - Advanced metastatic malignancy

Box 95.1 (*Contd.*)

- Infection
  - Septicemia, e.g., gram-negative or meningococcal; related to high metabolic requirements, reduced energy intake, and possibly cytokines from the inflammatory process
  - Malaria
- Starvation or malnutrition
  - Anorexia nervosa
  - Kwashiorkor or marasmus
- β-cell hyperplasia: very rare in adults
- Autoimmune
  - Antibodies to insulin (antibody-bound insulin dissociates leading to elevated free insulin; typically associated with postprandial hypoglycemia)
- Insulin receptor activating antibodies (rare, most common in middle-aged women; may require treatment with plasmapheresis or immunosuppression)
- Inborn errors of metabolism
  - Glycogen storage disease
  - Hereditary fructose intolerance
  - Maple syrup disease
- Hypoglycemias of infancy and childhood
- Reactive (postprandial) hypoglycemia: see p. 520

Epidemiology

Hypoglycemia is uncommon in adults, apart from patients with diabetes being treated with certain agents either alone or in combination (e.g., insulin, sulfonylureas, prandial glucose regulators, thiazolidinediones).

Pathophysiology

Physiology of glucose control

The liver is the major regulator (80–85%) of circulating blood glucose levels in healthy individuals and responds to changes in circulating insulin, growth hormone (GH), cortisol, glucagon, and adrenaline.

- *Postprandial state:* Hepatic glucose production is inhibited by both raised glucose and insulin concentrations.
- *Fasting state:* Serum glucose falls with a consequent decrease in insulin secretion, stimulating hepatic efflux of glucose (in the presence of cortisol, GH, and glucagon).

The brain is dependent on circulating glucose for its energy demands, which are high and comprise up to 50% hepatic glucose output.

Mechanisms of hypoglycemia

- *Excessive or inappropriate action of insulin or IGF-1:* inhibiting hepatic glucose production despite adequate glycogen stores, while peripheral glucose uptake is enhanced
- *Impaired neuroendocrine response,* with inadequate counterregulatory response (e.g., cortisol or GH) to insulin
- *Impairment of hepatic glucose production,* due to either structural damage or abnormal liver enzymes

Types of spontaneous hypoglycemia

- *Fasting hypoglycemia* occurs several hours (typically >5 hours) after food intake (e.g., early morning, following prolonged fasting or exercise) and almost always indicates underlying disease.
- *Postprandial (reactive) hypoglycemia* occurs 2–5 hours after food intake (⊞ see Post-prandial reactive hypoglycemia, p. 520).

Symptoms of hypoglycemia

- *Autonomic (adrenergic) symptoms:* sweats, pallor, tachycardia, tremor, hunger, anxiety
- *Neuroglycopenic symptoms:* poor concentration, drowsiness, double vision, irritability, perioral tingling, poor judgment, confusion, violent behavior, personality change, unexplained collapse, focal neurological signs, seizures, loss of consciousness, and death

Clinical features

Responses to hypoglycemia are sequential with the following:
- Deterioration in neuropsychological performance at plasma glucose 50–60 mg/dL
- Subjective perception of hypoglycemia at 50 mg/dL
- EEG changes at 35 mg/dL

Patients with recurrent hypoglycemia may not get symptoms until glucose concentrations are very low (so-called hypo-unawareness), whereas patients with poorly controlled diabetes mellitus may experience hypoglycemic symptoms at "normal" blood glucose levels.

Most symptoms of acute hypoglycemia are adrenergic, but neuroglycopenic symptoms occur with subacute and chronic hypoglycemia.

Investigation of fasting hypoglycemia

- Glucose strip: unreliable for low-glucose concentrations. If the level is <70 mg/dL, a laboratory glucose should be measured.
- Liver and renal function tests
- Fasting insulin, C-peptide, proinsulin, and glucose during hypoglycemia (Table 95.1)
- Inappropriately elevated insulin in the presence of hypoglycemia suggests insulinoma or self-administration of insulin or sulfonylurea.
- Presence of C-peptide indicates endogenous insulin release—either insulinoma or sulfonylurea.
- Insulinomas are often associated with elevated pro-insulin/insulin ratio.
- Consider an assay for presence of sulfonylureas.
- Ethanol concentration
- Cortisol (± cosyntropyn stimulation test)
- Fasting β-hydroxybutyrate (elevated in most causes of hypoglycemia, but suppressed if insulin is present, e.g., insulinoma, self-administration of insulin or sulfonylureas)
- Consider IGF-1 and 2: IGF-2 may be normal in NICH, but this is in association with suppressed IGF-1 and GH; the usual IGF-2/IGF-1 ratio is 3:1, ratio >10 is seen in NICH (see Box 95.2).
- Chest and abdominal radiographs/CT—?NICH source
- Consider insulin and insulin receptor antibodies.

Table 95.1 Biochemical features of insulinoma and factitious hypoglycemia

Plasma marker	Insulinoma	Sulfonylurea	Insulin injection
Glucose	↓	↓	↓
Insulin	↑	↑	↑
C-peptide	↑	↑	↓

Box 95.2 Non-islet cell tumor hypoglycemia (NICH)

Excess secretion of abnormal IGF-2 (↑ IGF-2) from tumors such as fibrosarcomas and mesotheliomas leads to hypoglycemia associated with the following:

- Suppressed insulin, C-peptide, and IGF-1
- Low GH
- Low β-hydroxybutyrate levels
- Autonomous IGFBP-2 secretion by tumors leads to suppression of GH secretion and reduced IGF-1 and IGFBPs and a high IGF-2/IGF-1 ratio.
- IGF-2 is usually IGFBP bound, which maintains it within the circulation.
- IGF-2 may therefore remain "free" in the circulation, with i tissue bioavailability, leading both to suppression of IGF-1 and GH and to hypoglycemia due to binding and stimulation of insulin receptors.

Definitive treatment is removal of the tumor.

High-dose glucocorticoids are the most effective medical therapy.

Therapy with GH replacement stimulates an increase in binding proteins (IGFBP-3) and IGF-1 and a reversal of hypoglycemia.

Further investigation of fasting hypoglycemia

Glucose and insulin

After a 15-hour fast, glucose <40 mg/dL and insulin >5 mU/L is inappropriate. This a good screening test if repeated 3 times.

72-hour fast

This is the most reliable test for hypoglycemia (detects 98% patients with insulinoma, compared with 71% at 24 hours).

The patient should remain active. Plasma glucose, insulin, C-peptide, and pro-insulin are measured q6h (unless the patient is symptomatic or the glucose level is <60 mg/dL when measurements are made every 1–2 hours). The test is terminated if the laboratory glucose is <40 mg/dL or after 72 hours. β-hydroxybutyrate should be measured at the end of the fast (its presence makes insulinoma unlikely).

Exercise test

This is used to precipitate hypoglycemia in patients with endogenous hyperinsulinism who might tolerate prolonged periods of fasting.

Blood is collected before and at 10-minute intervals during 30 minutes of intense exercise and for 30 minutes afterward.

Patients with spontaneous hypoglycemia become exhausted and their glucose concentration falls below 40 mg/dL.

Localization of tumor

📖 See Tumor localization (p. 473). This is only performed once an insulinoma is confirmed biochemically. MRI or spiral CT are usually first-line investigations (equal sensitivity 50–70%); endoscopic and intraoperative US have an improved resolution and sensitivity but are more invasive.

¹¹¹I Octreotide scan

This has 50% sensitivity and may detect metastases. It is less good for insulinomas than for other pancreatic tumors.

Selective angiography

Angiography with selective arterial calcium gluconate or secretin stimulation (rarely required) is done in centers with experienced radiologists, when biochemically proven insulinomas cannot be visualized on imaging.

Management

Acute hypoglycemia

If the patient is conscious, oral carbohydrate (ideally food and a sugary drink) should be administered as soon possible. A glucose-containing gel, which is absorbed by the buccal mucosa, may be used in drowsy, but conscious, individuals.

If the patient is unconscious, administer 25–50 mL 25% glucose IV into a large vein, followed by a saline flush, as the high concentration of glucose is an irritant and may even lead to venous thrombosis. A maintenance infusion of 5% or 10% dextrose is often required thereafter, especially if there is an ongoing risk of recurrent hypoglycemia (e.g., overdose of a long-acting insulin/analog).

A dose of 1 mg glucagon IM may be administered if there is no IV access. This increases hepatic glucose efflux, but the effect only lasts for 30 minutes, allowing other means of blood glucose elevation (e.g., oral), before the blood glucose falls again. It is

- Ineffective with hepatic dysfunction and if there is glycogen depletion, e.g., ethanol-related hypoglycemia.
- Relatively contraindicated in patients with known insulinoma, as it may induce further insulin secretion.
- Ineffective within 3 days following a previous dose of glucagon.

Secondary cerebral edema may complicate hypoglycemia and should be considered in cases of prolonged coma despite normalization of plasma glucose. Mannitol and/or dexamethasone may be helpful.

Recurrent chronic hypoglycemia

If definitive treatment of the underlying condition is unsuccessful or impossible, symptoms may be alleviated by frequent (e.g., q4h) small meals, including overnight.

Diazoxide, administered by mouth, is useful in the management of patients with chronic hypoglycemia from excess endogenous insulin secretion due to an insulinoma or islet cell hyperplasia.

Further reading

Gama R, Teale, JD, Marks V (2003). Clinical and laboratory investigation of adult spontaneous hypoglycemia. *J Clin Pathol* 56:641–646.

Service FJ (1997). Hypoglycemia. *Endocrinol Metab Clin North Am* 126(4):937–952.

Postprandial reactive hypoglycemia (PRH)

Definition
PRH is hypoglycemia following a meal due to an imbalance between glucose influx into (exogenous from food, and endogenous glucose production) and glucose efflux out of the circulation.

Pathophysiology and causes
- *Exaggerated insulin response* related to rapid glucose absorption, e.g., post-gastrectomy dumping syndrome. This results in a delayed insulin peak with respect to the peak blood glucose, probably related to an exaggerated GLP-1 (glucagons-like peptide 1) response.
- *Incipient diabetes mellitus* occasionally presents with postprandial hypoglycemia, possibly related to disordered insulin secretion.
- *Insulin resistance related hyperinsulinemia*, e.g., obese subjects with or without impaired glucose tolerance
- *Increased insulin sensitivity* with deficiency of counterregulatory hormones, glucagon, and adrenaline (rapid action), as well as cortisol and GH (delayed action, up to 12 hours)
- *Impaired glucagon sensitivity and secretion* in response to hypoglycemia are involved in the pathogenesis of PRH.
- *Renal glycosuria* accounts for up to 15% of patients with PRH.

Body composition
- 20% of very lean people are prone to PRH.
- Massive weight reduction increases the risk of PRH.
- Lower-body obesity (especially in women) is associated with high-normal insulin sensitivity and PRH.

Diet
- High-carbohydrate, low-fat diet, by ↑ insulin sensitivity
- Prolonged very low–calorie diets (>2 weeks), by reducing counterregulatory hormones, especially GH.

Alcohol
- Inhibits hepatic glucose output
- Increases insulin secretion in response to glucose and sucrose

There are also idiopathic causes of PRH.

Investigation
Prolonged oral glucose tolerance test is not physiological; 10% of the normal (asymptomatic) population has a positive response with blood glucose levels <47 mg/dL.

The *mixed-meal test* is more physiological; 47% of patients with suspected PRH have a positive test vs.1% of asymptomatic subjects.

Ambulatory glucose sampling is gaining favor, as it may correlate symptoms with low sugar readings, and improvement of symptoms with recovery from hypoglycemia.

Management

Diet

- Frequent, small, low-carbohydrate, high-protein meals
- Avoid rapidly absorbed carbohydrates
- Avoid sugary drinks, especially in combination with alcohol
- Addition of soluble dietary fibers, e.g., 5–10 g guar gum, or pectin, or hemicellulose per meal, delays absorption and lowers the glycemic and insulinemic indices (especially effective in rapid gut transit time).

Drugs

- Acarbose, an intestinal α-glucosidase inhibitor, delays sugar and starch absorption, thus reducing the insulin response to a meal.
- Metformin 500 mg can be useful with meals.
- Supplemental chromium is reported to down-regulate β-cell activity and increase glucagon secretion.
- In exceptional cases, with debilitating PRH, diazoxide (side effects are water retention, hypertrichosis, digestive disorders), or somatostatin analogs may be required.
- Propranolol and calcium antagonists have been used; however, controlled studies are lacking.

Further reading

Brun JF, Fedou C, Mercier J (2000). Postprandial reactive hypoglycemia. *Diabet Metab* 26:337–351.

Gama R, Teale JD, Marks V (2003). Clinical and laboratory investigation of adult spontaneous hypoglycemia. *J Clin Pathol* 56:641–646.

Teale JD, Wark G (2004). The effectiveness of different treatment options for non-islet cell tumour hypoglycemia. *Clin Endocrinol* 60:457–460.

Obesity

Definition

Obesity is defined as an excess of body fat (adiposity) sufficient to adversely affect health. In the almanac of direct measurements of body fat mass, body mass index (BMI) is a commonly used surrogate marker (see Box 96.1).

- Obesity is often defined in terms of BMI.
- BMI does not take body build or fat distribution into consideration, and thus can be misleading in the presence of large muscle mass.
- Lower cutoff values may be applicable to non-Caucasian ethnic groups.
- Fat distribution: central (abdominal) obesity ("apple shape") vs. gluteofemoral obesity ("pear shape").
- Apple-shaped people have an ↑ cardiovascular risk compared to that of pear-shaped people.
- Adverse consequences of central obesity may reflect ↑ visceral (intra-abdominal fat) stores, (blood draining into the portal vein may expose the liver directly to the effluent from visceral fat).

Assess fat distribution using waist circumference (see Boxes 96.2 and 96.3).

Box 96.1 BMI

BMI (kg/m^2) = weight (kg) / [height (m)]^2

Classification

BMI (kg/m2)	WHO class
<18.5	Underweight
18.5–24.9	Healthy
25.0–29.9	Pre-obese (overweight)
30.0–34.9	Obese class I (obese)
35.0–39.9	Obese class II (obese)
>40.0	Obese class III (severely obese)

Box 96.2 Waist circumference

Suggested indicators of central obesity (and ↑ cardiovascular risk):

Waist circumference
- Men >40 in (102 cm)
- Women >35 in (88 cm)

Another study suggested a waist circumference of <100 cm makes insulin resistance unlikely (irrespective of sex).

Waist circumference cutoffs should be adjusted for individuals of certain racial and ethnic backgrounds.

Box 96.3 Measurement of waist circumference

Measurements should be recorded over underwear or light clothing. The subject should stand with their arms by their sides.

The position of the waist is midway between the lower rib margin and the iliac crest.
1. Identify the bony landmarks in the mid-axillary line.
   a. The lower rib margin (bottom of the rib cage)
   b. The iliac crest (highest bony part of the pelvis)
2. Measure the vertical distance between them. Note the midpoint.
3. Ask the subject to stand with their feet 23–30 cm apart.
4. Ensure that the tape measure is at the same level around the body at the midpoint. Gently tighten the tape measure so that it is taut but not too tight.
5. Ask the subject to breathe normally and record the measurement at the end of normal expiration.
6. Record waist circumference.

Epidemiology

There has been a rapid increase in obesity in both the developed and developing worlds.

In the United States, the prevalence of obesity has increased—in 1980, 12% of men and 16% of women were obese. By 2004, the figures had increased to 31% and 33%, respectively. Now, 2/3 of the population is either overweight or obese.

Prevalence in children has also increased rapidly (17% of adolescents in 2004) with an attendant risk of type 2 diabetes.

In some ethnic populations, prevalence of overweight is >75%.

Prevalence varies with age (peak prevalence at 50–70 years) and socioeconomic class.

Etiology

Genetic factors

Monogenic
This is rare.
- Leptin deficiency or resistance (massive obesity and hyperphagia in early childhood) (see Box 96.4)
- Prader–Willi syndrome (obesity, learning difficulties, chromosome 15)
- Lawrence–Moon–Biedl syndrome (obesity, polydactyly, learning difficulties, retinitis pigmentosa)
- Melanocortin 4 receptor (MC4R) deficiency (obesity, hyperphagia, dominant inheritance (see Box 96.5)

Box 96.4 Leptin

- First hormone described to be secreted from adipose tissue
- Encoded by *Lep* gene (chromosome 7q31.3)
- Synthesized in and secreted by adipose tissue
- Affects the hypothalamus to decrease food intake and increase energy expenditure (by sympathetic activation)
- Primary role in humans may be to indicate nutritional depletion or fasting and for falling leptin levels to indicate insufficient energy reserves for growth and reproduction
- Exerts potent anti-obesity effects in animals such as the *ob/ob* (leptin deficient) mouse
- Leptin therapy benefits humans with congenital leptin deficiency and leptin-deficient partial lipodystrophy.
- Most obese humans do not have abnormalities of the leptin gene. Plasma leptin ↑ in obese humans, and obese humans appear to be leptin resistant. Reduced leptin transport to the brain has been suggested as a potential mechanism of leptin resistance in humans.
- Trials in humans with polygenic obesity are equivocal (high doses of SC leptin lead to more weight loss than placebo, but long-term consequences of supraphysiological doses are unknown; sympathetic activation for weight loss by other agents has unwanted side effects).
- Loss of function mutations in the leptin receptor gene is associated with hyperphagia and early-onset obesity; serum leptin levels do not predict leptin receptor mutations.
- Leptin is stimulated by glucocorticoids.

Box 96.5 Melanocortin peptides

- Melanocortin peptides are derived by cleavage from pro-opiomelanocortin (POMC).
- Mutations result in ACTH deficiency, obesity, and pale skin (and no hair in Caucasians).
- Mutations in the receptor (MC4R) are the most common mongenic causes of obesity found—1% of adults with BMI >30 kg/m^2 and 5–6% of overly obese children under the age of 10.
- MC4R mutations are dominantly inherited.

Polygenic

Estimates of heritability range from 40 to 80%, thus genetic factors play a major role in obesity.

Environmental factors

Excess energy intake or ↓ energy expenditure due to physical inactivity are major determinants of obesity in genetically susceptible individuals.

Secondary causes

These include Cushing's disease or syndrome, hypothyroidism, and hypothalamic lesions (↑ appetite).

Pathophysiology

There is complex regulation of appetite and energy expenditure that is still not fully understood. Understanding has not yet been translated into therapeutic modalities (perhaps reflecting that long-term attempts to change one pathway leads to compensatory changes in other pathways).

Long-term signals associated with body-fat stores are provided by leptin and insulin. These circulating molecules also modulate short-term signals that determine meal initiation and termination.

Short-term information about hunger and satiety is provided by gut hormones, such as cholecystokinin, ghrelin (Box 96.6), and peptide YY_{3-36} (PYY), and signals from vagal afferent neurons within the GI tract that respond to mechanical deformation, macronutrient balance, pH, tonicity, and hormones.

Neural and humoral signals from specific regions of the hypothalamus, brain stem, and neural networks are involved in regulation of energy homeostasis and are regulated by peripheral signals such as leptin, which regulates neuropeptides and neurotransmitters expressed in these brain areas.

In *fat vs. carbohydrates*, overall, there is close regulation of metabolism and storage of carbohydrates, but not of fat.

In terms of *weight homeostasis*, overeating increases both fat-free mass (FFM) and fat mass (~1 kg FFM gain for ~2 kg fat gain). FFM is the major determinant of resting energy expenditure.

Box 96.6 Ghrelin

- Plasma concentrations inversely proportional to degree of obesity
- Peptide (28 amino acids) from oxyntic cells in the stomach fundus
- Acts on GH secretagogue receptors to increase release of GH from the pituitary
- Also important in energy homeostasis
- Appears to regulate pre-meal hunger and meal initiation
- Circulating ghrelin concentrations increase preprandially and decrease postprandially.
- Ghrelin increases food intake through the stimulation of ghrelin receptors on hypothalamic neuropeptide Y–expressing neurons and agouti-related protein-expressing neurons (📖 see Box 96.7).
- Patients with Prader–Willi syndrome have disproportionately elevated levels of ghrelin, although the relevance of this finding is unclear.

Box 96.7 Neuropeptide Y (NPY)

- Synthesized in the arcuate nucleus of the hypothalamus and transported axonally to the hypothalamic paraventricular nucleus
- A potent appetite stimulant and reduces sympathetic output, thus reducing energy expenditure
- ↑ By insulin and glucocorticoids, and ↓ by leptin and estrogen
- Genetic studies have not shown any association between the genes for NPY or its receptor in human obesity.

Consequences of obesity

Increased body fat is associated with ↑ morbidity and mortality, but the causal link is unclear. For example, low cardiorespiratory fitness is an independent predictor of cardiovascular disease, irrespective of body fat.

Standardized mortality rates rise sharply at BMI of 30 kg/m^2.

Diseases associated with obesity include the following:

- Type 2 diabetes (BMI >40 in <55-year-old leads to ↑ risk 18-fold in men, 13-fold in women)
- Hypertension (BMI 25–29.9 leads to ↑ risk 1.6-fold; BMI >40 leads to ↑ risk 5.5-fold)
- Dyslipidemia (moderate relationship with total cholesterol, closer relationship with ↑ triglycerides, ↓ HDL cholesterol)
- Cardiovascular disease (BMI >29 leads to ↑ risk 4-fold)
- Gall bladder disease (men, BMI >40 leads to ↑ risk 21-fold; women, BMI >40 leads to ↑ risk 5-fold).
- Osteoarthritis, varicose veins, obstructive sleep apnea, some cancers (e.g., endometrium, breast, ovary, prostate, colon)

However, obesity protects against osteoporosis.

Evaluation of an obese patient

- Weight history from birth on (early onset is associated with genetic syndromes)
- Previous treatment or management strategies and their success
- Current eating habits and activity levels
- Triggers for eating
- Family history of obesity
- Comorbidities such as cardiovascular disease, diabetes, psychological issues (depression, low self-esteem), osteoarthritis, obstructive sleep apnea, polycystic ovarian syndrome
- Assess for coexistent cardiovascular risk factors such as smoking and diabetes, family history of cardiovascular disease.
- Look for eruptive xanthomata (hypertriglyceridemia), acanthosis nigricans (insulin resistance), skin tags (insulin resistance), striae (Cushing's syndrome), and fat distribution (Cushing's, partial lipodystrophy—probably underdiagnosed).

Consider a secondary cause if there are additional clinical features:
- Hypothyroidism (measure TSH)
- Cushing's syndrome (measure 24-hour urinary free cortisol and consider dexamethasone suppression testing)
- Hypothalamic disorder (uncontrolled appetite—MRI)
- Prader–Willi syndrome
- Lawrence–Moon–Biedl syndrome

Consider coexistent conditions, e.g., polycystic ovary syndrome.

Box 96.8 Metabolic syndrome

- A clustering of metabolic risk factors: hyperinsulinemia, impaired glucose tolerance or frank diabetes, ↑ triglycerides, ↓ HDL cholesterol, hypertension, and central obesity
- Associated with ↑ risk of vascular disease. Data suggest that >95% of centrally obese patients have some risk factors; <50% of subcutaneously obese patients do as well.

Different diagnostic criteria exist. A typical definition is three of the following criteria:
- Abdominal obesity (see abdominal circumference cutoff values)
- Raised plasma triglyceride concentrations
- Low plasma HDL-cholesterol concentrations
- Raised blood pressure
- Impaired fasting glucose

Investigations

Consider the following:
- CBC (polycythemia)
- Electrolytes
- Liver function tests (LFTs) (nonalcoholic steatohepatitis, subsequent cirrhosis)
- Glucose (impaired fasting glucose, diabetes)
- Fasting lipid profile (raised triglycerides, total and LDL-cholesterol, lowered HDL cholesterol)
- TSH (hypothyroidism)
- Urine dipstick (glycosuria with diabetes, proteinuria with glomerular hyperfiltration)
- ECG (coronary vascular disease, left ventricular hypertrophy)
- Waist circumference
- Height and weight

Management

Weight normalization and maintenance rarely occurs. Even in the best weight management programs about 10% of weight is lost, but most people regain 2/3 of the lost weight in a year, and 95% of it is gained in 5 years. A weight loss of 5–10% of the initial body weight reduces the health risks associated with obesity.

The aims should be modest weight loss maintained for the long term, with treatment methods and goals being decided for each individual after careful assessment of the degree of overweight and any associated comorbid conditions. See Box 96.9.

There is a limited range of treatments available. The first-line strategy for weight loss and its maintenance is a combination of supervised diet, exercise, and behavior modification.

Diet

Diet alone does not usually maintain weight loss, and most dieters regain weight within 3 years.

Reduce calorie intake to 500 kcal below current intake. Reduce fat intake—standard dietary advice is to limit fat intake to 20–35% of total calorie intake. Reduction of fat intake can lead to weight loss, often without a conscious reduction in calorie intake.

Extreme diets may have problems:

Very low–calorie diets (<600–800 kcal/day) are used occasionally for up to 26 weeks in specialized centers in combination with high-quality proteins (daily intake of 1 g/kg of ideal body weight), electrolytes, vitamins, and trace elements. These can produce weight loss of ~2 kg/week (more in the first week as glycogen-bound fluid is lost).

Weight is often regained after stopping the diet. Side effects include fatigue, malaise, and electrolyte disturbances.

Very high–carbohydrate/low-fat diets have been associated with hypertriglyceridemia and lower LDL-cholesterol concentrations.

Box 96.9 Effects of losing weight

- *Diabetes:* weight loss of 5 kg
  - Halves the risk of developing type 2 diabetes
  - Improves glycemic control
- *Hypertension:* weight loss of 1 kg reduces blood pressure by 1–2 mmHg.
- *Dyslipidemia*: weight loss of 1 kg:
  - Lowers LDL cholesterol by 0.77 mg/dL
  - Lowers triglycerides by 1.33 mg/dL
  - Raises HDL cholesterol by 0.35 mg/dL
- *Obesity-related cancers:* weight loss of 0.5–9 kg is associated with a 53% reduction in cancer-related deaths.
- *Osteoarthritis and obstructive sleep apnea:* weight loss has significant mechanical benefits.
- *Gallstones:* weight loss (or weight gain) can provoke gallstone formation by altering the cholesterol saturation of bile.

Low-carbohydrate/high-protein diets (>25% of calories as protein) have little or no long-term safety data (especially on renal disease, ischemic heart disease; diets tend to be high in saturated fat and cholesterol). Side effects include constipation, renal stones, and ↑ urinary calcium losses.

They can be effective in inducing weight loss. They probably work by ↑ sense of satiety, leading to a ↓ calorie intake.

Exercise

Exercise is the most effective method of maintenance of weight loss when combined with calorie restriction and behavioral modification. It promotes the preservation of FFM (the major determinant of resting energy expenditure) in the face of weight loss.

Current recommendations are 20+ minutes exercise 3–5 times/week.

Regular exercise induces cardiorespiratory fitness and leads to a beneficial effect on other risk factors, with a reduction in blood pressure and improvement in lipid profile.

Interestingly, nonvoluntary activity ("fidgeting") is a significant determinant of resting energy expenditure. Factors controlling nonvoluntary activity are unclear.

Behavioral interventions

Few relevant data are available, but these should probably include self-monitoring of behavior and progress, stimulus control, goal setting, slowing rate of eating, social support, problem solving, assertiveness, cognitive restructuring (modifying thoughts), reinforcement of changes, relapse prevention, and strategies for dealing with weight regain.

A formal psychological assessment of patients with eating disorders (a minority of obese patients) is helpful.

Drug treatment

This should be used in combination with other treatments (exercise, calorie restriction, behavior modification).

It is for the following patients:
- Those at medical risk from obesity (BMI >30kg/m²); *or*
- Those with BMI >27 with established comorbidities (e.g., diabetes, heart disease, severe respiratory problems, dyslipidemia).

Use drug treatment only after dietary and lifestyle modifications have been unsuccessful (defined as not achieving a 10% weight reduction after at least 3 months of supervised care).

Not all obese patients respond to drug therapy.
- Stop drug treatment if 5% weight reduction is not achieved.
- If a 5% weight loss is attained, treatment may be continued, provided body weight is continually monitored and weight is not regained.
- Rapid weight regain is common after short-term use of anti-obesity drugs (12 weeks or less).

Fat-absorption inhibitors

Orlistat
- Intestinal pancreatic lipase inhibitor; reduces fat absorption

- Increases dietary fat loss to 30% (compared to <5% on placebo)
- Average weight loss of 5–10%
- Licensed for use up to 2 years.
- Contraindications: cholestasis, malabsorption syndromes
- Drug interactions with warfarin (possible ↓ vitamin K absorption) and cyclosporine (reduced serum drug levels)
- No data on patients aged >75 years
- Dosing: 60–120 mg with main meals
- Consider vitamin supplementation (especially vitamin D) if there is concern about fat-soluble vitamin deficiency.

Side effects include flatus (24%), oily rectal discharge, fatty stool (20%), fecal urgency (22%), fat-soluble vitamin deficiency, and incontinence (8%). Side effects are limited by dietary fat reduction (to <35% of energy).

Appetite-suppressant drugs
Phentermine
- Centrally acting noradrenergic/dopamine release inhibitor
- Decreases food intake
- Average weight loss 5%
- Cautions: hypertension, vascular disease
- Drug interactions: sympathomimetics, MAO inhibitors, other anorexants
- Side effects: increased BP and HR, insomnia, agitation, dry mouth, headache, tremor
- Approved for only 3 months use only
- Dosing between 15 and 37.5 mg daily

Other appetite-suppressant drugs, such as fenfluramine and dexfenfluramine, have been withdrawn because of associations with valvular heart disease and pulmonary hypertension.

Surgery

Bariatric
- Associated with significant weight loss for at least 8 years
- Improves QoL, hypertriglyceridemia, and hyperuricemia, and reduces the incidence of type 2 diabetes
- Data on benefit to BP and cholesterol concentrations unclear
- Jejunoileal bypass and jaw wiring are not recommended.
- Only indicated in severely obese (>100% above ideal weight, BMI >40 or BMI >35 with serious comorbidities) adults (>18 years)
- Failure to lose weight before surgery is not a contraindication.
- Candidates for surgery should be thoroughly assessed with multidisciplinary assessment (including a biopsychosocial assessment).
- Long-term follow-up is required.

Malabsorptive bariatric surgery:
- Shortening the length of gut so that the amount of food absorbed by the body is reduced

- Most common procedure now is Roux-en-Y gastric bypass. Jejunoileleal or biliopancreatic diversions are less common and associated with dumping syndrome or recurrent hypoglycemia.

Restrictive bariatric surgery:
- Induces early satiety, limits rate of food intake, or both
- E.g., laparoscopic gastric banding (reduction in functional capacity of stomach by partitioning off part of the body of the stomach)

Liposuction
The benefit of liposuction on metabolic parameters is equivocal.

One study has shown that removal of 10 kg SC abdominal adipose tissue by liposuction failed to improve parameters such as BP, plasma glucose, and insulin concentrations.

Further reading

Brennan AM, Mantzoros CS (2006). Drug insight: the role of leptin in human physiology and pathophysiology—emerging clinical applications. *Nat Clin Pract Endocrinol Metab* 2(6):318–327.

Kahn R, Buse J, Ferrannini E, et al. (2005). The metabolic syndrome: time for a critical appraisal joint statement from the American Diabetes Association and the European Association for the Study of Diabetes. *Diabetes Care* 28(9):2289–2304.

National Institute for Health and Clinical Excellence (NICE) Clinical guideline 43: Obesity guidance on the prevention, identification, assessment, and management of overweight and obesity in adults and children. http://www.nice.org.uk/page.aspx?o=91525

Rucher D, Padwal R, Li SK, et al. (2007). Long term pharmacotherapy for obesity and overweight: updated meta-analysis. *BMJ* 335(7631):1194–1199.

Sjöström L, Narbo K, Sjöström CD, et al. (2007). Effects of bariatric surgery on mortality in Swedish obese subjects. *N Engl J Med* 357(8):741–752.

Endocrinology and aging

Introduction

Aging causes changes in many hormonal axes. How much of this change is normal physiology associated with aging and how much represents true endocrine dysfunction and thus warrants treatment is unclear.

Concomitant disease and polypharmacy are common in the elderly population, with frequent secondary effects on the endocrine system.

Fluid and electrolyte homeostasis in the elderly

Elderly patients are particularly prone to fluid and electrolyte disturbances due to changes associated with aging, concomitant disease, and drug usage.

Elderly patients have ↓ renal function compared with that of younger patients:
- ↓ Glomerular filtration rate (GFR) with creatinine clearance ↓ by 8 mL/min/1.73 m^2 per decade after age 30
- ↑ Renovascular disease
- ↓ Renal sensitivity to circulating hormones
  - Aldosterone
  - Vasopressin
  - Atrial natriuretic peptide (probable)
- ↓ Ability to dilute or concentrate urine

Elderly patients have ↓ renin levels with secondary decreases of aldosterone levels (both basal and stimulated levels). Aldosterone levels may be <50% normal by 70 years of age. Increased renal sensitivity to aldosterone may result in isolated mineralocorticoid deficiency (distal renal tubular acidosis [type 4] with hyponatremia, hyperkalemia, hyperchloremia, and normal anion gap acidosis); this is more common with diabetes mellitus.

Vasopressin and ADH

Unlike many other hormones, vasopressin (ADH) responses are potentiated in elderly patients with ↑ release from the neurohypophysis in response to an osmotic stimulus and less effective suppression.

Normal vasopressin release is a balance of inhibitory and stimulatory effects at baroreceptors and osmoreceptors. It may be that loss of inhibition with aging due to degenerative changes results in relatively unopposed stimulation of ADH and a ↓ ability to suppress ADH release.

In addition, altered renal sensitivity to vasopressin results in ↓ ability to excrete free water.

Hypernatremia and dehydration

Perception of thirst is altered in elderly persons (in younger people, thirst is perceived at plasma osmolalities >292 mOsm/kg, whereas in older people, thirst is perceived at plasma osmolalities >296 mOsm/kg). Elderly patients may also be unable to ingest fluids because of other disabilities and/or effects of medications.

Thus, elderly persons are particularly susceptible to dehydration (e.g., during hot summers).

Hyponatremia

This is particularly common in elderly patients (prevalence of 2–20%). In hospital patients, overall incidence of hyponatremia (Na <137mmol/L) is 7%, but in geriatric facilities it is 18–22%, with 53% incidence of one or more episodes of hyponatremia at any time during admission to geriatric care facilities.

Mortality rates in hospitalized elderly patients with hyponatremia are high (in patients aged >65 years, 16% mortality in those with hyponatremia compared with 8% without hyponatremia).

Hyponatremia is often associated with medication (e.g., diuretics). It is the most common electrolyte disturbance in cancer (📖 see SIADH due to ectopic vasopressin production, p. 550).

Symptoms include confusion, lethargy, coma, and seizures.

The overall approach to investigation and management is similar to that for hyponatremia in younger patients (📖 see Hyponatremia, p. 156).

Mild idiopathic hyponatremia is also recognized in elderly patients, without necessarily having a sinister cause or consequence, and is thought to be secondary to an altered threshold for ADH secretion.

Bone disease

Osteoporosis

Osteoporosis is not an inevitable part of aging but it is a common disease in elderly people and is associated with high morbidity and mortality in both males and females. 📖 See Osteoporosis (p. 405).

Vitamin D deficiency and osteomalacia

This is very common in the elderly. Vitamin D insufficiency (evidence of secondary hyperparathyroidism, ↑ bone turnover, BMD loss) occurs at levels of 25OH-vitamin D <50 nmol/L.

Vitamin D deficiency is usually defined at levels <30 nmol/L (with additional problems of myopathy, ↑ sway, ↓ psychomotor function, and frank osteomalacia).

Vitamin D deficiency and/or insufficiency is common particularly in elderly institutionalized patients in extreme latitudes and in fracture patients. In a Danish study, 40% of postmenopausal women had vitamin D levels of 25–50 nmol/L, with a further 7% with frank deficiency (<25 nmol/L). 80% of elderly men and women (aged >65 years) have vitamin D insufficiency. 44% of nursing home patients have severe vitamin D deficiency (25OH vitamin D <12 nmol/L). In patients with hip fracture, 75% have vitamin D insufficiency, 25% have vitamin D deficiency, and 5% have severe vitamin D deficiency (25OH vitamin D <12.5 nmol/L).

Supplementation with 800 IU vitamin D and 1200 mg calcium daily in institutionalized elderly patients reduces falls and fractures Supplementation in free-living elderly patients (>65 years of age) also ↓ fracture risk.

Vitamin D is known to have an antitumor effect with ↓ proliferation, ↑ differentiation of cells, and ↑ apoptosis of malignant cells. Vitamin D may also boost the immune response with further antitumor effect.

Vitamin D insufficiency and/or deficiency may contribute to higher rates of malignancy in elderly patients (e.g., breast, colon, and prostate). Therapeutic use of vitamin D in malignant disease is limited by hypercalcemia.

Primary hyperparathyroidism

Prevalence of primary hyperparathyroidism is 10/100,000 in women <40 years old, rising to 190/100,000 in women >65 years old. Half of all cases of primary hyperparathyroidism occur in women >60 years old.

Elderly people are more prone to symptoms (weakness, fatigue, confusion) at relatively mild levels of hypercalcemia (2.8–3.0 mmol/L).

Other causes of hypercalcemia must be excluded.

Coexisting vitamin D insufficiency and deficiency is common.

Management is similar to that described in 📖 Chapter 68, Hypercalcemia (p. 376). Surgery is not contraindicated by age alone.

Paget's disease

📖 See Chapter 73, Paget's disease (p. 421).

Further reading

Mosekilde L (2005). Vitamin D and the elderly. *Clin Endocrinol* 62:265–281.

GH and IGF-1 in the elderly

Many of the features of aging resemble growth hormone deficiency. Changes in body composition include ↓ lean body mass (d body water, ↓ muscle mass, and ↓ bone mass) and ↑ total body fat and visceral fat mass, associated with abnormal lipid profile (↑ total and LDL cholesterol, ↑ TGs), insulin resistance, and cardiovascular disease.

Overall, integrated GH concentrations show a decrease with age with ↓ GH pulse amplitude and duration, but pulse frequency unchanged.

IGF-1 falls with ↑ age (reflected in age-adjusted normative ranges). IGF-BP3 also falls with age (and is also GH dependent).

Older patients with GH deficiency related to pituitary disease are usually easily differentiated from other subjects with age-related decline in IGF-1 using standard provocative testing (GH response to insulin-induced hypoglycemia, arginine, or glucagon). Treatment with GH in patients with clear GH deficiency results in ↑ lean body mass and bone mineral density, and ↓ adipose tissue, as well as possibly psychological and functional improvement.

Small, frequently open-label studies of supraphysiological doses of GH given to healthy older persons have shown that GH may result in improved body composition (improved physiological function has not been observed). Side effects are frequently observed in the treated group (edema, arthralgias, carpal tunnel syndrome, glucose intolerance) and theoretical concerns of malignancy related to raised IGF-1 levels remain.

GH is not approved for healthy elderly people without clear evidence of GH deficiency.

Gonadal function in the elderly

Women

The mean age of menopause is 51 years (range 35–58 years) and is defined retrospectively after 12 months of amenorrhea as the permanent cessation of menstruation due to loss of ovarian follicular activity.

- FSH 10–15 × higher than premenopausal levels
- LH 3–5 × higher
- Estrogen 10% of previous level (often lower than those of men of similar age)
- Inhibin is often undetectable.

The adrenal gland is the major source of sex steroids postmenopausally, with estrogen production mainly from aromatization of adrenal androgens (androstenedione) in adipose tissue.

Low FSH/LH may indicate hypopituitarism, although gonadotropins may be depressed by serious illness.

📖 See Chapter 51, Menopause (p. 264) for further discussion.

Men

Men may remain potent and fertile until their death. However, sexual activity, libido, and potency decline gradually and progressively from midlife.

As with GH, there is an overlap between clinical features of hypogonadism and normal aging (loss of lean body mass and muscle function, increase in fat mass, loss of virility, loss of libido, and ↓ sexual and overall well-being). Functional secondary hypogonadism is common in serious chronic illness, especially when associated with malnutrition and debilitation.

Normal ranges for testosterone in men of different ages have not been well established.

Free testosterone levels decrease slowly with age, but there is significant intra- and interindividual variation. SHBG increases with age. Testicular weight, Leydig cell function, and FSH/LH response to GnRH stimulation all decrease with age.

The extent to which lower testosterone per se and/or a lower free androgen index explain the age-related decline in sexual function is not clear. Although testosterone levels may be lower than in younger men, testosterone levels are still sufficient for normal libido and sexual function. Profoundly low testosterone levels (<230 ng/dL in an A.M. blood sample) in the appropriate clinical setting should prompt investigation for hypoandrogenism.

Gonadotropins should be raised in primary testicular failure. Low levels associated with low testosterone should prompt a search for secondary causes, although gonadotropins may be low because of other serious disease.

Fat body mass increases more than lean body mass with age. Thus there is ↑ aromatization of androgens to estrogens. The effects of this are unclear.

Hypoandrogenism may also result from hyperprolactinemia due to pituitary/hypothalamic disease, renal dysfunction, hypothyroidism, or drugs (psychotropic and antidopaminergic agents), all more common in the elderly population.

Testosterone therapy
There are a few small studies in elderly men, either as replacement in patients with clear hypogonadism or in healthy men.

Data point toward a positive effect on well-being, muscle mass, and strength and in ↓ fat mass in elderly patients, the greatest effect being in patients with clear hypogonadism.

Risks include secondary polycythemia, liver dysfunction (particularly if testosterone is taken orally), prostatic hyperplasia, exacerbation of prostate adenocarcinoma, and possibly dyslipidemia.

Erectile dysfunction
This is common in elderly men; 50% of men >60 have erectile dysfunction; 90% of these men have concurrent medical problems or are on medication potentially causing impotence.

Etiology is often multifactorial:
- Atherosclerosis—most common cause with both macro- and microvascular disease
- Penile denervation—autonomic neuropathy (most commonly due to diabetes mellitus); pelvic surgery (including prostatectomy—30% of men >75 develop erectile dysfunction after prostatectomy [cf. 7% of younger men after prostatectomy])
- Drugs (β-blockers, calcium channel antagonists, other antihypertensive agents, psychotropic drugs)
- Psychogenic

Delayed or absent ejaculation
Increased incidence is common with age, due to autonomic nerve dysfunction, drugs, previous surgery, and is usually the harbinger of erectile dysfunction.

Evaluation is similar to that of younger patients (🕮 see Evaluation, p. 308).

Management is similar to that for younger patients, with the caveat that phosphodiesterase inhibitors may interact with nitrates and antihypertensive agents.

Fertility
Spermatogenesis persists into old age. There are very few data regarding spermatozoa number, motility, and morphology in elderly men.

However, errors in DNA replication increase with age, as reflected in paternal age effects in some genetic disorders.

Adrenal function in the elderly

Cortisol

Overall, cortisol secretion in elderly persons is generally very similar to that in younger persons.

Dynamic testing shows more prolonged release of ACTH and cortisol to stress (physiological, insulin-induced hypoglycemia, and/or CRH administration) and slower inhibition of ACTH secretion by cortisol.

Dehydroepiandrosterone sulfate

DHEA and DHEAS levels peak in humans aged 20–30 years and thereafter decline with age (20% of peak values in men and 30% of peak values in women by age 70 years). Responsiveness to ACTH-stimulated secretion also reduces with age.

The physiological relevance of the fall of DHEA and DHEAS levels with age is not established.

Replacement in otherwise healthy elderly patients has not consistently demonstrated improved longevity, well-being, bone density, cognitive function, body mass composition, or cardiovascular status in double-blind placebo-controlled trials, despite many Internet claims to the contrary.

Aldosterone

📖 See Fluid and electrolyte homeostasis in the elderly (p. 535).

Thyroid disease

Thyroid disease is twice as common in the elderly as in younger patients.

Goiter

Diffuse goiter becomes less frequent with age in both men and women (found in 31% of women aged <45 years compared with 12% of women aged >75 years on clinical examination).

Multinodular goiter as assessed by both clinical and US examination increases with age (incidence of US-detected multinodular goiter is 90% of women >70 years, 60% of men >80 years).

Management is similar to that of multinodular goiter in younger patients (📖 see Multinodular goiter and solitary adenomas, p. 44).

Abnormal thyroid function tests

Concomitant disease and polypharmacy are common in the elderly and may alter the interpretation of results. For example, glucocorticoids (prescribed to 2.5% of the population aged 70–79 years) cause decreased TSH, ↓ thyroid hormone release, ↓ concentration of thyroid hormone binding proteins, and ↓ T_4-to-T_3 conversion.

Sick euthyroid syndrome is more common in the elderly because of frequent, concurrent nonthyroidal illness, with reduced free tri-iodothyronine (FT_3), ↑ reverse free tri-iodothyronine, and (less commonly) reduced free thyroxine (FT_4), along with inappropriately normal or suppressed TSH levels.

Hypothyroidism

This is the most common thyroid problem in elderly people, affecting 2–7% of elderly people. The male-to-female ratio increases with aging.

The most common causes are autoimmune thyroiditis, previous surgery, or radioiodine therapy.

Only 25% present with classical symptoms of hypothyroidism. An insidious decline in health and mobility is more common than cold intolerance, hair loss, or skin coarsening.

The elderly are more susceptible to hypothyroid (myxedema) coma than younger people; it remains rare, however.

Hypothyroidism should be considered in elderly patients with increased CK or transaminases, ↓ Na, macrocytic anemia, or dyslipidemia.

Thyroid replacement therapy should be done cautiously as ischemic heart disease may be unmasked or exacerbated, e.g., 12.5–25 mcg/day of levothyroxine ↑ by 12–25 mcg increments every 3–8 weeks until TSH is normalized.

Total replacement T_4 dosage is lower in the elderly than in younger patients (in younger patients approximately 1.6 mcg/kg is required but older patients may require 20–30% less).

Hyperthyroidism

This affects 2% of elderly people. Presentation is often atypical, often with few signs or symptoms.

Commonly, symptoms are mainly in a single, vulnerable organ system, e.g., depression, lethargy, anxiety, confusion and agitation; muscle wasting and weakness; heart failure, arrhythmias, atrial fibrillation; weight loss; and osteoporotic fracture.

An isolated suppressed TSH concentration is associated with an ↑ cardiovascular mortality and a 3-fold higher risk of atrial fibrillation in the next 10 years. From 2 to 24% of elderly patients with atrial fibrillation are hyperthyroid and 9–35% of elderly patients with hyperthyroidism have atrial fibrillation.

The underlying cause may be toxic multinodular goiter or Graves' disease.

Treatment options are similar to those in younger patients (📖 see Treatment p. 21).

Radioactive iodine is favored because it is definitive and it avoids risks of surgery. Hypothyroidism is common after radioiodine therapy.

Thyroid cancer

The total incidence rate for all thyroid cancers is unchanged in the elderly, but the relative frequencies are altered. Papillary carcinoma is more common in young and middle-aged patients, but the prognosis is poorer in the elderly. Follicular carcinoma is more common with aging.

Anaplastic thyroid carcinoma occurs almost exclusively in patients >65 years. It presents with a rapidly growing hard mass that is often locally invasive and may be associated with metastatic lesions. The prognosis is poor.

Sarcomas and primary thyroid lymphomas are more common in elderly patients.

Overall evaluation and treatment are similar to that of younger patients, but accurate preoperative histology is very important, as tumors not treated surgically (e.g., anaplastic carcinoma and lymphoma) are relatively more common.

Glucose homeostasis

Elderly patients have impaired glucose homeostasis and are more likely to manifest hyperglycemia in response to acute illness and stress (e.g., post–myocardial infarction).

Further reading

Grimley Evans J, Williams TF, Michel J-P, et al. (eds.) (2000). *Oxford Textbook of Geriatric Medicine*. Oxford, UK: Oxford University Press.

Vermeulen A (Ed.) (1997) Endocrinology of aging. *Baillieres Clin Endocrinol Metab* 11:223–250.

Endocrinology of critical illness

Endocrine dysfunction and AIDS

Wasting syndrome

Definition

This is the involuntary loss of >10% of baseline body weight in combination with diarrhea, weakness, or fever. Wasting is an AIDS-defining condition.

Cause

The cause is unknown but in part reflects ↓ calorie intake due to anorexia associated with secondary infection. Underlying ↑ resting energy expenditure is associated with HIV infection per se. Hypogonadism is common in men with wasting syndrome.

Treatment

Highly active antiretroviral therapy (HAART)

HAART is associated with overall weight gain, though lean body mass may remain unchanged.

Nutritionally based strategies

Adequate caloric intake is required to meet metabolic demands. Efficacy is limited as refeeding generally increases fat body mass with little or less effect on lean body mass.

Appetite stimulants

Megestrol acetate increases caloric intake and weight compared to placebo, although most of the weight gain is due to ↑ fat mass. Dronabinol stimulates appetite but weight gain is minimal.

Exercise

Although exercise can increase total and lean body mass in patients with AIDS, its role in patients with wasting syndrome is not known.

Androgen therapy

In hypogonadal male patients with wasting syn-drome, testosterone increases overall weight and in particular lean body mass. Both IM and transdermal testosterone are effective. Testosterone therapy not indicated in eugonadal men with wasting.

Growth hormone therapy

Patients with the wasting syndrome generally have GH resistance, as suggested by high serum GH and low IGF-1 levels. The most likely cause for this is undernutrition.

High-dose GH has shown improvements in lean body mass and protein balance in patients with acquired GH deficiency or severe catabolic states.

Side effects (peripheral edema, arthralgias, myalgias) are common due to the high doses required. GH may improve fat redistribution that occurs with refeeding.

Cytokine modulators

Although many inflammatory cytokines are ↑ during acute illness and sepsis, their specific role in wasting syndrome is not known. Thalidomide, a potent inhibitor of tumor necrosis factor (TNF), can increase body weight and reduce protein catabolism but has a very high rate of serious side effects and is contraindicated in women of childbearing age due to phocomelia.

Lipodystrophy

Loss of SC fat occurs, particularly in the face, peripheries, and buttocks, in some cases with concomitant SC fat deposition, particularly in the abdominal area, neck, dorsocervical area ("buffalo hump"). Visceral fat deposition also occurs.

Lipodystrophy is associated with dyslipidemia with hypertriglyceridemia, low HDL cholesterol, insulin resistance, glucose intolerance, and (less commonly) frank diabetes mellitus. There is ↑ cardiovascular mortality from myocardial infarction.

It is also associated with HIV-1 protease inhibitors (PIs), used as part of HAART. 40% of patients treated with PIs will develop lipodystrophy by 1 year. HIV PI-naive patients have similar body composition and fat distribution to that of non-HIV-infected men. Indinavir may be less potent in inducing lipodystrophy than ritonavir and saquinavir.

Abnormal body composition and hypertriglceridemia may be part of the refeeding phenomenon following improved well-being and loss of anorexia.

Nucleoside reverse transcriptase inhibitors may be associated with fat loss and accumulation as well, but this may be a separate phenome-non from that seen with PIs.

Management

- Observation in mild cases
- Very low–fat diets and exercise (particular resistance exercise)
- Withdrawal or switching of PIs in some circumstances may be warranted.
- Anabolic agents (testosterone, GH) are not effective.
- Liposuction from areas of fat accumulation; fat pad insertions for areas of lipoatrophy also used
- Standard lipid-lowering agents for hypertriglyceridemia (e.g., gemfibrozil)
- HMG CoA reductase inhibitors metabolized by P4503A4 (which is inhibited by PIs) so risk of myopathy may be ↑
- The role for thiazolidinediones is unclear.

Adrenal

Adrenal insufficiency

This is uncommon (<4% of patients with AIDS). In patients with clinical signs suggestive of adrenal insufficiency (hyponatremia, and hypovolemia), there is a 30% incidence of inadequate response to Cortrosyn.

Causes
Infection

This is histologically common. Adrenal function is usually maintained, since 10% of residual adrenal tissue is adequate for normal function.

- CMV (adrenalitis found postmortem in 40–90% of patients dying of AIDS)
- *Mycobacterium avium intracellulare* (MAI) complex, tuberculosis
- *Cryptococcus*

Neoplasm
- Lymphoma, Kaposi's sarcoma

Hemorrhage

Drug induced
- Rifampicin induces ↑ hepatic metabolism of corticosteroids. In patients with already compromised adrenal reserve, this may precipitate an addisonian crisis.
- Ketoconazole inhibits cortisol synthesis.
- Megestrol acetate possesses glucocorticoid activity and may cause secondary adrenal insufficiency. Abrupt cessation after long-term treatment may precipitate an adrenal crisis.

Secondary adrenal insufficiency
- Drugs (megestrol acetate)
- Hypopituitarism secondary to toxoplasmosis, *Cryptococcus*, CMV
- Idiopathic anterior pituitary necrosis

Hypercortisolism

Mild hypercortisolemia is common in all stages of HIV infection, without clinical manifestation of Cushing's syndrome.

Possible causes
- Chronic stress
- Proinflammatory cytokines
- Binding protein dysfunction
- Glucocorticoid resistance

Gonads
Males

Testosterone deficiency is common in male patients with AIDS (6% of patients with asymptomatic HIV infection compared with 50% of patients with AIDS).

Hypogonadism is associated with wasting, ↓ muscle mass, fatigue, loss of libido, and impotence. Hypogonadism may be primary or secondary; up to 75% of patients with hypogonadism have low or inappropriately normal gonadotropins.

Causes

Primary hypogonadism
- *Testicular destruction/infiltration:* due to infection (CMV most commonly, MAI, toxoplasma, TB) or neoplasm (lymphoma, Kaposi's sarcoma, germ cell tumors)
- *Drug induced:* ketoconazole (inhibits steroidogenesis causing lowered testosterone levels); megestrol acetate, other glucocorticoids

Secondary hypogonadism
This is due to malnutrition, severe acute illness, destructive disorders of pituitary/hypothalamus (CMV, toxoplasmosis, lymphoma), and medications such as megestrol acetate (glucocorticoid-like action causes hypogonadotropic hypogonadism).

Females
Hypogonadism in women as evidenced by oligo- and amenorrhea is less common than in men unless there is advanced disease. Fertility rates are not affected until there is advanced disease.

Hypoandrogenism (testosterone, DHEA) is common in women with wasting syndrome.

Electrolyte disturbance due to endocrine pertubation in HIV/AIDS

Hyponatremia
This is very common in advanced disease and is due to SIADH in 50%. Adrenal insufficiency also a common cause.

Calcium disorders
Hypocalcemia
- Common (18% of patients with AIDS). Main cause is vitamin D deficiency. Other causes include severe illness; hypomagnesemia; altered PTH secretion/metabolism; malabsorption of calcium and vitamin D due to GIT opportunistic infection; and medications (foscarnet [complexes with calcium], pentamidine [induces renal magnesium wasting and secondary PTH deficiency]).

Hypercalcemia
- Rare. It may relate to lymphoma or granulomatous disease.

Thyroid

Overt thyroid dysfunction is uncommon. The most common thyroid dysfunction is sick euthyroid syndrome (nonthyroidal illness). Increased thyroid-binding globulin is often observed (significance is unknown).

Subclinical hypothyroidism may occur during HAART.

Infections
These are rare and are usually postmortem diagnoses. Thyroid function is usually euthyroid or sick euthyroid.
- *Pneumocystis jirovecii* (may also cause a thyroiditis)
- Mycobacteria

- *Cryptococcus neoformans*
- *Aspergillosis*

Neoplasm

This is rare and is usually euthyroid or sick euthyroid. It may be hypothyroid due to infiltrative destruction.

- Kaposi's sarcoma
- Lymphoma

Pituitary

- Anterior hypopituitarism is very rare.
- Posterior pituitary dysfunction causing diabetes indipidus (DI) is common.
- Infection, toxoplasmosis, TB
- Neoplasm, cerebral lymphoma

Cancer

Chemotherapy and radiotherapy may have endocrine effects.

Anticancer chemotherapy

There are three types of anticancer chemotherapeutic agents.

Cytotoxics

These have no direct hormonal sequelae. Alkylating agents are more likely to induce permanent male sterility (without affecting potency) and in women they may induce premature menopause, which may increase the likelihood of osteoporosis.

Immunomodulators

Prednisolone in excess causes Cushing's syndrome, and acute withdrawal may precipitate adrenal insufficiency. *Cyclophosphamide* in particular may cause early menopause.

Thyroid dysfunction has been reported rarely with tacrolimus and interferon-α and -β therapy.

Hormones

Progestogens are used in breast cancer. Of these, *megestrol acetate* has potent glucocorticoid activity and thus may cause Cushing's syndrome in excess or adrenal insufficiency if abruptly withdrawn.

Aromatase inhibitors such as aminoglutethimide may cause adrenal insufficiency and corticosteroid replacement is necessary.

Trilostane, which inhibits 3β-hydroxysteroid dehydrogenase, may also cause adrenal insufficiency.

Gonadorelin analogs, used for prostatic cancer and breast cancer, cause an initial increase in LH levels and then suppression and cause side effects similar to those of orchiectomy in men and menopause in women.

Antiandrogens used in prostatic cancer have predictable side effects such as gynecomastia, hot flashes, impotence, and impaired libido.

Radiotherapy

Cranial radiotherapy whose field encompasses the hypothalamic–pituitary area may result in hypopituitarism (see Chapter 13, Hypopituitarism, p. 94).

Head and neck irradiation may result in hypothyroidism and hypoparathyroidism.

After 5 or more years of follow-up, 50% of patients treated with radiotherapy only for laryngeal and pharyngeal carcinoma will develop hypothyroidism. Combined surgery and radiotherapy results in roughly 90% of patients developing hypothyroidism. The rates for hypoparathy-roidism are 88% and 90%, respectively.

Radiotherapy affects the testes dose dependently. Fertility is affected much more than androgensynthesizing capacity, so most men have normal testosterone levels unless given testicular doses >20–30 Gy.

The effects of radiotherapy to both ovaries are amplified with age. Premature menopause may be elicited by doses >10 Gy.

Syndromes of ectopic hormone production

Definition

The secretion into the systemic circulation, of a hormone or other biologically active molecule, by a neoplasm (benign or malignant) that has arisen from tissue that does not normally produce that hormone or molecule, results in a clinically significant syndrome. See Table 98.1 for common syndromes associated with ectopic hormone production.

SIADH due to ectopic vasopressin production

Diagnosis

- Hyponatremia (Na <130 mmol/L)
- Dilute plasma (serum osmolality <270 mmol)
- Inappropriately concentrated urine (in the face of hyponatremia and plasma hypoosmolality, any urine osmolality >plasma osmolality is inappropriate)
- Persistant renal Na excretion
- Euvolemia (or very mild hypervolemia)
- Normal renal, adrenal, and thyroid function

Plasma urea and uric acid levels can be helpful markers of plasma dilution.

The most common tumors causing SIADH are tumors with neuroendocrine features, most commonly small-cell lung carcinoma and carcinoid tumors. Small-cell lung carcinomas have usually metastasized by the time SIADH is present.

Lung diseases and neurological disorders (including malignancies) may cause SIADH due to aberrant hypothalamic vasopressin release rather than vasopressin release from the tumor per se. In SIADH due to ectopic hormone secretion, release of vasopressin from the neurohypophysis may be suppressed.

Other causes of SIADH must be excluded (□ see Syndrome of inappropriate ADH, p. 159).

Management

Hyponatremia

The initial management is fluid restriction with daily monitoring of the plasma sodium and osmolality. Hyponatremia has usually developed gradually, and its correction should be similarly gradual. Fluid restriction to 500 mL total fluid intake per day may be needed for several days.

Urate levels can be useful as a marker of water intoxication and its resolution. As hyponatremia is corrected, fluid restriction can be relaxed depending on the plasma sodium; 1500–2000 mL/day is usual.

For patients in whom fluid restriction is insufficient or not possible, demeclocycline (150–300 mg daily) can be used to produce a nephrogenic diabetes insipidus to achieve a normal plasma sodium. Demeclocycline can result in photosensitivity,thus patients should be warned to avoid prolonged exposure to sunlight.

Life-threatening hyponatremia (e.g., convulsions) may rarely require hypertonic saline and furosemide. However, rapid correction of hyponatremia may

Table 98.1 Common syndromes associated with ectopic hormone production

Syndrome	Ectopic hormone	Typical tumor types
Hypercalcemia of malignancy	PTHrP	Squamous cell lung carcinoma Other squamous cell carcinoma (skin, esophagus, head, and neck) Renal cell carcinoma Breast adenocarcinoma Adult T-cell lymphoma associated with HTLV-1
	1,25(OH)$_2$ cholecalciferol	Lymphomas
SIADH	Vasopressin/ADH	Small-cell lung carcinoma Squamous-cell lung carcinoma Bronchial carcinoid Mesothelioma Pancreatic or gut carcinoid Adenocarcinoma of the duodenum, pancreas, prostate Pheochromocytoma Medullary thyroid carcinoma Hematopoietic malignancies (lymphoma, leukemia)
Cushing's syndrome	ACTH (most commonly)	Small cell lung carcinoma Thymic carcinoid tumor Bronchial carcinoid tumor Pancreatic endocrine tumors (including carcinoid tumors) Carcinoid tumors of the gut Pheochromocytoma Medullary thyroid carcinoma Other lung cancers (adenocarcinoma, squamous cell carcinoma)
	CRH (rarely)	Carcinoid tumor
	Ectopic expression of receptors for GIP; LH	Macronodular adrenal hyperplasia
Non–islet cell hypoglycemia	IGF-2	Mesenchymal tumors Mesothelioma Fibrosarcomas
Oncogenic osteomalacia	FGF-23	Sarcomas Hemangiomas Fibromas Prostate adenocarcinoma Osteoblastomas
Male feminization	hCG	Testicular neoplasms (seminomas, teratomas) Germinomas Choriocarcinomas
Acromegaly	GHRH	Pancreatic islet cell tumors Carcinoid tumors
	GH	Lung, pancreatic islet cell tumors

result in central pontine myelinolysis and in the vast majority of cases, water restriction is safe, effective, and sufficient.

Management of the underlying tumor

Curative surgery will also cure the SIADH, as will curative chemotherapy and/or radiotherapy. Chemotherapy and radiotherapy may have an important palliative role, as the tumor is usually incurable by the time hyponatremia is detected.

Humeral hypercalcemia of malignancy

Hypercalcemia is a common complication of malignancy. It may be due to ectopic hormone secretion (PTHrP; rarely 1,25(OH)$_2$ cholecalciferol), cytokine and inflammatory mediators that activate osteoclastic bone resorption (such as IL-6 and RANK-L production by myeloma cells), or bone destruction by metastases.

Parathyroid hormone-related peptide (PTHrP)

PTHrP binds to and activates PTH/PTHrP receptor type 1, resulting in osteoclast-mediated bone resorption and reduced renal excretion of calcium.

The biochemical picture of hypercalcemia and hypophosphatemia may be indistinguishable from that of primary hyperparathyroidism. However, PTH levels are suppressed in PTHrP-mediated hypercalcemia (primary hyperparathyroidism can coexist with malignancy).

PTHrP secretion by metastatic cells within bone also causes hypercalcemia by causing local osteolysis.

PTHrP can be measured directly and is elevated in 80% of cancer patients with hypercalcemia.

Tumors that metastasize to bone are more prone to produce PTHrP than tumors that do not metastasize to bone (50% of primary breast cancer express PTHrP compared with 92% of metastases of breast cancer to bone). This may be due to induction of PTHrP secretion by the bone microenvironment; alternatively PTHrP production by tumor cells may enhance their ability to metastasize to bone.

📖 For tumors associated with humoral hypercalcemia see Table 98.1.

Management

This is as per normal management of hypercalcemia (📖 see Other causes of hypercalcemia, p. 385).

Glucocorticoids may be particularly effective in treatment of hypercalcemia associated with malignancy. This may be due to direct effects of glucocorticoids on the tumor cells (e.g., hemopoietic malignancies) and/or down-regulation of production of 1,25(OH)$_2$ cholecalciferol.

Bisphosphonates may also have antitumor effects in myeloma as well as control osteoclastic destruction of bone.

Cushing's syndrome due to ectopic ACTH production

Ectopic ACTH production is responsible for 10–20% of all endogenous Cushing's syndrome.

The most common tumor types are those with neuroendocrine features. Half of ectopic ACTH-secretion is due to small-cell lung carcinoma. Carcinoid tumors are also very common (thymic carcinoid 15%; pancreatic endocrine tumors including pancreatic carcinoids 10%; bronchial carcinoid 10%).

Diagnosis

Despite often extremely high cortisol levels, patients often do not manifest central weight gain, due to the underlying malignant process with its rapid progress and associated cachexia.

Hypertension, hypokalemia, and metabolic alkalosis are common features (overwhelming of the 11B-hydroxysteroid dehydrogenase enzyme resulting in exposure of the mineralocorticoid receptor to high circulating glucocorticoids).

Glucose intolerance, susceptibility to infection, thin skin, poor wound healing, and steroid-associated mood disturbance are all common features.

Patients may be pigmented from MSH arising from high POMC levels.

ACTH levels may be extremely high (usually >100 pg/mL).

In 90% of ectopic ACTH-secreting tumors, high-dose dexamethasone testing (2 mg qds) shows a failure of cortisol levels to drop to 50% of baseline values, due to a lack of any normal physiological feedback on ACTH production. However, some carcinoid tumors may behave indistinguishably from pituitary-dependent ACTH production. CRH testing and/or inferior petrosal sinus sampling may be necessary to distinguish these conditions.

Ectopic ACTH-producing tumors can be extremely difficult to localize and may require multiple modalities of imaging.

Management

Excision of the underlying tumor may be possible. Other options include medical management using metyrapone and/or ketoconazole, although very high doses may be needed.

Bilateral adrenalectomy with glucocorticoid and mineralocorticoid replacement is also an option.

Macronodular adrenal hyperplasia

- A rare cause of ectopic Cushing's syndrome
- Most commonly due to synthesis of ectopic GIP receptors in adrenal tissues
- GIP secretion associated with meals results in activation of adrenal glands and food-related hypercortisolemia.
- Other ectopic receptors reported include B-adrenergic receptors and LH receptors.

Carcinoid tumors and ectopic hormone production

📖 See p. 465 and Table 98.1 (p. 551).

Liver disease

Sex hormones—males

See Table 98.2.

Hypogonadism occurs in 70–80% of men with chronic liver disease. There is a combination of primary testicular failure and failure of hypothalamo–pituitary regulation.

Alcohol acts independently to produce hypogonadism, leading to a combination of primary testicular failure and failure of hypothalamic–pituitary regulation.

The effects of elevated estrogens result in ↑ loss of the male escutcheon, loss of body hair, redistribution of body fat, palmar erythema, spider nevi, and gynecomastia.

The ↑ conversion of testosterone and androstenedione to estrone is attributed at least in part to portosystemic shunting. In addition, the large increase in SHBG concentration will increase the estrogen/testosterone ratio as testosterone has a higher affinity for SHBG.

Spironolactone may result in iatrogenic feminization by inhibiting testosterone action.

There is no evidence that exogenous administration of androgens reverses hypogonadism in chronic liver disease.

Sex hormones—females

See Table 98.2.

Alcoholism increases the frequency of menstrual disturbances and spontaneous abortion but does not affect fertility. Liver dysfunction of whatever etiology is associated with an early menopause.

Alcohol rather than liver disease is the prime cause of hypogonadism. Nonalcoholic liver disease is only associated with hypogonadism in advanced liver failure when it is accompanied by encephalopathy and impaired GnRH secretion.

Table 98.2 Sex hormone changes in liver disease

Hormone	Level
Testosterone	↓↑
SHBG	↑
Estrone	↑
Estradiol	↑/normal
LH	Inappropriately low/normal
FSH	Inappropriately low/normal
Prolactin	↑/normal
IGF-1	↓
IGFBP-3	↓

Table 98.3 Thyroid function changes in liver disease

Hormone	Acute hepatitis	CAH/PBC	Cirrhosis
T_4	↑↓	↑	↓
fT_4	↑ →	→	↑
T_3	↓	↑	↓
fT_3	↓	↓	↓
rT_3	↑	→	↑→
TSH	↑	↑	↑→
TBG	↑	↑	→

CAH, chronic active hepatitis; PBC: primary biliary cirrhosis.

Plasma testosterone and estrone concentrations are usually normal, androstenedione concentration is increased, and dehydroepiandros-tene-dione and dehydroepiandrostenedione sulfate levels are reduced.

Thyroid

The liver synthesizes albumin, T_4-binding prealbumin (TBPA), and T_4-binding gobulin (TBG), all of which bind thyroid hormones covalently and reversibly.

Thyroid function tests (TFTs) must be interpreted with caution in patients with liver disease. In acute liver disease, e.g., acute viral hepatitis, TBG levels are increased, which increases the measured total circulating T_4 and T_3 levels.

In biliary cirrhosis and chronic active hepatitis, TBG may be increased. In other chronic liver disease and in hepatomas, TBG is also increased.

In severe cases of acute liver disease, TBG may be low due to reduced synthesis. The liver deiodinates T_4 to T_3 and this is impaired in liver disease. The T_4 is preferentially converted to rT_3 and there is an increase in the rT_3/T_3 ratio. In liver cirrhosis, TBG, T_4, and T_3 are low.

Table 98.3 summarizes the changes in TFTs with liver disease. Free T_4 and T_3 assays are essential for the accurate interpretation of thyroid status in liver disease.

Adrenal hormones

Patients who abuse alcohol may develop a clinical phenotype of Cushing's syndrome with moon faces, centripetal obesity, striae, and muscle wasting, and may have increased plasma cortisol concentrations. This is termed *pseudo-Cushing's syndrome.*

Reversible (on abstention) adrenocorticorticoid hyperresponsiveness occurs in alcoholics. In liver disease, cortisol metabolism may be impaired, leading to elevated plasma cortisol levels, loss of diurnal cortisol variation, and failure to suppress with dexamethasone.

Further reading

Malik R, Hodgson H (2002). The relationship between the thyroid gland and the liver. *Q J Med* 95:559–569.

Renal disease

Calcitriol

There is impaired renal conversion of 25-hydroxyvitamin D_3 to 1,25 $(OH)_2D_3$ in end-stage renal failure (ESRF) leading to metabolic bone disease.

Parathyroid hormone and renal osteodystrophy

Serum parathyroid hormone (PTH) secretion is stimulated by low serum calcium in ESRF. This is due to the following:

- ↓ Renal phosphate clearance (resulting in ↑ cacium/phosphate mineral ion product, precipitation of vascular calcification with consequent hypocalcemia triggering PTH release). Vascular calcification is a major contributor to vascular death in ESRF. High phosphate may increase PTH secretion directly, but evidence of the mechanism for this is lacking.
- Impaired renal calcitriol secretion

As renal function declines, an elevated PTH and a ↓ calcitriol can be detected with creatinine clearance of 50 mL/min. This rise in PTH is initially sufficient to maintain the serum calcium in the normal range.

In ESRF, patients are markedly hyperphosphatemic and hypocalcemic. The degree of hyperparathyroidism progresses inversely with the fall in renal function. Tertiary hyperparathyroidism occurs when PTH secretion becomes autonomous, and hypercalcemia will persist even after renal transplantation.

Hyperparathyroid bone disease and osteomalacia are the main mechanisms behind the development of high-turnover bone disease in renal osteodystrophy. Hypogonadism is also common in both men and women with ESRF. Adynamic bone disease also contributes, probably due to direct toxic effects from urea and other nitrogenous compounds on bone cells. Renal osteodystrophy causes bone pain and fractures.

Treatment of renal osteodystrophy

The goals are maintenance of normal phosphate levels with phosphate binders (such as calcium carbonate) and treatment of osteomalacia. The ↑ use of calcium carbonate has been suggested as the cause of the ↑ incidence of adynamic renal osteodystrophy, but intensive vitamin D therapy and peritoneal dialysis are probably also contributory.

Calcitriol (which does not require renal 1α-hydroxylation) is effective in treating osteomalacia. A dose of 1–2 mcg/day is used for established renal osteodystrophy. Lower doses of calcitriol (0.25–0.5 mcg/day) are used in early ESRF to prevent the devel-opment of renal osteodystrophy.

Parathyroidectomy is advocated in bone disease uncon-trolled by vitamin D therapy or the development of tertiary hyperpara-thyroidism.

Cinacalcet acts directly at the calcium-sensing receptor to lower PTH secretion. This markedly improves secondary hyperparathy-roidism, calcium and phophate levels, and renal osteodystrophy. Improvement in mortality due to ↓ vascular calcification has not yet been demonstrated.

Prolactin

Hyperprolactinemia is common in ESRF but is usually mild, i.e., <100 mcg/L. The cause is both ↑ secretion and ↓ renal clearance.

Gonadal function

Hypogonadism—clinical and biochemical—is common in ESRF.

In men, there is impaired pulsatile release of LH, although basal LH levels are usually elevated because of impaired renal clearance. Serum FSH is usually normal or mildly elevated.

In women, levels of estradiol, progesterone, and FSH are reported to be within the normal range in the early follicular phase but fail to show the usual cyclical changes. Menstrual disturbance is common. Amenorrhea, polymenorrhea, and menorrhagia can also occur on dialysis. Infertility is the rule, and conception on dialysis is the exception.

Sexual dysfunction is common in both sexes but has been better studied in men. 60% of men have some degree of impotence and examination yields 80% to have testicular atrophy and 14% to have gynecomastaia.

Treatment of hypogonadism in ESRF is suboptimal. Testosterone therapy is not associated with any clinical benefit in men.

Growth hormone and growth retarda-tion

Basal GH levels are normal, but there is impaired secretion following an adequate hypoglycemic stimulus in 40–70% of patients with ESRF.

There is impaired growth in children, particularly during periods of greatest growth velocity, and puberty is delayed. This combination leads to short stature. The improved growth velocity after renal transplantation is often too little too late in order to attain a normal stature.

Recombinant human GH (rhGH) has been shown to be an effective treatment for growth retardation in children with stable chronic kidney disease (CKD) and ESRF as well as after renal transplantation.

Thyroid

The "euthyroid sick" finding is common in CKD (☐ see Sick euthyroid syndrome, p. 15).

Adrenal

The adrenal axis is not impaired clinically by CKD.

There is evidence of blunted cortisol response to hypoglycemia but this is not relevant clinically.

Patients with amyloidosis are at risk of hypoadrenalism due to adrenal amyloid infiltration.

Endocrinology in the critically ill

📖 See Table 98.4.

ACTH and cortisol

CRH, ACTH, and cortisol increase rapidly during all forms of acute illness. Low albumin and CBG cause free cortisol to be substantially higher. This physiological adaptation results in the following:

- Provision of substrates for major organ energy expenditure (via catabolism)
- Hemodynamic advantages (enhanced sensitivity to angiotensin II, ↑ vaso-pressor and inotropic response to catecholamines
- Prevention of an ex-cessive immune response

Inflammatory cytokines result in ↑ cortisol metabolism and reduced receptors, i.e., peripheral cortisol resistance.

After moderate to severe injuries, plasma cortisol starts to fall af-ter a day or two but only reach normal levels after a week.

Table 98.4 Endocrine and other changes seen in critical illness

Acute illness	
ACTH/CRH	↑↑↑
Albumin/CBG	↓
Free cortisol	↑↑
Catabolism	↑
Immune response	↓
Inflammatory response	↑
Cortisol resistance	↑
Glucose	↑
Insulin resistance	↑
TSH	→
FT$_4$ and FT$_3$	↓
IGF-1, IGFBPs, GHBPs	↓
Prolonged critical illness	
ACTH/CRH	↑↑
Free cortisol	or ↑
TSH, total T$_4$	↓
rT$_3$	↑
LH/FSH/T/estradiol	↓
GH	↓
Response to GHRH	↓

Cortisol is elevated for at least 2 weeks in patients with severe burns.

Prolonged critical illness results in low CRH and ACTH with a normal or slightly raised cortisol, perhaps driven by an alternative pathway involving endothelin.

Cortisol deficiency should be suspected in an acutely ill patient with a plasma cortisol of <20 mcg/dL, or an increment of <9 mcg/dL on a 250 mcg cortrosyn test.

Drugs used in intensive care may contribute to adrenal insufficiency by
• Reducing cortisol metabolism, e.g., etomidate (frequently used in induction of anesthesia) and ketoconazole.
• Promoting cortisol metabolism, e.g., phenytoin, carbamazepine, and rifampicin.

Metabolism

Hyperglycemia is common in critical illness (even in non-diabetic subjects) due to ↑ cortisol, catecholamines, GH, and glucagon. These hormones and inflammatory cytokines also contribute to insulin resistance.

IV insulin titrated to maintain normoglycemia (glucose <6.1mmol/L) reduces mortality by >40%.

TSH and thyroid hormones

TSH levels usually remain stable in acute injury. Total T_4 and T_3 tend to fall but may remain within the normal range.

Thyroid hormone metabolism is enhanced by increased activity of liver deiodinase type 3 (peripheral hormone deactivator).

With prolonged illness, the total T_4 tends to fall below the normal range. The FT_4 remains in the normal range.

Total and free T_3 levels fall after injury and may remain suppressed for 2–3 weeks after a severe injury. The rT_3 level rises.

In prolonged critical illness, the thyroid function conforms to the "sick euthyroid syndrome" (📖 see Euthyroid sick syndrome, p. 15).

Gonadotropins and gonadal steroids

In prolonged illness hypogonadotropic hypogonadism occurs.

Growth hormone

In critical illness, the GH axis is profoundly affected with initially raised GH secretion, but low IGF-1, IGFBPs, and GHBP related to peripheral GH resistance. Prolonged critical illness >5–7 days results in low GH and a blunted response to GHRH.

Recombinant GH was proposed as a beneficial agent for critical illness, but the evidence is lacking, and there are reports of a detrimental effect.

Hormone replacement and critical illness

There is no evidence that, other than insulin, hormonal supplementation in the critically ill improves outcome.

Further reading

Elleger B, Debaveye Y, Van den Berghe G (2005). Endocrine interventions in the ICU. *Eur J Intern Med* 16:71–82.

Isidori AM, Kaltsas GA, et al. (2006). The ectopic adrenocorticotropin syndrome: clinical features, diagnosis, management, and long-term follow-up. *J Clin Endocrinol Me-tab* 91(2):371–377.

Perioperative management of endocrine patients

Transsphenoidal surgery/craniotomy

Preoperative assessment

Confirm the following:

- Anterior and posterior pituitary function is normal or on adequate replacement:
  - Cortrosyn stimulation test (CST; note both the 0- and 30-minute values) and/or normal ACTH/cortisol before 9 A.M. Patients with recent loss of LFTH will have a normal response to CST, as adrenal atrophy will not have evolved. If there is in any doubt, replace with glucocorticoids.
  - FT_4
  - LH, FSH, estradiol, or testosterone
  - Prolactin
  - Serum and urine osmolality and electrolytes if polyuric
- Recent (<3 months) MRI pituitary
- Formal visual field perimetry and visual acuity assessment
- Document extraocular muscle movements
- Urea and electrolytes (<1 week presurgery)
- Group and save serum

Methicillin-resistant *Staphylococcus aureus* (MRSA) screen should be done at least 2 weeks prior to admission for surgery if the patient has been in the hospital within the last year.

Record therapeutic options discussed with patient:

- Risks of surgery (e.g., CSF leakage, meningitis, bleeding, partial or total hypopituitarism including diabetes insipidus and potential effects on fertility and visual deterioration)
- Risk of recurrence requiring further surgery or radiotherapy

Warn patients that a sample of fat may be taken from their thigh or abdomen for packing of the pituitary fossa. Reiterate the need for lifelong follow-up.

Ensure antibiotic prophylaxis is given prior to surgery (the precise regimen may vary depending on the center and patient. Some surgeons advocate a prolonged course of antibiotics if CSF leakage occurs, whereas others recommend close surveillance and prompt treatment if concern about possible meningitis [lower threshold for patients with Cushing's disease]).

MRSA-positive patients require prophylaxis with IV vancomycin.

If the patient is steroid-deficient, steroid reserve is unknown, or a patient has Cushing's disease (inadequate stress response), give hydrocortisone 20 mg orally with morning premedication.

Postoperative (Table 99.1)

Consider steroid status; if the patient requires steroid coverage:

- Start IV hydrocortisone (HC), 50–100 q6–8h, postoperatively.
- Convert to oral glucocorticoids once patient is eating and drinking.
- After nasal packs are removed (following transsphenoidal surgery), stop glucocorticoids (usually <48 hours).
- Check 9 A.M. cortisol level the following two mornings, having omitted the evening dose for the preceding day. Continue off steroids if patient is asymptomatic, however if symptomatic only omit the evening dose.

In patients with Cushing's disease, 9 A.M. cortisol (x2) <1.8 mcg/dL indicates cure; occasionally, cortisol takes a few days to fall to undetectable levels.

See Table 99.1 for patients without Cushing's disease.

If the patient is acutely unwell with postural BP drop when hydrocortisone is stopped, check random cortisol and restart HC without delay.

Fluid balance—watch for diabetes insipidus:

- Review the clinical status of the patient at regular intervals (euvolemic, hypovolemic, hypervolemic).
- Record fluid input and output assiduously (fluid replacement in surgery may be excessive, therefore always include perioperative fluids in fluid balance charts and note sodium content).
- Check plasma electrolytes and plasma and urine osmolalities on a regular basis (at least once daily and more frequently if there are clinical concerns).
- Postoperatively, restrict to 2 L total fluid input (IV and PO).
- Record fluid input and output assiduously.

Table 99.1 Postoperative glucocorticoid management of patients without Cushing's disease*

9 A.M. cortisol level	Action
>20 mcg/dL	Stay off hydrocortisone
15–20 mcg/dL	Advise to start hydrocortisone if unwell (give patient supply of oral and parenteral hydrocortisone to take home with appropriate written advice)
<15 mcg/dL	Start regular oral hydrocortisone (10mg/5mg/5mg)

*In female patients who have stopped estrogen replacement therapy <6 weeks before surgery, interpret results with caution (potential confounding effect of raised CBG levels).

- If the patient becomes polyuric, i.e., >200 mL/h for ≥3 consecutive hours (in the context of a 2 L/24-hour fluid restriction), urgently check plasma electrolytes, plasma and urine osmolalities, and urinary sodium. While waiting for results allow free fluids; the aim is to replace the fluid deficit. (Fluid replacement in surgery may be excessive, always include perioperative fluids in fluid balance sheets.)
- If diabetes insipidus is confirmed by the results, give a single dose of desamino-D-arginine vasopressin (desmopressin) (1 mcg SC).
- When the fluid deficit has been replaced (usually orally), restart 2–3 L fluid restriction (again include IV and PO routes).
- If polyuria recurs, treat as before.
- Regular plasma electrolytes and plasma and urine osmolalities are required.
- If polyuria continues to recur up to and after 96 hours postoperatively, consider regular DDAVP orally or intranasally, if possible (not if a transsphenoidal approach is used).

Hyponatremia occurring 1 week after a transsphenoidal adenectomy is most commonly due to SIADH; rarely, cerebral salt wasting may occur. Check urinary sodium and assess fluid status (cerebral salt wasting causes very high urinary sodium and is associated with dehydration).

Check thyroid function (FT_4) between days 5 and 7 postoperatively.

Check for CSF leakage.

Recheck visual acuity and visual field perimetry and eye movements formally prior to discharge.

Thyroidectomy

Preoperative

Ensure euthyroidism.

If surgery is required in the presence of hyperthyroidism, give potassium iodide (60 mg 3x a day for 10 days); this reduces thyroid hormone release and probably decreases perioperative blood loss. The radiographic contrast agent iopanoic acid, which is rich in iodine, provides a useful alternative, and has the additional benefit of potently inhibiting the 5-deiodinase, thus reducing T_4 to T_3 conversion.

Oral propranolol (30–120 mg 3x a day) reduces clinical manifestations of thyrotoxicosis.

Check vocal cord function by indirect laryngoscopy.

Warn of postoperative risks: recurrent laryngeal nerve damage <1%, keloid scarring, hemorrhage, permanent hypoparathyroidism <0.5%, and hypothyroidism (10% of partial thyroidectomy patients).

Postoperative

There is a risk of hemorrhage in first 24 hours, particularly major hemorrhage deep to the strap muscles, leading to airway compression. Watch for stridor, respiratory difficulties, and wound swelling. Drainage from wound drains is unhelpful. Treat by evacuating the hematoma, and consider intubation or a tracheostomy. Clip removers and artery forceps should be kept to hand on the ward.

Recurrent laryngeal nerve damage is permanent in <1% and transient in 2–4%. The patient's voice is often husky for about 3 weeks postoperatively and may be treated with lozenges and humidified air.

Symptomatic unilateral damage can be treated by stabilization of the affected cord in adduction by submucosal Teflon® injection under direct laryngoscopy.

Bilateral damage leads to unopposed adductor action of the cricothyroid muscle, which causes glottis closure and airway obstruction. Treatment involves reintubation, paralysis, hydrocortisone (100 mg 4x a day IM for edema), and extubation at 24 hours. If that fails, a tracheostomy should be performed.

If recurrent laryngeal nerve damage is persistent at 9 months, an attempt can be made to resuture the nerve.

Monitor calcium. Transient hypoparathyroidism is usually evident within 7 days. 📖 See Hypoparathyroidism (p. 394) for treatment.

Following total thyroidectomy for malignancy, thyroid hormone withdrawal may be necessary prior to postoperative radioiodine ablation (📖 see Follow-up of papillary and follicular thyroid carcinoma, p. 76). Alternatively, recombinant TSH can be used.

If total thyroidectomy is performed for hyperthyroidism, levothyroxine (~1.5 mcg/kg) should be started 4–5 days postoperatively, as during the operation, handling of the thyroid results in release of stored thyroid hormones and levothyroxine has a long t½. Check TSH in 6–8 weeks.

Following partial thyroidectomy, transient biochemical hypothyroidism may occur during the first 2 months and does not warrant treatment unless the patient is symptomatic or it becomes persistent.

Parathyroidectomy

Parathyroidectomy of one or two glands undertaken for primary hyper-parathyrodism may result in transient and self-limited hypocalcemia.

Total parathyroidectomy (e.g., for MEN1 or as part of surgical management of advanced head and neck malignancy) may be complicated by severe and permanent hypocalcemia, which may be very difficult to manage.

Postoperative care for patients undergoing parathyroidectomy of 1–2 glands

Check calcium, phosphate, magnesium, and albumin on the evening of surgery and daily thereafter. Calcium begins to fall postoperatively after about 4–12 hours; the nadir is usually reached by 24 hours. Calcium may recover spontaneously, however 1/3 of patients will require calcium support perioperatively.

With the advent of minimally invasive parathryoidectomy and short hospital stays (<24 hours) many centers advocate prophylactic calcium and vitamin D replacement in all cases in the immediate aftermath of surgery. This treatment is continued until the patient is reviewed 1–2 weeks later in the outpatient clinic.

Symptoms of hypocalcemia (mainly due to neuromuscular irritability) include perioral parasthesias, Chovstek's sign, Trousseau's sign, tetany, laryngospasm, bronchospasm, seizures, prolonged QT interval on ECG, extrapyramidal movement disorders, and delirium. Calcium levels are often <7.0 mg/dL before symptoms manifest, although rapid changes in calcium result in more pronounced symptomatology.

Magnesium deficiency is common due to previous hyperparathyroidism (causes renal wasting of magnesium). Chronic magnesium deficiency impairs release of PTH and causes functional hypoparathyroidism and hypocalcemia.

Causes of hypocalcemia after 1–2 gland removal

Functional hypoparathyroidism

This is common. Causes include delayed recovery of the other parathyroid glands due to long-term suppression, parathyroid gland ischemia, parathyroid gland "stunning" by intraoperative handling, and hypomagnesemia.

The PTH level will be detectable; phosphate should be normal. It usually improves spontaneously over days to weeks.

Management of symptomatic hypocalcemia (Ca usually <7.2 mg/dL) is with calcium (up to 2 g/day in divided doses). Add in vitamin D and vitamin D metabolites for persistent hypocalcemia. Replace magnesium as necessary.

Gradual withdrawal of therapy is needed to assess recovery.

Hungry bone syndrome

This is due to extensive skeletal remineralization once the skeleton is released from PTH excess. There is ongoing ↑ alkaline phosphatase (ALP), ↓ calcium, ↓ PO_4, and ↓ Mg. PTH levels may be normal or high. Pre-existing vitamin D deficiency will exacerbate hypocalcemia.

The patient may require large doses of calcium and vitamin D and vitamin D metabolites for weeks to months.

Permanent hypoparathyroidism.
This is rare (<2% of cases). Check PTH level after day 3; the level will be undetectable (<1 pg/mL). Replace with oral calcium and vitamin D and vitamin D metabolites long term.

Other complications
- Recurrent laryngeal nerve palsy (<1%)
- Failure to correct hypercalcemia

Overall, both minimally invasive and conventional parathyroidectomy are very safe operations with low morbidity and mortality.

Calcium management following total parathyroidectomy

Hypocalcemia is inevitable unless management is instituted.

Preemptive treatment is worth considering (e.g., calcitriol 1–2 mcg/day—this dose may be insufficient to completely prevent hypocalcemia but may prevent life-threatening hypocalcemia and is unlikely to cause serious toxicity in the short term).

Acute management is required in patients with life-threatening hypocalcemia (e.g., Trousseau's sign, laryngospasm, seizures):
- 10 mL of 10% calcium gluconate diluted 1 in 10 in normal saline or dextrose 5% infused into a large vein over 10 minutes. Monitor cardiac rhythm.
- Repeat as necessary to control acute emergency.
- Patients will need ongoing calcium replacement: 100 mL of 10% calcium gluconate in 1 L of 5% dextrose or 0.9% sodium chloride infused over 24 hours (monitor calcium regularly (q4–6h) and adjust rate as necessary).
- Start oral vitamin D analogs and oral calcium.

Vitamin D analogs (calcitriol)
These are potent and effective in acute hypocalcemia because of the rapid correction of calcium. The short half-lives allow rapid and careful titration of a dose in response to calcium levels. There is a narrow therapeutic window (hypercalcemia is much shorter-lived if it develops).

Reassess often (at least every 1–2 days) in the early stages of management. Longer-term options include ergocalciferol or colecalciferol, but hypercalcemia will be more prolonged if it develops.

Calcium
Give 1–2 g/daily in divided doses. A maximum daily absorbable dose of calcium is probably 3 g/day.

Absorption may vary from different types of calcium salts and may be greater when calcium is given away from food.

The long-term aim is to manage without calcium just on vitamin D or vitamin D metabolites.

The long-term goal of management is to prevent symptoms of hypocalcemia without toxicity. Aim for the lower half of normal range (8.0–9.2 mg/dL) with normal urinary calcium excretion (to minimize risk of nephrolithiasis and nephrocalcinosis.

Pheochromocytoma

Preoperative

Check for bilateral disease or metastases: MRI chest and abdomen and an MIBG scan (10% multiple).

Ensure adequate α- and β-blockade once the diagnosis is made. Start α-blockade before β-blockade (unopposed β-blockade can lead to marked vasoconstriction, ischemic damage, and hypertension).

- *α-blockade:* Start *phenoxybenzamine* (10–20 mg, orally, 3–4x day), an irreversible α-blocker. Adequacy of dosage can be assessed by monitoring hematocrit and postural drop in BP (reflects BP vasodilation).
- Start treatment at least 1 week, ideally >3 weeks, before surgery.
- *β-blockade:* Start *propranolol* (20–80 mg, orally, 3x day) at least 48 hours after initiating phenoxybenzamine.

To control BP, α- and β-blockers are often sufficient. If not, add a calcium channel blocker or ACE inhibitor; α-methyltyrosine 1–4 g/day (a false catecholamine precursor that inhibits tyrosine hydroxylase, the rate-limiting step for catecholamine synthesis) is rarely used to control BP.

Some centers advocate the use of additional IV phenoxybenzamine (0.5–1.0 mg/kg in 250 mL 5% dextrose given over 2 hours) for the 3 days prior to surgery (titrate the dose according to BP; often 0.5 mg/kg is sufficient).

Group and save serum, and cross-match 2 units of blood.

Ensure that the patient is well hydrated (if necessary, use an IV infusion of saline) prior to going to surgery.

Postoperative

Watch for ↓ BP: sudden withdrawal of catecholamines leads to marked arterial and venous dilatation. This is worsened by inadequate volume loading and should initially be treated with volume replacement rather than by pressor agents.

If hypertension persists 2 weeks postoperatively, residual tumor or metastases must be considered.

Long-term monitoring is required as approximately 14% recur.

If bilateral adrenalectomy is performed, see the next section.

Bilateral adrenalectomy

Give hydrocortisone (100 mg, 4x day, IM) postoperatively. This will provide adequate mineralocorticoid and glucocorticoid coverage. Continue this until the patient is eating and drinking (often <48 hours). Monitor electrolytes.

From day 3, give hydrocortisone PO (double usual replacement dose, e.g., 20 mg/10 mg/10 mg) and add fludrocortisone PO (100 mcg daily).

Long-term replacement is with hydrocortisone 10/5/5 and fludrocortisone 50–150 mcg daily.

Pheochromocytoma in pregnancy (see p. 364)

This is a rare condition. It may present as paradoxical supine hypertension, with pressure from the gravid uterus causing release of catecholamines, and normal blood pressure in the supine and erect positions.

Start α-blockade then β-blockade, phenoxybenzamine can cross the placenta but is generally safe for the fetus (may cause perinatal CNS depression and transient hypotension).

Surgery is more controversial, although some authors advocate surgery in the first and second trimesters up to 24 weeks' gestation.

Caesarian section is advocated with a combined tumor resection. Vaginal delivery carries a significant maternal risk.

Syndromes of hormone resistance

Definition

In these syndromes there is reduced responsiveness of target organs to a particular hormone, usually secondary to a disorder of the receptor or distal signaling pathways. This leads to alterations in feedback loops and elevated circulating hormone levels.

Thyroid hormone resistance

📖 see Resistance to thyroid hormones (p. 37).

Androgen resistance

📖 see Androgen insensitivity syndrome (p. 335).

Glucocorticoid resistance

Autosomal dominant and recessive forms have been described.

Diminished sensitivity to glucocorticoid leads to reduced glucocorticoid feedback on CRH and ACTH, leading to ↑ CRH, ACTH, and cortisol concentrations.

The clinical features are not due to excess glucocorticoid, as there is reduced peripheral tissue sensitivity. However, elevated ACTH leads to ↑ secretion of mineralocorticoid (e.g., deoxycorticosterone) and androgen (DHEA and DHEAS). This may lead to hypertension and hypokalemic alkalosis, hirsutism, acne, oligomenorrhea in females, and sexual precocity in males.

Glucocorticoid resistance may be differentiated from Cushing's syndrome because, despite evidence of ↑ urinary cortisol, abnormal suppression with dexamethasone, and ↑ responsiveness to CRH, the diurnal rhythm of cortisol secretion persists, there are no clinical features of Cushing's syndrome, BMD is normal or ↑, and there is a normal response to insulin-induced hypoglycemia.

Low-dose dexamethasone treatment (2 mg/day) may efficiently suppress ACTH and androgen production.

ACTH resistance

This is a rare autosomal recessive disorder in which the adrenal cortex fails to respond to ACTH in the presence of an otherwise normal gland. (mineralocorticoid secretion is preserved under angiotensin II control).

The presenting clinical features include hypoglycemia, which is often neonatal, neonatal jaundice, ↑ skin pigmentation, and frequent infections.

Occasionally, ACTH resistance is a component of the triple-A syndrome of alacrima (absence of tears), achalasia of the cardia, and ACTH resistance.

Biochemical features include undetectable or low 9 A.M. cortisol, with grossly elevated ACTH (often >1000 ng/mL), and normal renin, aldosterone, and electrolytes, and impaired response to the cortrosyn stimulation test.

Treatment is with steroid replacement.

Mineralocorticoid resistance

Also known as type 1 pseudohypoaldosteronism, this is a rare inherited disorder that usually presents in children with failure to thrive, salt loss, and dehydration. Both autosomal dominant and recessive forms have been described.

Biochemical features are as follows:
- ↓ Serum sodium
- ↑ Serum potassium (hyperkalemic acidosis)
- ↑ Urinary sodium (despite hyponatremia)
- ↑ Plasma and urinary aldosterone
- ↑ Plasma renin activity

Diagnosis requires proof of unresponsiveness to mineralocorticoids (no effect of fludrocortisone on urinary sodium).

Treatment with sodium supplementation has been used successfully. With time, treatment can often be weaned, and salt wasting is unusual following childhood.

Further reading

Charmandari, E, Kino T, Ichijo T, et al. (2008). Generalized glucocorticoid resistance: clinical aspects, molecular mechanisms, and Implications of a rare gentic disorder. *J Clin Endocrinol Med* 93:1563–1572.

Differential diagnosis of possible manifestations of endocrine disorders

Sweating

- Menopause/gonadal failure
- Thyrotoxicosis
- Pheochromocytoma
- Acromegaly
- Hypoglycemia
- Diabetes mellitus
- Autonomic neuropathy (gustatory sweating)
- Renal cell carcinoma
- Chronic infection (e.g., TB)
- Hematological malignancy (e.g., lymphoma)
- Anxiety
- Idiopathic
- Drugs, e.g., fluoxetine

Investigation of sweating

- History
- Clinical examination
- Thyroid function tests
- Serum gonadotropin levels
- Blood glucose level
- Specific investigations according to clinical suspicion

Management of sweating

- Treat the underlying cause, where possible
- Antiperspirants
- Topical aluminum chloride ± ethanol
- Anticholinergics—glycopyrronium bromide (oral or topical)
- Clonidine—taken at night to avoid sedation
- Iontophoresis
- Botulinum toxin A injections into affected areas (inhibits the release of acetylcholine at the synaptic junction of local nerves)
- Local excision of axillary sweat glands
- Sympathetic denervation
  - Video-assisted endoscopic thoracic sympathectomy
    - Excision
    - Radioablation
  - Sympathotomy (chain disconnection between T2 ganglion and stellate ganglion)

Palpitations (often associated with sweating)

- Thyrotoxicosis
- Hypoglycemia (insulinoma)
- Pheochromocytoma
- Anxiety states
- Cardiac arrhythmia

- Caffeine excess
- Alcohol or drug withdrawal

General malaise, tiredness
- Addison's disease
- Hypo- or hyperthyroidism
- Hypogonadism
- Hypopituitarism or GH deficiency
- Osteomalacia
- Diabetes mellitus
- Cushing's syndrome
- Anemia
- Drugs (prescription and recreational drugs)
  - Antihistamines
  - Antidepressants
  - Antihypertensives (β-blockers, methyl-dopa, clonidine)
  - Neuroleptics
  - Corticosteroids
- Malignancy
- Chronic fatigue syndrome (may be associated with reduced cortisol output both basally and in response to a variety of challenges)
- Chronic illness (cardiac, respiratory, hepatic)
- Fibromyalgia
- Depression
- Sleep disorders (obstructive sleep apnea)
- Infection
- Musculoskeletal or neurological disease (mysthenia gravis)
- Toxins
- Idiopathic

Investigation of fatigue
- Careful history-taking
  - Duration, onset, recovery, and type of fatigue
  - Person's usual activity level
- Clinical examination
- Serum electrolytes
- Hemoglobin ± serum ferritin level
- Inflammatory markers (ESR, CRP)
- Liver function tests
- Serum calcium and phosphate levels
- Thyroid function tests
- Cosyntropin stimulation test

Flushing
- Gonadal failure (with flushing and sweats)
- Drugs
  - Chlorpropamide
  - Nicotinic acid
  - Antiestrogens
  - LHRH agonists

- Carcinoid (dry flushing—no sweats)
- Mastocytosis
- Medullary thyroid cancer
- Anaphylaxis
- Pancreatic cell carcinoma
- Pheochromocytoma (more often pallor)
- Fever
- Alcohol
- Autonomic dysfunction
- Some foods
  - Fish
  - Tyramine containing food (cheese)
  - Nitrites (cured meat)
  - Monosodium glutamate
  - Spicy food
- Gustatory flushing
- Benign cutaneous flushing
- Idiopathic

Initial evaluation of patients with flushing

- Careful history
- Physical examination (ideally during a flush, although this is not often possible)
  - Examine skin carefully
  - Pulse rate
  - BP
  - Thyroid examination
  - Respiratory examination (wheeze)
  - Careful abdominal examination
- Biochemistry
  - Gonadotrophin levels
  - 2x 24-hour urinary 5HIAA measurements
  - Serum chromogranin A
  - 2x 24-hour urinary catecholamine measurements
  - Plasma metanephrines (if high level of suspicion)
  - Serum tryptase level (if suspecting mastocytosis)
  - Calcitonin level (if suspecting medullary thyroid cancer)
  - Plasma VIP (if suspecting pancreatic carcinoma)
  - Immunoglobulin levels (raised IgE may suggest allergies)
- Specific investigations according to suspected diagnosis

Management of flushing

- Treat the underlying cause.
- Nadolol (nonselective β-blocker) effective in some cases of benign cutaneous flushing.
- Somatostatin analogs can be used to treat flushing associated with carcinoid syndrome.
- Antihistamines may be effective in some histamine-secreting carcinoid tumors.

Further reading

Cleare A (2003). The neuroendocrinology of chronic fatigue syndrome. *Endocr Rev* 24(2):236–252.

Cornuz J, Guessous I, Favrat B (2006). Fatigue: a practical approach to diagnosis in primary care *CMAJ* 174(6):765–767.

Eisenach J, Atkinson J, Fealey R (2005). Hyperhidrosis: evolving therapies for a well-established phenomenon. *Mayo Clin Proc* 80(5):657–666.

Izikson L, English J, Zirwas M (2006). The flushing patient: differential diagnosis, workup and treatment. *J Am Acad Dermatol* 55(2):193–208.

Stress and the endocrine system

Definition

Stress may be considered as a state of threatened or perceived as threatened homeostasis. The principal effectors of the stress response are corticotropin-releasing hormone (CRH), glucocorticoids (GCs), catecholamines, arginine vasopressin (AVP), and POMC-derived peptides (especially β-endorphins).

Allostasis is a state of dyshomeostasis occurring from an inadequate, excessive, or prolonged adaptive stress response.

Endocrine effects of stress

Hypothalamic–pituitary axis
- ↑ Amplitude of synchronized pulsatile release of CRH and AVP (potent synergistic factor of CRH) into the hypophyseal portal system
- ↑ Stimulated ACTH production
- ↑ Adrenal glucocorticoid and androgen secretion

GCs also play a role in termination of the normal stress response by negative feedback at the pituitary, hypothalamus, and extrahypothalamic regions.

Growth hormone axis
GCs suppress GH production and inhibit the effects of IGF-1 (thus, children with anxiety disorders may have short stature).

CRH increases somatostatin production, inhibiting GH production.

GH response to IV glucagon is blunted.

Thyroid axis
GCs reduce the production of TSH and limit the conversion of T_4 to the more active T_3 by reducing deiodinase activity.

Somatostatin suppresses both TRH and TSH release.

📖 See Sick euthyroid syndrome (p. 15).

Reproductive axis
CRH reduces GnRH secretion.

GCs suppress GnRH neurons and pituitary gonadotropes and render the gonads resistant to gonadotropins. GCs also render peripheral tissues resistant to estradiol.

Chronic stress leads to amenorrhea in females and low LH and testosterone in males.

Estrogens increase CRH expression via an estrogen response element in the promoter region of the CRH gene. This may account for the sex-related differences in the stress response and HPA axis activity.

CRH is produced by the ovary, endometrium, and placenta during the latter half of pregnancy leading to physiological hypercortisolism.

Metabolism

GCs via their direct effect, and via reduced GH and sex hormone activity, result in muscle and bone catabolism and fat anabolism.

Chronic activation of the stress system is associated with ↑ visceral adiposity, ↓ lean body mass, and suppressed osteoblastic activity (which may ultimately lead to osteoporosis).

GCs induce insulin resistance and other features of the metabolic syndrome.

Further reading
Charmandari E, Tsigos C, Chrousos G (2005). Endocrinology of the stress response. *Annu Rev Physiol* 67:259–284.

Alternative or complementary therapy and endocrinology

Introduction

Many patients use natural products alongside or instead of conventional therapy. Products and information are available from many sources, particularly the Internet.

Patients need to be asked specifically about usage.

Hospital pharmacists can be extremely helpful in sourcing information about natural products, including interactions with conventional medicines.

Quality control of natural products is usually poor, with content ranging anywhere from 0% of stated level to several-fold higher.

Safety data are often absent or inadequate.

Discussion of any natural products listed here is not intended **in any way** to imply efficacy or safety of these products or to recommend their usage but rather to illustrate the compounds being promoted for these conditions by alternative information sources.

Alternative therapy used in patients with diabetes mellitus

A major concern with natural products used by patients with diabetes mellitus is of interaction with conventional medicines placing the patient at risk of hypoglycemia.

Hypoglycemic agents

These work by ↑ insulin secretion from the pancreas or through direct insulin-like action at the insulin receptor.

Banaba (Lagerstroemia speciosa)—crepe myrtle

Banaba extracts contain corosolic acid and ellagitannins, which may have direct insulin-like effects at insulin receptors.

Bitter melon (Momordica charantia)

This contains a polypeptide with insulin-like effects. It is used as juice, powder and extracts and in fried food. It is often part of Asian and Indian foods.

Fenugreek (Trigonella foenum-gracum)

This is used as powder, seeds, or part of a dietary supplement. It may enhance insulin release and may also decrease carbohydrate absorption due to a laxative effect. It may also inhibit platelets and thus increase bleeding diathesis.

Gymnema (Gymnema sylvestre)

Gurmar in Hindi means "sugar destroying". The extract GS4 is also used. Gymnema may increase endogenous insulin secretion (↑ C-peptide levels noted in users). In some preliminary studies, gymnema improved HbA1c and ↓ insulin or OHA requirements.

Insulin sensitizers

Cassia cinnamon (Cinnamomum aromaticum)

This is also known as Chinese cinnamon. It may increase insulin sensitivity and lower fasting blood glucose levels. It appears to be safe and well tolerated.

Chromium

Chromium deficiency is associated with impaired glucose tolerance, hyperglycemia, and ↓ insulin sensitivity. Chromium forms part of a glucose tolerance factor complex, thus supplements are sometimes labeled "chromium GTF."

In patients with diabetes and chromium deficiency, addition of chromium improves glycemic control. However the role of chromium in patients without deficiency is not clear.

The American Diabetes Association (ADA) only recommends chromium usage in patients with documented chromium deficiency. Excessive chromium may cause renal impairment.

Vanadium

Vanadium is thought to stimulate hepatic glycogenolysis; inhibit gluconeo-genesis, lipolysis, and intestinal glucose transport; and increase skeletal muscle glucose uptake, utilization, and glycogenolysis. High-dose vanadium (taken as vanadyl sulfate) may improve insulin sensitivity and glycemic control in patients with type 2 diabetes, with large doses of elemental vanadium required for these effects. However, doses >1.8 mg/day vanadium may cause renal impairment.

Ginseng

This includes both Panax ginseng and American ginseng (*Panax quinquefolius*). They both contain ginsenoisides, which may improve insulin sensitivity. Efficacy and safety are not established.

Prickly pear cactus (Opuntia ficus-indica)

Also called *opuntia* or *nopals* (referring to the cooked leaves of the cactus, this agent is prominent in Mexican folk medicine as a treatment for diabetes. *Opuntia streptacantha* stems may improve glycemic control by either acting as an insulin sensitizer or slowing carbohydrate absorption; however this is not observed with other prickly pear cactus species.

Carbohydrate absorption inhibitors

Soluble fiber increases viscosity of intestinal contents, thus slowing gastric emptying time and carbohydrate absorption, resulting in lower postprandial blood glucose levels.

The following products have some evidence of reducing postprandial blood glucose levels and may also improve total and LDL cholesterol levels in patients. They may also interfere with absorption of drugs and thus should not be taken at the same time as conventional medicines:

- Blond psyllium seed (*Plantago ovata*)
- Guar gum (*Cyamopsis tetragonoloba*)
- Oat bran (*Avena sativa*)
- Soy (*Glycine max*) —contains both soluble and insoluble fiber and may improve insulin resistance, fasting basal metabolism, lipid profile, and HbA1c in type 2 diabetes

Insoluble fiber. Glucomannan (*Amorphophallus konjac*)—can delay glucose absorption.

Other products used by patients with diabetes mellitus

- α-Lipoic acid. Antioxidant. May improve insulin resistance. It may help symptoms of diabetic neuropathy (?mechanism).
- Stevia (*Stevia rebaudiana*) may enhance insulin secretion. It may be toxic.

Alternative therapy used in menopause

Phytoestrogens

The main types are isoflavones (which are the most potent and most widespread), lignans, and coumestans.

Sources include the following:

- Isoflavones: legumes (soy, chickpea, garbanzo beans, red clover, lentils, beans). The main active isoflavones are genistein and daidzein.
- Lignans: flaxseed, lentils, whole grains, beans, many fruits and vegetables
- Coumestans: red clover, sunflower seeds, sprouts

Other phytoestrogens include chasteberry (vitex agnus-castus)

These agents are not structurally similar to estrogen or to selective estrogen receptor modulators (SERMs) but contain a phenolic ring that allows binding to estrogen receptors-α and -β. Effects of binding depend on ambient estrogen levels, relative ratio and concentration of ER-α and ER-β, and tissue type and location. Phytoestrogens are relatively much less potent than endogenous estrogen (by 100- to 10000-fold).

Phytoestrogens in vitro stimulate proliferation of normal human breast tissue and of estrogen-sensitive breast tumor cells. Theoretically, phytoestrogens may stimulate ER+ breast cancer and other estrogen-sensitive tumors. Phytoestrogens may also antagonize the effects of tamoxifen or other SERMs.

Phytoestrogens have not been shown to stimulate endometrial growth; however, they are not usually taken with progestogenic compounds. It is not known whether the other serious side effects of conventional estrogens (e.g., DVT, pulmonary emboli, IHD, stroke) occur with phytoestrogen use. Many sources of phytoestrogens (e.g., coumestans) interfere with warfarin.

Soy protein (20–60 mg/day; containing 34–76 mg isoflavones) modestly decreases frequency and severity of vasomotor symptoms in a proportion of menopausal women.

Synthetic isoflavones (ipriflavone) do not have antivasomotor activity.

Phytoestrogens from red clover have not shown consistent improvement in vasomotor symptoms. Other sources of phytoestrogens have not shown improvement in menopausal symptoms.

📖 For use in osteoporosis, see Alternative therapy used by patients with osteoporosis (p. 582).

Other compounds with estrogenic activity

- Kudzu (*Pueraria lobata*)
- Alfalfa (*Medicago sativa*)
- Hops (*Humulus lupulus*)
- Licorice (*Glycyrrhiza glabra*)
- Panax ginseng (ginseng)—in vitro evidence of stimulation of breast cancer cells

Other substances used

Black cohosh (*Actaea racemosa*, formerly *Cimicifuga racemosa*) is not to be confused with blue cohash and white cohash, which are entirely separate plants. Black cohash is widely used in menopause. Although often advertised as such, black cohash does not bind to estrogen receptors or have estrogen effects and there is little evidence for efficacy for hot flashes.

Dong quai (*Angelica sinensis*)—it is not clear if it is estrogenic. There is in vitro evidence of promotion of breast cancer cells.

Alternative therapy used by patients with osteoporosis

Calcium

There are hundreds of preparations available.

Several types of calcium salts are available (including citrate, carbonate, lactate, gluconate, and phosphate) with little evidence of superiority of absorption between the different compounds, other than calcium citrate, which is useful in patients with low gastric acidity (e.g., on concomitant proton pump inhibitors or H2 antagonists).

Magnesium

Magnesium is necessary for release of PTH.

It is not effective alone in treating osteoporosis unless patients are deficient in magnesium.

Fluoride

Fluoride increases bone density but not strength—bones are less elastic, and more brittle, with resultant ↑ fracture rate.

Trace elements

Examples are manganese, zinc, boron, and copper.

While many trace elements are important for multiple enzyme systems including those in bone, most patients are not deficient, thus supplements have negligible positive effect on osteoporosis. Moreover, many minerals in high doses cause serious side effects (e.g., manganese doses >11 mg/day can cause extrapyramidal side effects).

Vitamin D

Multiple preparations are available, mainly as ergocalciferol or colecalciferol (vitamin D metabolites require prescription).

Isoflavones

📖 See Alternative therapy used in menopause (p. 580), for more detail about phytoestrogens' mechanism of action.

Soy protein in doses >80 mg/day may improve bone mineral density but no studies of soy have shown improvement in fracture rate. There are possible adverse effects on estrogen-sensitive tissues such as ER-positive breast cancer.

Ipriflavone—semisynthetic isoflavone—is produced from daidzein. There are no estrogenic effects. There is no evidence of improved fracture outcome. Some studies of ipriflavone with calcium have reported improved BMD, although other studies have not shown an improvement. Ipriflavone can cause serious lymphopenia (<1 x 10^9 mL), which may take up to a year to recover.

Tea

Tea consists of green tea (unfermented), oolong tea (partially fermented), and black tea (completely fermented). All teas contain fluoride and have high isoflavonoid content in addition to caffeine.

Coffee (with a high caffeine content) has been associated with ↑ hip fracture risk. However, tea drinking of all types of has been associated with higher BMD, although no fracture outcome has been reported.

DHEA

📖 See Miscellaneous (p. 203).

Wild yam

Wild yam contains diosgenin, which is used commercially as a source for DHEA synthesis; however this does not occur in humans.

Other compounds used by patients for osteoporosis

- Flaxseed (alphalinolenic acid and lignans)
- Gelatin
- Dong quai
- *Panax ginseng*
- Alfalfa
- Licorice

There is no evidence of a positive effect on bone of these compounds.

Miscellaneous

Iodine and the thyroid

Sources include kelp and shellfish-derived products.

Effects include iodine-induced goiter or hypothyroidism, particularly in patients with underlying thyroid disease (may have a Wolff–Chaikoff effect in patients with Graves' disease, causing inhibition of iodide organification and thus thyroid hormone production).

Iodine-induced hyperthyroidism occurs in areas of endemic goiter and iodine deficiency.

DHEA—"elixir of youth"

DHEA is reported to slow or improve changes associated with aging, including general well-being, cognitive function, sexual function, energy levels, body composition, and muscle strength, and to aid weight loss and treat the metabolic syndrome.

The mechanism of action is that DHEA is secreted by the adrenal glands and interconverted to DHEAS. Both DHEAS and DHEA are converted to androgens and estrogens that then act directly at their receptors.

DHEA and DHEAS may play a role in replacement of adrenal androgens in patients with adrenal insufficiency, resulting in improved well-being, particularly with respect to sexual function.

It is not proven in controlled trials to improve health in other patients without adrenal insufficiency.

There are risks of androgenic effects in women when taken at high doses (100–200 mg/DHEA daily). DHEA has a theoretical risk of promoting hormone-sensitive cancers such as prostate and breast cancers. DHEA may also interfere with antiestrogen effects of anastrazole and other aromatase inhibitors.

Further information

Natural Medicines Comprehensive Database. Available at www.naturaldatabase.com (requires subscription).

Part 11

Diabetes

Boris Draznin

Classification and diagnosis

Background

Diabetes mellitus (DM) is characterized by an elevated blood glucose. The classification of diabetes gives an idea of the underlying cause or defect.

Currently, 4–7% of the U.S. population has diabetes, with about half that many still undiagnosed. In 2003, worldwide, 189 million people were known to have diabetes; this figure may reach 324 million by 2025.

Diagnosis

DM is a biochemical diagnosis based on fasting and postprandial glucose levels. The venous plasma glucose levels for this are shown in Table 103.1.

In 1997, the American Diabetes Association (ADA) suggested lowering the normal fasting plasma glucose level to <110 mg/dL and the diabetic level to >126 mg/dL. A fasting glucose is therefore the diagnostic test of choice. Only pregnant woman are expected to have a 2-hour postprandial level checked routinely.

A diagnosis of diabetes is made in any symptomatic person with a random blood glucose >200 mg/dL. Asymptomatic patients or those with intercurrent illness still require a further abnormal result before a diagnosis of diabetes can be made.

Table 103.1 WHO classification

Status	Measurement condition	Venous plasma glucose (mg/dL)
Normal	Fasting *and*	<110
	2-hour postprandial	<140
Diabetes	Fasting *or*	>126
	2-hour postprandial	>200
Impaired glucose tolerance (IGT)	Fasting *and*	<126
	2-hour post-prandial	140–200
Impaired fasting glucose (IFG)	Fasting	110–126

Classification

The first accepted classification of diabetes was drawn up by the WHO and modified in 1985 (📖 see Table 103.1). The original classification into insulin-dependent DM (IDDM), or type 1, and non–insulin-dependent DM (NIDDM), or type 2 (Table 103.2), is now no longer used but is still seen in non-diabetes literature.

The current classification includes both clinical stage and etiology and has been used since 1997. The clinical staging is from normal glucose tolerance through impaired glucose tolerance (IGT) and/or impaired fasting hyperglycemia (IFG) and on to frank DM, which is split into non-insulin requiring, insulin requiring for control, and insulin requiring for survival. The etiological groups are listed in Box 103.1.

Table 103.2 Differences between type 1 and type 2 diabetes

Factor	Type 1 diabetes	Type 2 diabetes
Peak age of onset	12 years	60 years
U.S. prevalence	0.25–0.7%	5–7% (10% of those >65 years)
Etiology	Autoimmune	Combination of insulin resistance, β-cell destruction, and β-cell dysfunction
Initial presentation	Polyuria, polydypsia, and weight loss with ketoacidosis	Hyperglycemic symptoms but often with complication of diabetes
Treatment	Diet and insulin from outset	Diet with or without oral hypoglycemic agents or insulin

Box 103.1 Classification of diabetes

Type 1 (5–10% of cases): pancreatic islet β-cell deficiency
- Autoimmune—associated with autoantibodies to islet autoantigens (glutamate decarboxylase (GAD), IA-2 and insulin)
- Idiopathic

Type 2 (80–95% of cases): defective insulin action or secretion
- Insulin resistance
- Insulin secretory defect

Others

Genetic defects of β-cell function
- Maturity-onset diabetes of the young (MODY)
- Chromosome 20, HNF4β (MODY 1)
- Chromosome 7, glucokinase (MODY 2)
- Chromosome 12, HNF1α (MODY 3)
- Chromosome 13, IPF-1 (MODY 4)
  - Mitochondrial DNA 3242 mutation
  - Mutations associated with neonatal diabetes (KIR6.2, SUR)
- Others

Genetic defects of insulin action
- Type A insulin resistance
- Leprechaunism (type 2 diabetes, intrauterine growth retardation + dysmorphic features)
- Rabson–Mendenhall syndrome (DM + pineal hyperplasia + acanthosis nigricans)
- Lipoatrophic diabetes
- Others

Diseases of the exocrine pancreas
- Pancreatitis
- Trauma or surgery (pancreatectomy)
- Neoplasia
- Pancreatic destruction, e.g., cystic fibrosis, hemochromatosis
- Others

Endocrinopathies
- Cushing's syndrome
- Acromegaly
- Pheochromocytoma
- Glucagonoma
- Hyperthyroidism
- Somatostatinoma
- Others

Box 103.1 *(Contd.)*

Drug or chemical induced
Infections
- Congenital rubella or cytomegalovirus (CMV)
- Others

Uncommon forms of immune-mediated diabetes
- Anti-insulin receptor antibodies
- Stiff man syndrome (type 1 diabetes, rigidity of muscles, painful spasms)
- Others

Other genetic syndromes associated with diabetes
- Down syndrome
- Klinefelter syndrome
- Lawrence–Moon–Biedl syndrome
- Myotonic dystrophy
- Prader–Willi syndrome
- Turner syndrome
- Wolfram syndrome (or DIDMOAD – **d**iabetes **i**nsipidus, **DM**, **o**ptic **a**trophy + sensorineural **d**eafness)
- Others

Gestational diabetes

Genetics

Type 1 diabetes

The overall lifetime risk in a Caucasian population of developing type 1 diabetes is only 0.4%, but this rises to

- 1–2% if your mother has it.
- 3–6% if your father has it.
- 6% if siblings have it.
- Monozygotic twins have a 40% concordance rate.

Islet cell antibodies are seen in only 0.3% of the general population but in 40–50% of monozygotic twins and 5% of siblings of type 1 patients. A genetic predisposition is therefore suggested, but this also highlights the importance of environmental triggers, as not all those with antibodies go on to develop diabetes. Genetic predisposition accounts for 1/3 of susceptibility to type 1 diabetes.

Although several different regions of the human genome are linked to the development of type 1 diabetes, the most common are the major histocompatibility complex (MHC) antigens and human leukocyte antigens (HLA). In the United States, more than 90% of patients with type 1 diabetes have HLA-DR3, DR4, or both.

Certain variants of the *DQB1* or *DQA1* gene result in expression of susceptible alleles of DR3/DR4. This association is not true in all races, notably the Japanese.

There are currently 10 distinct genetic areas (IDDM1–IDDM10) known to be linked to type 1 diabetes; some relate to MHC genes, others to the insulin gene region. MHC antigens commonly found in those with type 1 diabetes and felt to predispose to it are B15, B8, and DQ8. The DR2, DQ6, and DQ18 genes appear to be protective.

Linkage studies have suggested type 1 susceptibility genes on the following chromosomes:

- 6q (also known as IDDM5)
- 11p (IDDM2)
- 11q (IDDM4)
- 15q (IDDM3)

These genetic variations may help explain susceptibility, but their link to ↑ levels of islet cell antibodies, antiglutamate decarboxylase (GAD) antibodies, and antityrosine phosphatase antibodies (anti-IA-2 antibodies) often seen soon after diagnosis is less clearly decided.

If all of these three antibodies are present in a nondiabetic individual, the person has an 88% chance of developing type 1 diabetes within the next 10 years.

Maturity-onset diabetes of the young (MODY)

The genes known to be involved in MODY are gradually ↑ as our understanding of insulin signaling and receptors expands.

MODY 1 (HNF4α)

- Accounts for <0.0001% of all type 2 patients and about 5% of cases of MODY
- Usually presents in adolescence or early adulthood, <25 years of age
- Can give severe hyperglycemia, with 20% needing insulin therapy and 40% needing oral agents
- Results in a high frequency of microvascular complications
- Inherited as an autosomal dominant disorder with a defect on chromosome 20q, resulting in altered activity of the hepatic nuclear factor (HNF)4α gene, which is a positive regulator of HNF1α. This is a transcription factor found in the liver and β cells of the pancreas, where it acts as a transactivator of the insulin gene in rat models.

MODY 2 (glucokinase)

- Accounts for <0.2% of type 2 patients and 10–14% of cases of MODY
- Presents in early childhood
- Gives only mild hyperglycemia and thus infrequent microvascular complications, with 90% of patients being controlled on diet alone and insulin usually only needed when becoming pregnant
- Autosomally dominantly inherited with a defect in the glucokinase gene on chromosome 7. This results in altered glucose sensing in the β cells of the pancreas and impaired hepatic production of glycogen.

MODY 3 (HNF1α)

- Affects 1–2% of type 2 patients and accounts for 70% of MODY patients
- Presents in adolescence or early adulthood (peaks around 21 years of age)
- Causes severe hyperglycemia and frequent microvascular complications; 1/3 require insulin therapy and 1/3 require oral agents
- Linked to a mutation on chromosome 12q24 that directly alters HNF1α activity. How this causes type 2 diabetes is not fully understood.

MODY 4 (IPF-1)

- Accounts for <1% of cases of MODY
- A mutation occurs in transcription factor gene *IPF-1,* which in its homozygous form leads to total pancreatic agenesis.
- MODY 5 (HNF1-β)
- Accounts for 3% of cases of MODY
- Average age of presentation is 22 years, with renal cysts (RCAD—renal cysts and diabetes) and often uterine abnormalities, gout, and insulin resistance

Type 2 diabetes

In patients with type 2 diabetes, the concordance between monozygotic twins for diabetes is much higher (60–100% vs. 40% for type 1), but the rate among dizygotic twins is much less, suggesting a much stronger genetic element in its etiology than for type 1 diabetes. Unlike patients with type 1 diabetes, however, those with type 2 do not seem to have the same HLA-linked genes.

In most families this appears to be polygenic, although the much less common MODY is autosomal dominant but only accounts for a few percent of all type 2 patients.

MODY is currently split into four types, with type 4 accounting for 15% of cases and for those cases that do not fit into types 1–3, although a chromosome 13 defect in the insulin promoter factor 1 gene may fall into this group.

Other recognized genetic subtypes of type 2 diabetes include *mitochondrial diabetes*, which affects 1–3% of type 2 patients and is maternally transmitted. It is associated with deafness and other neurological abnormalities.

Insulin resistance is an important part of type 2 diabetes, and rare genetic defects causing this are recognized. A 40% reduction in the biological effect of any given insulin molecule is suggested by clamp studies in type 2 patients, but these rarer genetic syndromes may result in a more severe picture.

Further reading

Alberti KG, Zimmet PZ, for the WHO consultation (1998). Definition, diagnosis and classification of DM and its complications. Part 1: Diagnosis and classification of DM. Provisional report of a WHO consultation. *Diabet Med* 15:539–553.

Alcolado JC, Thomas AW (1995). Maternally inherited DM: the role of mitochondrial DNA defects. *Diabet Med* 12(2):102–108.

Hattersley AT (1996). Maturity onset diabetes of the young (MODY). *Bailliere Clin Paediatr* 4(4):663–680.

Robinson S, Kessling A (1992). Diabetes secondary to genetic disorders. *Bailliere Clin Endocrinol Metab* 6:867–898.

World Health Organization (1985). *Diabetes Mellitus: Report of a WHO Study Group* (Technical Report Series no. 727). Geneva: World Health Organization.

World Health Organization (1999). *Definition, Diagnosis and Classification of Diabetes Mellitus and its Complications. Report of a WHO Consultation. Part 1, Diagnosis and Classification of Diabetes Mellitus.* Geneva: World Health Organization.

General management and treatment

Background

After diagnosis, all patients with diabetes need to see a dietitian and have a full medical assessment. The first priority is to decide whether this is a person with type 1 or type 2 diabetes, as the former needs insulin immediately whereas the later needs initial dietary advice. Such advice should always take into account the patient's circumstances and culture and be individually tailored to be achievable.

Assessment of the newly diagnosed patient

History
- Duration of symptoms, e.g., thirst, polyuria, weight loss
- Possible secondary causes of diabetes, e.g., acromegaly
- Family history
- Presence of complications of diabetes
- Risk factors for developing complications, e.g., smoking, hypertension, hyperlipidemia

Examination
- BMI
- Clues for secondary causes
- Cardiovascular system—especially BP + peripheral pulses
- Signs of autonomic and peripheral neuropathy
- Eyes—for retinopathy
- Feet

Investigations
Initial investigations will be modified by the history and examination but as a minimum should include the following:
- Blood tests for urea and electrolytes, liver and thyroid function, and a full lipid profile
- Urine tests for ketones, macro- and (if negative) microalbuminuria
- An ECG in all patients with type 2 diabetes

Treatment
In patients with type 1 diabetes, insulin therapy is mandatory, along with dietary advice and standard diabetes education. The education of all newly diagnosed patients is intended to provide an incentive for good compliance. A full education package should include the following:
- An explanation of what diabetes is and what it means to the patient
- Aims of treatment, e.g., rationale of reducing complications and exact values to aim for
- Types of not just drugs but also dietary advice and lifestyle modification, such as ↑ physical activity, stopping smoking, and reducing alcohol intake
- Self-monitoring, the reasons for doing it, and what to do with the results
- An idea of some chronic complications of diabetes and what to watch for, e.g., a podiatrist's input and review is advised, especially for those with type 2 diabetes.

All patients with type 2 diabetes should be considered for such an educational package.

In most patients the next step is to try diet, exercise, and weight reduction (if obese, which most will be) before initiating drug therapy if control is not adequate. If this fails to improve control adequately after 1–2 months, consider oral therapy with *metformin* in the overweight and *sulfonylureas* in the lean if there are no contraindications.

After the initial assessment, all patients should be put into a formal review system, whether by their PCP or an endocrinologist, for further education, maintenance of good control, and complication screening.

Dietary advice

In the overweight patient (e.g., BMI >27), a reduction in total calorie intake to aid weight reduction is also required. A standard diabetic diet should aim to have the following:

- <10% of its energy in the form of saturated fat (<8% if hyperlipidemic)
- <30% from all fats
- 50% as carbohydrate, which is mostly complex high fiber
- Sodium content <6 g/day in most people or <3 g/day if hypertensive

Alcohol is a significant source of calories; reduced intake is advised in the overweight or hypertriglyceridemic patient.

The current "standard" diet for a person with diabetes is a weight-reducing low-fat, low–glycemic index diet with reduced sodium content. Most patients will have type 2 diabetes and are slightly overweight, so this diet needs to be modified to the individual.

Oral hypoglycemic agents

Sulfonylureas (Table 104.1)

These agents are used as first-line treatment in non-obese patients with type 2 diabetes. The first-generation agents, *chlorpropamide*, *tolbutamide*, and *tolazamide*, are rarely used today.

Second-generation agents such as *glibenclamide*, *gliclazide*, and *glipizide* are more commonly used. Third-generation agents such as *glimepiride* are also available.

Mode of action

Sulfonylureas act by stimulating a receptor on the surface of β cells, closing a potassium channel, and opening a calcium channel with subsequent

Table 104.1 Properties of sulfonylureas

Sulfonylurea	Length of action	Begins working within	Daily dose (mg)
Glibenclamide	16–24 hours	2–4 hours	2.5–15
Gliclazide	10–24 hours	2–4 hours	40–320
Glipizide	6–24 hours	2–4 hours	2.5–20
Chlorpropamide	24–72 hours	2–4 hours	100–500
Tolbutamide	6–10 hours	2–4 hours	500–2000
Glimepiride	12–24 hours	2–4 hours	1–6

insulin release. A doubling of glucose-stimulated insulin secretion can be expected with both first- and second-phase insulin secretion affected. This results in a 1–2% reduction in HbA1c over the long term.

Side effects

These are hypoglycemia and weight gain. The elderly are particularly at risk of hypoglycemia with the longer-acting agents such as glibenclamide, and these should be avoided in this age group.

Occasional skin reactions, alterations in liver function tests, and minor GI symptoms may occur. Also avoid sulfonylureas in porphyria.

Biguanides (Table 104.2)

Metformin is first-line therapy in obese or overweight people with type 2 diabetes. It is also used in some insulin-treated, insulin-resistant, overweight subjects to reduce insulin requirements.

The UK Prospective Diabetes Study (UKPDS) showed significantly better results from metformin for complications and mortality compared to other therapies in overweight patients with type 2 diabetes. Although a 1–2 kg weight loss is seen initially, UKPDS data suggest metformin does not significantly alter weight over a 10-year period.

Mode of action

Metformin works by ↓ hepatic gluconeogenesis and ↑ muscle glucose uptake/metabolism, thus increasing insulin sensitivity. With long-term use a 0.8–2.0% reduction in HbA1c can be expected.

Side effects and contraindications

Metformin is contraindicated in patients with renal (creatinine >1.4), hepatic, or cardiac impairment or those who consume significant amounts of alcohol.

GI side effects include nausea, epigastric discomfort, and diarrhea and occur in up to 30% of patients in the first 1–2 weeks of treatment but are usually transient. If the starting dose is low (e.g., 500 mg once daily), most people develop a tolerance to these and are able to take higher doses; <5% are totally intolerant.

Rarely, skin rashes may occur. When seen, they usually occur in patients with hepatic, renal, or cardiac impairment.

Use of radiological contrast media with metformin is associated with an ↑ risk of lactic acidosis. Therapy should be stopped at the time of or prior to such investigations and restarted 2 days after the test unless renal

Table 104.2 Biguanides and prandial glucose regulators

Drug	Length of action	Begins working within	Daily dose (mg)
Metformin	24–36 hours	2.5 hours	500–2000
Repaglinide	4–6 hours	<1 hour	0.5–16
Nateglinide	4 hours	<1 hour	180–540

function has been affected by the procedure, in which case this should be resolved first.

Lactic acidosis occurs very infrequently, e.g., 0.024–0.15 cases/1000 patient years in a Swedish study. Although it is known to reduce folic acid and vitamin B_{12} absorption, this is not usually a significant problem clinically with metformin.

Prandial glucose regulators (Table 104.2)

These agents can be used in type 2 patients who have inadequate control on diet or metformin. They predominantly target postprandial hyperglycemia because of their short duration of action.

Repaglinide, a carbamoylmethyl benzoic acid derivative, is a non-sulfonylurea oral hypoglycemic agent that stimulates the secretion of insulin from pancreatic β cells. It works on separate parts of the β-cell sulfonylurea receptor from the sulfonylureas.

Its use results in an approximate 0.6–2% reduction in HbA1c levels. Its very short duration of action reduces the risk of hypoglycemia compared to that with some sulfonylureas.

It has an insulinotropic effect within 30 minutes of oral administration and a return to normal insulin levels within 4–6 hours (elimination half-life is around 1 hour). It should not, however, be used in patients with renal or hepatic impairment and may result in hepatic dysfunction, so periodic liver function test monitoring is required.

Nateglinide is a D-phenylalanine derivative with an insulinotropic effect within 15 minutes of oral administration and a return to normal insulin levels by 2 hours (elimination half-life 1.5 hours), thus reducing the risk of subsequent hypoglycemia. Efficacy is similar to that of repaglinide.

α-glucosidase inhibitors (Table 104.3)

These are used in type 2 patients who have inadequate control on diet or other oral agents alone. When taken with food, acarbose reduces

Table 104.3 Oral hypogylcemwic agents: summary

Class	Mechanism of action	Expected reduction in HbA1c (%)
Sulfonylureas	Stimulate pancreatic insulin secretion	1.5–2.5
Biguanides	Increase muscle glucose uptake and metabolism; decrease hepatic gluconeogenesis	0.8–2.0
Prandial glucose regulators	Stimulate pancreatic insulin secretion	0.5–1.9
α-Glucosidase inhibitors	Inhibit a digestive enzyme	0.4–0.7
Thiazolidinediones	Activate PPAR-γ receptor	0.6–1.5

postprandial glucose peaks by inhibiting the digestive enzyme α-glucosidase, which normally breaks carbohydrates into their monosaccharide components, thus retarding glucose uptake from the intestine and reducing postprandial glucose peaks.

Some improvement in lipids has also been reported.

These undigested carbohydrates then pass into the large intestine where bacteria metabolize them. This may explain the common side effects of postprandial fullness or bloating, abdominal pain, flatulence, and diarrhea.

Thiazolidinediones (Table 104.3)

This class of drugs acts as insulin-sensitizing agents by activating the peroxisome proliferator activated receptor (PPAR-γ), which stimulates gene transcription for glucose transporter molecules such as Glut 1 and Glut 4. The first of this class was *troglitazone*, which was withdrawn soon after its launch because of reports of hepatotoxicity.

Other agents, such as *rosiglitazone* and *pioglitazone*, are available, giving a 0.6–1.5% drop in HbA1c. These do not seem to have the same problem with hepatotoxicity, and there is often an improvement in liver function, especially with nonalcoholic steatohepatitis (NASH).

Although the risk of hepatic dysfunction is not high, initial checks of liver function and monitoring of liver function test are still currently advised. In view of the more common problem with fluid retention, avoidance of use in patients with heart failure is also strongly suggested.

Recent studies suggest a link with osteoporosis with both the currently available agents. The weight gain seen with both agents is also an important factor when considering the best therapy for any patient.

Indications
- Type 2 diabetes, oral combination with metformin or a sulfonylurea or a meglitinide

Dose
- Rosiglitazone 4–8 mg/day (combination metformin and rosiglitazone tablets are also available, either 2 mg or 4 mg rosiglitazone with 500 mg or 1 g metformin per tablet)
- Pioglitazone 15–45 mg/day (combination metformin and pioglitazone as 15 mg pioglitazone and 850 mg metformin per tablet)

Side effects
- Fluid retention
- Weight gain
- Hepatotoxicity

The incretin system (GLP-1 mimetics and DPP4 inhibitors)

Glucagon-like polypeptide-1 (GLP-1) and gastric inhibitory polypeptide (GIP), also known as glucose-dependent insulinotropic peptide, are hormones made in the L- and K-cells of the jejunum and ileum in response to a food load entering the GI tract. These incretin hormones stimulate glucose-dependent insulin secretion, suppress glucagon secretion, and slow gastric emptying, with an improvement in insulin sensitivity.

Exenatide is a GLP-1 mimetic. Dipeptidyl peptidase-4 (DPP-4) breaks down GIP and GLP-1. This enzyme can be inhibited by oral drugs such as sitagliptin and vildagliptin (i.e., DPP-4 inhibitors) with a resultant 0.4–0.7% reduction in HbA1c over a 12-month period. They are weight neutral if not help in reducing weight.

Liver monitoring with vildagliptin is currently recommended. The GLP-1 mimetic exenatide is available and is taken as a twice-daily injection of 5 mcg or 10 mcg per dose. It yields a 0.6–0.8% reduction in HbA1c after 30 weeks' use and a 1.6–2.8 kg weight loss over the same period.

Several depot preparations of GLP-1 analogs/mimetics are in development. Long-acting GLP-1analogs are coming to the market as well.

Indications
- Sitagliptin/vildagliptin—type 2 diabetes, combination with metformin or thiazolidinediones
- Exenatide—type 2 diabetes, combination with metformin or sulfonylurea or both

Dose
- Sitagliptin 100 mg/day orally
- Vildagliptin 100 mg/day orally
- Exenatide 5–10 mcg twice daily by injection

Side effects
- Sitagliptin—GI disturbance, upper respiratory tract infection, nasopharyngitis, peripheral edema
- Vildagliptin—as sitagliptin + abnormal liver function tests
- Exenatide
  - GI upset with nausea, vomiting, abdominal distension, diarrhea
  - Headache, dizziness and increase sweating
  - Injection site reactions

Insulin

Insulin is required in all patients with type 1 diabetes and in some with type 2, for the preservation of life; in other patients with type 2 diabetes it is needed to achieve better glycemic and metabolic control or for the relief of hyperglycemic symptoms (see Table 104.4 for detailed aims of treatment). Most insulin is in a biosynthetic human form (from yeast or bacteria) at a standard concentration: U100 (100 units/mL).

Insulin can be given by IV or SC route. More recently, short-acting insulin was also given as an inhaled formulation, but this was withdrawn. Standard insulins come as 10 mL vials for use with a 0.5 mL or 1.0 mL syringe or as 3.0 mL cartridges for use in pen devices.

The insulin itself is unmodified/neutral or mixed with agents such as protamine or zinc to alter its onset of action, peak effect, and duration of action (see Table 104.5 for a summary of insulins).

Analogs of human insulin to give more rapid onset or greater duration of action are also widely available and used. There are >30 types of insulin

Table 104.4 Suggested aims of treatment

Fasting blood glucose	<7 mmol/L
HbA1c	<7.2% (or <6.5% in those with significant complications)
Blood pressure	<140/80 mmHg
Body mass index	20–25 ideally
Home monitoring	Capillary blood glucose estimates taken fasting, pre-meal, 2 hours postprandially, and before bed. These will need to be frequent enough to allow alterations in treatment and assessment of adequate control. Often this monitoring 3× week in stable type 2 patients and daily in stable type 1 patients is adequate.

Table 104.5 Insulin: summary

Type of insulin	Examples	Peak activity (h)	Duration of action (h)
Insulin analog	Humalog® (insulin lispro)	0–2	3–4
	(NovoRapid®) Insulin Aspart	1–3	3–4
Short acting	Human Actrapid®	1–3	6–8
	Humulin® R	2–3	6–8
Intermediate acting	Human Insulatard®	2–8	10–16
	Humulin® N	2–8	10–16
	Human Monotard®	3–12	18–24
Long acting	Humulin® Zn	4–8	<24
	Human Ultratard®	6–24	<36

preparation available, which should allow full 24-hour cover for a wide variety of lifestyles.

The main problems with all insulin regimens are weight gain and hypoglycemia. The latter condition occurring overnight can be troublesome, especially as the patient may not know it has occurred and may react to the morning hyperglycemia by increasing their evening insulin dose. Occasional checks of 3 A.M. blood glucose levels may help sort this out.

Types of insulin

Short-acting (soluble/neutral) insulins

Humulin® and Novolin® are two regular insulins that have an onset 30 minutes after injection, with a peak onset at 2–4 hours, and a duration of up to 6–8 hours. They are rarely used now in the United States.

Insulin analogs

Insulin *lispro* (Humalog®), insulin *aspart* (NovoRapid®), and insulin *glulisine* (Apidra®) have been modified to allow injecting and eating to occur simultaneously. They have a more rapid onset of action and earlier peak effect with peak blood insulin levels approximately 1.5–2.5 times that from the same dose of regular human insulin.

The duration of action is also shorter at 5 hours. This may cause problems if there are long gaps between meals.

Long-acting analogs, insulin *glargine* (Lantus®) and insulin d*etemir* (Levemir®), are also available. These have a flatter profile with a duration of action of 22–24 hours. They can be used as part of a basal bolus regimen with short-acting analogs or regular insulins.

They appear to have less hypoglycemia than other background insulins and may reduce the risk of nocturnal hypoglycemia. Their use as a once-daily insulin alone or in combination with oral agents, such as glimepiride or the prandial glucose regulators, is also proving popular in the elderly type 2 patient.

While insulin glargine has a slightly longer duration of action, making it a popular once-daily preparation insulin detemir, because of its albumin-binding properties is reported to give less between-dose variability in the same individual. With a duration of action of 20–22 hours, it may be used in similar situations, although a significant proportion of people need to use this twice daily.

Intermediate-acting (isophane) insulins

Insulin action can be extended by addition of protamine to give isophane insulin, with an onset of action 1–2 hours after injection, a peak at 4–6 hours, and duration of action of 8–14 hours. Different preparations have slightly different profiles in terms of peak effect and maximal insulin concentrations, as with soluble preparations.

Biphasic/mixed insulins

Combinations of soluble/neutral or short-acting analogs with isophane insulins are extremely popular. The amount of soluble insulin present varies from 10 to 50%, with 30% being the most popular.

Depending on its monocomponents, onset is normally at 30 minutes, peak effect at 2–6 hours, and duration 8–12 hours. Insulin analog biphasic preparations have an onset, peak, and duration all slightly shorter than these.

Insulin regimens

Twice-daily free mixing

Historically, these were very popular, although now they are used less. The usual starting regimen was 2/3 isophane, 1/3 soluble, and 2/3 of the total daily dose was given pre-breakfast and 1/3 before the evening meal.

The main problems are mixing them and pre-lunch hypo- or hyperglycemia. If on the same doses twice daily, watch for pre-evening meal hyperglycemia and increase the morning isophane dose to compensate for this. A reduction in the morning soluble is often needed to reduce pre-lunch hypoglycemia.

Twice-daily fixed mixture
This is most commonly a 30% soluble/70% isophane mixture. Although this is not ideal for pre-lunch control or alterations in diet and exercise that are not preplanned, it is indicated in type 2 patients with poor control, those with significant osmotic symptoms, and those in whom there is no room to increase oral agents.

A suitable starting regimen is a 30/70 mixture with 2/3 pre-breakfast and 1/3 pre-evening meal. The exact doses tend to vary widely depending on insulin sensitivity, but a reasonable starting regimen may be 10–15 units pre-breakfast and 5–10 units pre-evening meal.

Basal bolus regimen
This is regular insulin (rarely) or an insulin analog given 3 × day pre-meal with a pre-bed isophane or long-acting analog. It may have more flexibility with meal times, portions, and exercise than that of previous regimens. The larger number of injections and more frequent capillary blood glucose measurements needed make it less popular with some patients.

If starting this as the first type of insulin, 3 equal pre-meal doses should be given and altered as required, e.g., 4–6 units is a reasonable starting dose, with 6–8 units of isophane pre-bed. If converting to a basal bolus regimen from a twice-daily biphasic regimen, the total daily insulin dose needs to be reduced by up to 10%.

Initially, 30–50% of the total daily insulin needed is given as a pre-bedtime isophane or long-acting analog and split the remaining insulin evenly between meals as soluble or short-acting analog insulin. Once the patient is on this regimen, the evening isophane or analog often needs to be increased to maintain adequate fasting sugars.

In patients using short-acting insulin analogs and, less often, those on standard soluble insulins, a 2 × daily isophane or a long-acting analog is occasionally needed, especially if there is a long gap between lunch and the evening meal.

Continuous SC insulin infusion (CSII)
Insulin pumps are used infrequently in patients with type 1 DM. Potential problems are pump failure, ketoacidosis, and cannula site infections, although with improvements in technology these are less common problems. Intensive diabetes education is a must.

Insulin and oral agent mixtures
In type 2 patients, several combinations are occasionally used. The two most popular ones are bedtime insulin + daytime tablets, and more frequent insulin + metformin.

In the first mixture, oral agents continue during the day with a pre-bed isophane or long-acting insulin analog used to give acceptable fasting sugar levels pre-breakfast. Although patients often start at 10 units/night, doses 5–6 times that are not infrequently needed.

In the second regimen, up to 2 g/day of metformin is added to any standard insulin regimen in order to reduce insulin requirements and improve control without the problem of further weight gain often seen if the insulin is continually increased.

Further reading

Alberti KGMM, Gries FA, et al. (1994). A desktop guide for the management of non-insulin dependent diabetes mellitus (NIDDM): an update. *Diabet Med* 11:899–909.

American Diabetes Association (1994). ADA position statement. Nutrition recommendations and principles for people with diabetes mellitus. *Diabet Care* 17:519–522.

Bailey CJ, Day C, Campbell IW (2006). A consensus algorithm for treating hyperglycaemia in type 2 diabetes. *Br J Diabet Vasc Dis* 6(4):147–148.

Bailey CJ, Turner RC (1996). Metformin. *N Engl J Med* 334:574–579.

Campbell IW (1990). Efficacy and limitations of sulphonylurea and metformin. In Bailey CJ, Flatt PR, (Eds). *New Antidiabetic Drugs*. Nishimura, Japan: Smith-Gordon, pp. 33–51.

Diabetes and Nutrition Study Group of the European Association for the Study of Diabetes (1995). Recommendations for the nutritional management of patients with diabetes mellitus. *Diabet Nutrit Metab* 8(3):186–189.

Nissen SE, Wolski K (2007). Effect of rosiglitazone on the risk of myocardial infarction and death from cardiovascular causes. *N Engl J Med* 356(24):2457–71. Erratum in *N Engl J Med* 357(1):100.

Ratner RE (1995). Rational insulin management of insulin-dependent diabetes. In Leslie RDG, Robbins DE (Eds) *Diabetes: Clinical Science in Practice*. Cambridge, UK: Cambridge University Press, pp. 434–449.

STOP-NIDDM Trial (2003). Acabose treatment and the risk of cardiovascular disease and hypertension in patients with impaired glucose tolerance. *JAMA* 290:486–494.

UK Prospective Diabetes Study (UKPDS) Group (1998). Intensive blood-glucose control with sulfonylureas or insulin compared with conventional treatment and risk of complications in patients with type 2 diabetes (UKPDS 33) *Lancet* 352:837–853.

UK Prospective Diabetes Study (UKPDS) Group (1998). Effect of intensive blood-glucose control with metformin on complications in overweight patients with type 2 diabetes (UKPDS 34). *Lancet* 352:854–865.

Diabetic eye disease

Epidemiology

Diabetic retinopathy remains the most common cause of blindness in the working population of developed countries. Currently, diabetic eye disease gives a person with diabetes a 10- to 20-fold ↑ risk of blindness. It is suggested that 84,000 of the 7.8 million North American patients with diabetics will develop proliferative retinopathy each year and another 95,000 will develop macular edema.

The prevalence of diabetic retinopathy depends on the duration of diabetes, glycemic control, BP control, and the racial mix of the group being examined. A prevalence of ~30% in a general diabetic population is often quoted.

In type 1 patients, <2% have any lesions of diabetic retinopathy at diagnosis and only 8% have any features of it by 5 years (2% proliferative). But 87–98% have abnormalities 30 years later, 30% of these having had proliferative retinopathy. In type 2 patients, 20–37% can be expected to have retinopathy at diagnosis; 15 years later, 85% of those on insulin and 60% of those not taking insulin will have abnormalities.

The 4-year incidence for proliferative retinopathy in a large North American epidemiological study was 10.5% in type 1 patients, 7.4% in older-onset/type 2 patients on insulin, and 2.3% in those not on insulin.

In the US, currently maculopathy is a more common and thus more significant sight-threatening complication of diabetes. It is suggested that 75% of those with maculopathy have type 2 diabetes, and there is a 4-year incidence of 10.4% in this group. Although type 2 patients are 10 times more likely to have maculopathy than type 1 patients, 14% of type 1 patients who become blind do so because of maculopathy.

Diabetic retinopathy, like many microvascular complications, is more common in ethnic minorities than in Caucasians. Cataracts are more common in people with diabetes and are actually the most common eye abnormality found. These occur in up to 60% of 30- to 54-year-olds.

Other abnormalities to look for include vitreous changes such as asteroid hyalosis, which occur in about 2% of patients. These are small spheres or star-shaped opacities seen in the vitreous that appear to sparkle when illuminated under an examining light and do not normally affect vision.

📖 See Box 105.1 for classification.

Box 105.1 Classification and features of diabetic retinopathy

Background retinopathy
- Microaneurysms
- Hemorrhages
- Hard exudates

Preproliferative retinopathy
- Soft exudates/cotton wool spots
- Intraretinal abnormalities (IRMAs)
- Venous abnormalities (e.g., venous beading, looping, and reduplication)

Proliferative retinopathy
- New vessels on the disc or within 1 disc diameter of it (NVD)
- New vessels elsewhere (NVE)
- Rubeosis iridis (± neovascular glaucoma)

Maculopathy (graded as M0 if none and M1 if present)
- Hemorrhages and hard exudates in the macula area
- Reduced visual acuity with no abnormality seen

Clinical features and histological features

The classification of diabetic retinopathy is based on ophthalmoscopic examination or retinal photographs. Several other changes not seen macroscopically may also explain some of these clinical findings.

One of the first histological changes seen is thickening of the capillary basement membrane and loss of the pericytes embedded in it. Both have been linked to hyperglycemia in experimental models; sorbitol accumulation and advanced glycation both have a role.

In normal retinal capillaries there is a 1:1 relationship between endothelial cells and pericytes. Pericytes may control endothelial cell proliferation, maintain the structural integrity of capillaries, and regulate blood flow. Altering these roles, along with the ↑ blood viscosity, abnormal fibrinolytic activity, and reduced red cell deformity also seen in diabetes, may lead to capillary occlusion, tissue hypoxia, and the stimulus for new vessel formation.

Exactly how locally produced growth factors, altered protein kinase C, alterations in oxidative stress responses, and alterations in the autoregulation of retinal blood flow combine to cause this remains unclear.

The natural progression is from background to preproliferative then to proliferative retinopathy/maculopathy and, ultimately, sight-threatening disease.

Background retinopathy

Capillary microaneurysms are the earliest feature seen clinically, as red dots. Small intraretinal hemorrhages, or "blots," also occur, as can hemorrhage into the nerve fiber layer, which are often more flame shaped. With ↑ capillary leakage, hard exudates, which are lipid deposits, can also be seen.

Preproliferative retinopathy

A *cotton wool spot* is an infarct in the nerve fiber layer that alters axoplasmic transport in ganglion cell neurons, giving an edematous infarct seen as a pale gray, fuzzy-edged lesion, which gives it its name. IRMAs are tortuous dilated hypercellular capillaries in the retina that occur in response to retinal ischemia.

A further change seen is alternating dilatation and constriction of veins (venous beading) as well as other venous alterations such as duplication and loop formation. Overall, there are large areas of capillary non-perfusion occurring in the absence of new vessels.

The Early Treatment of Diabetic Retinopathy Study (ETDRS) suggested that certain of these features matter and suggested a 4–2–1 rule:

- 4 quadrants of severe hemorrhages or microaneurysms
- 2 quadrants of IRMAs
- 1 quadrant with venous beading

If the patient has one of these features, there is a 15% risk of developing sight-threatening retinopathy within the next year; if two are present, the risk rises to 45%.

Proliferative retinopathy

New vessels are formed from the retina and can grow along, into, or out from it. A scaffolding for fibrosis then forms. There are two forms of new vessels: those on the disc or within 1 disc diameter of the disc (NVD) and new vessels elsewhere (NVE).

Both give no symptoms but can cause the problems of advanced retinopathy, such as hemorrhage, scar tissue formation, traction on the retina, and retinal detachment, which actually results in loss of vision. Thus panretinal photocoagulation, which can result in the regression of these new vessels, is used when such problems are seen.

Diabetic maculopathy

Edema in the macula area can distort central vision and reduce visual acuity. Any of the above changes can coexist with maculopathy. The changes seen can be as follows:

- *Edematous*—clinically it may just be difficult to focus on the macula with a hand-held ophthalmoscope.
- *Exudative*—with hemorrhages, hard exudates, and circinate exudates
- *Ischemic*—capillary loss occurs but clinically the macula may look normal on direct ophthalmoscopy but the unperfused area will show up on fluorescein angiography.
- Any combination of these

A ring or circinate pattern of lipid deposits suggest a focal defect that may be treated with focal laser therapy, whereas more diffuse problems may require more extensive treatment with a macula grid of laser.

Eye screening

Because so many patients can expect to develop eye complications, some of which are sight threatening but with treatment can be reduced, a suitable screening program is advisable. Patients with diabetes should undergo ophthalmic examination at least once a year. A full examination should include the elements discussed below.

Visual acuity

Use a standard chart for distance and check each eye separately. Let the patient wear their glasses for the test. If vision is worse than 20/30, also check with a pinhole as this will correct for any refractive (glasses) error.

If vison does not correct to 20/30 or better, consider more careful review; some maculopathy changes cannot be seen easily with a hand-held ophthalmoscope and an ophthalmology review may be needed. Cataracts are a more likely cause, so look carefully at the red reflex. If vision gets worse with a pinhole, assume maculopathy until proven otherwise.

High blood glucose readings can give myopia (difficulty in distance vision) and low blood glucose can produce hypermetropia (difficulty in reading), although this is not universal.

Eye examination

Dilate the pupil before looking into the eye.

- Use *tropicamide* 1% in most cases, as it dilates the pupil adequately in 15–20 minutes and lasts only 2–3 hours.
- In those with a dark iris, you may also need *phenylephrine* (2.5%) added soon after the tropicamide to give adequate views.
- The main reasons not to dilate are closed-angle glaucoma and recent eye surgery, although as such patients are usually under an eye clinic already, most people are suitable for dilatation.
- 1% *pilocarpine* drops can be used (although not routinely) if acuity is >20/40 after dilatation. They may speed up reversal and allow driving sooner.

Once the pupil is dilated, look at the red reflex to check for lens opacities. Examine the anterior chamber; although rare, rubeosis iridis is important to pick up. The vitreous is examined before examining the retina.

When examining the retina, use the optic disc as a landmark, follow all four arcades of vessels out from it, examine the periphery, and, at the end, examine the macula. This examination can be uncomfortably bright through a dilated pupil and if done at the start makes it difficult for anyone to keep their eye still enough to complete it adequately.

Retinal photographs

Although consultant diabetologists are more accurate than general practitioners, they still miss some cases of retinopathy, compared to the gold standard of an ophthalmologist.

One way to reduce the false-negative rate for a screening program is to use retinal photography and ophthalmoscopy. More than 90% of people can have good-quality photos performed. This was often performed using 35 mm slide film, although digital images are now of sufficiently good quality, require a less intense flash, and avoid the delay of having to develop the film.

A digital image should be used with a minimum of 27 pixels per degree and a 45° field of vision for each of the two images taken per eye (one centered on the macula the other on the optic disc).

The images obtained should then be graded and assessed by a trained observer with a quality assurance system to maintain consistency of grading.

When to refer

The physician performing eye screening will need consultation with an experienced ophthalmologist (see Box 105.2).

Box 105.2 Reasons for and timing of referral to an ophthalmologist

Immediate referral
- R3/proliferative retinopathy, as untreated NVD carries a 40% risk of blindness in <2 years and laser treatment reduces this
- Rubeosis iridis/neovascular glaucoma
- Vitreous hemorrhage
- Advanced retinopathy with fibrous tissue or retinal detachments

Early referral (<6 weeks)
- R2/preproliferative changes
- M1/maculopathy, for nonproliferative retinopathy involving the macula or for any hemorrhages/hard exudates within 1 disc diameter of the fovea
- Fall of >2 lines on a Snellen chart (regardless of what fundoscopy shows)

Routine referral
- Cataracts
- Nonproliferative retinopathy with large circinate exudates not threatening the macula/fovea

Other categories
- R0/no retinopathy—annual screening
- R1/background retinopathy—annual screening and inform diabetes care team

---

Treatment

Glycemic control

There is good epidemiological evidence for an association between poor glycemic control and worsening of retinopathy (see Box 105.3).

The Diabetes Control and Complications Trial (DCCT) looked at intensive glycemic control in type 1 patients over age 6.5 years and showed a 76% reduction in risk of initially developing retinopathy in the tightly managed group compared to the control group. The rate of progression of existing retinopathy was slowed by 54% and the risk of developing severe nonproliferative or proliferative retinopathy was reduced by 47%.

The UKPDS looked at type 2 patients over a 9-year period and showed a 21% reduction in progression of retinopathy and 29% reduction in the need for laser therapy in those with good glycemic control. The long-term benefits of improved glycemic control are therefore clear.

However, the DCCT, the UKPDS, and several previous studies also showed an initial worsening of retinopathy in the first 2 years in the groups with tight or improved glycemic control. Thus all patients need careful monitoring over this period. The long-term benefits outweigh this initial risk.

Blood pressure control/therapy

There is good evidence for an association between both systolic and diastolic hypertension and retinopathy in type 1 patients, but the link may only be with systolic hypertension in type 2 patients.

The UKPDS looked at BP control in type 2 patients and showed that the treatment group, with a mean BP of 144/82 mmHg, compared to the control group, which had a mean of 154/87 mmHg, had a 35% reduction in the need for laser therapy. Adequate BP control, e.g., <140/80 in type 2 patients, is therefore advocated.

Use of angiotensin converting enzyme (ACE) inhibitors as first-line therapy should be considered with caution in those with pre-existing renal

---

Box 105.3 Risk factors for development or worsening of diabetic retinopathy

- Duration of diabetes
- Type of diabetes (proliferative disease is more common in type 1 and maculopathy in type 2)
- Poor diabetic control
- Hypertension
- Diabetic nephropathy
- Recent cataract surgery
- Pregnancy
- Alcohol (variable results, which may be related to the type of alcohol involved, e.g., worse in Scotland than Italy)
- Smoking (variable results, but appears worse in young people with exudates and older women with proliferative disease)

disease, as these agents may cause hyperkalemia and may worsen renal function in those with undiagnosed renal artery stenosis.

Experimental evidence suggests these agents may have antiangiogenic effects by altering local growth factor levels and reducing blood pressure. Studies using *enalapril* and *lisinopril* have both shown a reduction in the progression of retinopathy in type 1 patients.

Lipid control/therapy

Experimental evidence suggests that oxidized low-density lipoprotein (LDL) cholesterol may be cytotoxic for endothelial cells. Epidemiological data also suggest an association between higher LDL cholesterol and worse diabetic retinopathy, especially maculopathy with exudates.

A total cholesterol of >270 mg/dL gives a 4-fold greater risk of proliferative retinopathy than a total cholesterol of <200 mg/dL. A worse outcome from laser therapy in those treated for maculopathy has also been seen if hyperlipidemia is present. Aggressive lipid lowering is therefore advocated, especially in patients with maculopathy.

Antiplatelet therapy

In view of the altered rheological properties of diabetic patients, these agents have been tried, but the results are variable. No evidence that they make things worse has been shown, and some studies suggest that *aspirin* and *ticlopidine* may slow the progression of retinopathy, although the benefit was small.

Lifestyle advice

Although stopping smoking reduces macrovascular risk, its effect on retinopathy is less clear. Alcohol consumption and physical activity also show no consistent effect.

Other therapies

The use of agents such as protein kinase-C inhibitors and vascular endothelial growth factor (VEGF) inhibitors (e.g., bevacizumab) are currently being investigated to see if they can delay the progression of diabetic retinopathy. Initial studies are encouraging.

Surgical treatment

Laser treatment

Up to 1500–7000 separate burns of 100–500 micron diameter, each taking about 0.1 seconds to apply, are needed for panretinal or "scatter" laser photocoagulation. For edematous/exudative maculopathy, a macula grid may use only 100–200 burns of 100–200 micron diameter separated by 200–400 micron gaps, avoiding the fovea.

Laser therapy is usually performed as 3–4 sessions of outpatient treatment on conscious patients. Topical local anesthetic drops allow a contact lens to be placed on the cornea and are often all that is needed.

In some patients, however, this procedure may be slightly uncomfortable. A retro-orbital injection (performed through the inside of the lower eyelid) can be given to anesthetize the eye.

The laser energy is absorbed by the choroid and the pigment epithelium, which lie below the neurosensory layer. This also absorbs the energy and heat and is destroyed.

In patients with severe proliferative retinopathy, panretinal photocoagulation reduces visual loss by >80%, wheras a macula grid reduces visual loss in maculopathy by >50%.

The aim of laser treatment is to prevent further visual loss, especially in maculopathy, not to restore vision, and this distinction must be emphasized to all patients requiring treatment. The benefits from laser therapy currently outweigh the risks, which include accidental burns to the fovea if the eye moves during therapy, a reduction in night vision, and, in a small number of patients, interference with visual field severe enough to affect the ability to drive.

Vitrectomy

If the vitreous contains scar tissue, hemorrhage, or any opacity, a vitrectomy to remove it may help restore vision and allows the possibility of intraoperative laser treatment or a better view for postoperative laser therapy. It can also help reduce retinal traction and allows retinal reattachment to be performed.

A success rate at restoring vision of 70% is seen, but the risk of worsening vision, detaching the retina, or worsening lens opacities should also be considered.

Cataract extraction

This is a common procedure with a slightly higher complication rate than that in the nondiabetic population. Approximately 15% of patients undergoing a cataract extraction can be expected to have diabetes.

A large lens implant should be considered, especially if laser therapy is going to be needed subsequently. Worsening of maculopathy after cataract extraction is also a risk that needs careful monitoring.

Further reading

British Multi-Centre Study Group (1983). Photocoagulation for diabetic maculopathy: a randomized controlled clinical trial using xenon. *Diabetes* 32:1010–1016.

Early Treatment Diabetic Retinopathy Study Research Group (1985). Photocoagulation for diabetic macular edema. *Arch Ophthalmol* 103:1796–1806.

Scottish Intercollegiate Guidelines Network (2001). Management of diabetes. http://www.sign.ac.uk/guidelines/fulltext/55/index.html

Diabetic renal disease

Background

Diabetic nephropathy is now a major cause of premature death in patients with all types of diabetes. Approximately 1/6 patients entering most renal replacement programs in developed countries have diabetes, at least 50% with type 2 diabetes.

Definition

Diabetic nephropathy is defined as albuminuria (albumin excretion rate >300 mg/24 hours, which equates to 24-hour urinary protein >0.5 g) and declining renal function in a patient with known diabetes who does not have a urinary tract infection, heart failure, or any other renal disease.

This is usually associated with systemic hypertension, diabetic retinopathy, or neuropathy. In the absence of these, the diagnosis needs to be carefully evaluated. 📖 See Box 106.1.

> **Box 106.1 Investigations of lipid abnormalities**
>
> - *Proteinuria*—urinary protein >0.5 g/24 hours
> - *Albuminuria*—urinary albumin excretion rate >300 mg/24 hours or >200mcg/min
> - *Microalbuminuria*—urinary albumin excretion rate 30–300 mg/day or 20–200 mcg/min

Epidemiology

Microalbuminuria has a prevalence of 6–60% of patients with type 1 diabetes after 5–15 years' duration of diabetes. Diabetic nephropathy occurs in up to 35% of patients with type 1 diabetes, more commonly in males and in those diagnosed <15 years of age, with a peak incidence approaching 3%/year 16–20 years after the onset of diabetes.

Of those type 1 patients who develop proteinuria, 2/3 will subsequently develop renal failure. In the UK, 15% of all deaths in diabetic patients <50 years old are due to nephropathy.

In type 2 patients there are more obvious racial differences, with up to 25% of Caucasians and 50% of Asians expected to develop nephropathy, giving a prevalence in a general clinic of 4–33%. The duration of diabetes before development of clinical nephropathy is also often shorter in type 2 than in type 1 patients. This may be due to an initial delay in diagnosis of type 2 diabetes.

Making the diagnosis

A urine positive on dip testing for protein (i.e., >0.5 mg/L protein or >300 mg/L albumin) suggests diabetic nephropathy. A timed urine collection either overnight or over 24 hours will confirm proteinuria or albuminuria, but other causes of proteinuria must be excluded before labeling this diabetic nephropathy.

Proteinuria from nondiabetic renal disease occurs in up to 10% of type 1 and 30% of type 2 patients. Urinary tract infections, acute illness, heavy exercise, and cardiac failure are the most common causes to exclude (Box 106.2). The absence of hypertension or diabetic retinopathy would also put the diagnosis in question; confirmation from a renal biopsy may be required.

If the urine is standard dip test negative for albumin, microalbuminuria should be looked for. The implementation group for the St. Vincent Declaration recommends that all patients with negative protein on conventional urinalysis be annually screened for microalbuminuria.

A urinary albumin/creatinine ratio >2.5 mg/mmol in males and >3.5mg/mmol in females or a positive urine dip test (urine albumin >20 mcg) should be followed by a timed urine collection repeated 3× with at least two being abnormal.

Box 106.2 False positives for microalbuminuria

- Exercise
- Urinary tract infection
- Menstruation
- Semen

Pathology

Although macroscopically there is an increase in kidney size, microscopically there is thickening of the glomerular basement membrane, expansion of glomerular supporting tissues (the mesangium), and fibrotic changes in both efferent and afferent arterioles. If localized, this is termed *nodular glomerular sclerosis* (Kimmelstiel–Wilson nodules) and if more widespread, *diffuse glomerular sclerosis*.

The thickened basement membrane initially results in alteration in its electrical charge but not in pore size, which allows ↑ passage of albumin into the glomerular ultrafiltrate, seen clinically as microalbuminuria.

Pathogenesis

Hyperglycemia

As with all microvascular diabetic complications, hyperglycemia has been implicated in the pathogenesis of diabetic nephropathy via metabolic alterations. The DCCT showed a reduction in the development of microalbuminuria in patients with better glycemic control, which would support this.

The UKPDS showed similar improvements. These metabolic alterations may be due to sorbitol accumulation from the polyol pathway, which in turn is the result of the accumulation of advanced glycation end-products (AGE) or an as-yet unknown mechanism.

AGE have been linked to the extracellular matrix accumulation known to occur in nephropathy. The use of aminoguanidine to block renal AGE accumulation and an associated slowing in the progression of albuminuria and mesangial expansion would support their role in the pathogenesis of nephropathy.

The evidence for the polyol pathway's importance comes from aldose reductase inhibitor trials, the results of which are more variable. Ongoing studies (e.g., Action 1 and Action 2 for aminoguanidine) will examine whether any agents are useful clinically.

Hemodynamic alterations

Increased intraglomerular pressures can be associated with elevations in systemic blood pressure (85% of type 1 patients with nephropathy are hypertensive), ↑ vasoactive hormones (e.g., angiotensin-II, endothelin), or altered levels of specific growth factors (e.g., TGF-β, IGF-I, and VEGF).

Hormonal and growth factor alterations have been suggested as important in the initial hyperfiltration phase seen in type 1 patients who progress to nephropathy. A role for angiotensin-II in the accumulation of extracellular matrix has also been postulated. Whether these changes are secondary to or independent of hyperglycemia is not certain.

Genetic predisposition

There is an increase in red blood cell sodium–lithium countertransport activity in nephropathic patients and their parents in some populations, and an ↑ incidence of hypertension in the relatives of diabetic patients with nephropathy.

An association between nephropathy and polymorphisms of the ACE gene has also been noted.

Smoking

A consistent link between cigarette smoking and nephropathy has been known for some time, but an etiological mechanism is not yet known.

Natural history

In 20–40% of type 1 diabetic patients there is initially a period of glomerular hyperfiltration. The first sign of nephropathy, however, is microalbuminuria, usually occurring 5–15 years after the onset of type 1 diabetes but possibly present at the time of diagnosis in those with type 2 diabetes. Associated with this is often the development of hypertension, a reduction in high-density lipoprotein (HDL) cholesterol, and an increase in LDL cholesterol and triglycerides.

This progresses to the next stage of frank proteinuria or albuminuria, which has a peak incidence ~17 years after the diagnosis of type 1 diabetes. This is the start of overt nephropathy; in both type 1 and type 2 patients an approximate 10 mL/min^{-1} 1.73 m^{-2} reduction in glomerular filtration rate (GFR) occurs each year once the albumin excretion rate has reached 300 mg/day, although in some patients the deterioration may be more rapid, and treatment may reduce it.

Once serum creatinine concentration reaches 200 µmol/L, a fall of 1 mL/min per month in GFR is expected. This leads to end-stage renal failure (ESRF) with uremia and potentially death 7–10 years after onset of albuminuria. A plot of the reciprocal of creatinine against time is a relatively straight line showing the projected rate of deterioration.

Patients with diabetes and persistent proteinuria/albuminuria have a high mortality rate, due to cardiovascular disease in 40% of cases. Nephropathy carries a 20–100 × greater mortality than that in age-matched diabetic patients without proteinuria. See Box 106.3.

Box 106.3 Risk factors for development of microalbuminuria

- Duration of diabetes
- Poor long-term glycemic control
- Hypertension
- Dyslipidemia
- Hyperfiltration
- Parents with renal disease

Treatment

Treatment options for ESRF are either renal dialysis (hemodialysis or ambulatory peritoneal dialysis) or renal transplantation, but life expectancy with either is no better than that of some common malignancies. Several other therapies can, however, delay the progression to this stage.

Blood pressure

Controlling hypertension reduces the progression to microalbuminuria and from this to albuminuria and subsequent progression to ESRF. BP should be reduced to <130/85 mmHg, with avoidance of hypotension, although if proteinuria is >1 g/day, a better target is <120/75 mmHg. Weight loss, alcohol restriction, and reduced salt intake help, but drugs are usually needed to achieve this.

Studies show benefits from β-blockers, furosemide, hydralazine, and calcium channel blockers, but the ACE inhibitors are currently the preferred first-line agent in both microalbuminuric and albuminuric patients as they also have an effect on kidney function independent of their hypotensive action. Several studies suggest, however, that more than one agent will be required to control BP adequately.

Large studies with several ACE inhibitors have confirmed their benefit in hypertensive patients. These agents delay the progression of microalbuminuria to albuminuria and then to ESRF. There is no documented benefit in treating normotensive patients without microalbuminuria.

Captopril (50 mg 2× day) for 2 years in type 1 patients with microalbuminuria reduced progression to albuminuria by 68%.

Enalapril (10 mg daily) given to type 2 patients with microalbuminuria for 5 years reduced progression to albuminuria by 67%. When used for 4 years in type 1 patients with nephropathy, captopril (50 mg 2× day) reduced the risk of death, dialysis, and transplantation by 50% and slowed the reduction in creatinine clearance.

The EUCLID study looked at treating normotensive microalbuminuric type 1 patients. In this study, *lisinopril* reduced the albumin excretion rate by nearly 20% compared to placebo, but there was a 3 mmHg lower BP in the treatment group. From this result it was suggested that normotensive type 1 patients be treated with ACE inhibitors. An *enalapril* study in normotensive type 2 patients showed similar results.

Angiotensin II receptor antagonists can also reduce progression of microalbuminuria and ESRF from trials with losartan (RENAAL) and irbesartan (IDNT, IRMA-II).

Glycemic control

Correction of hyperglycemia can reverse glomerular basement membrane thickening and mesangial changes. Studies looking at progression to microalbuminuria and subsequent progression to frank albuminuria (e.g., the Steno 1 and II Studies, the KROC Study) also suggest a clinical benefit from improving glycemic control. In the DCCT, tight glycemic control of type 1 patients was shown to reduce progression to microalbuminuria by 30% and subsequent progression to albuminuria by 54%.

Not all trials confirm this finding (e.g., the Microalbuminuria Collaborative Study Group Trial), and not all patients with good control in the above trials gained benefit. Even so, the current treatment aim is to normalize or significantly reduce HbA1c (<7.2%) while avoiding any weight gain or hypoglycemia associated with the increased use of both oral agents and insulin needed to do so.

Dietary protein restriction

High dietary protein can damage the kidney by increasing renal blood flow and intraglomerular pressures in experimental situations. For microalbuminuric type 1 patients, in small studies, reducing dietary animal protein intake appears to reduce both hyperfiltration and micralbuminuria, and the benefit in more severe renal impairment is more evident.

In type 2 patients, the UKPDS showed an initial reduction in microalbuminuria with dietary modification, which may in part be related to protein reduction. A dietary protein content <0.8 g/kg is suggested.

Lipid lowering

Although diabetic nephropathy is not shown to reduce the progression of microalbuminuria to albuminuria or renal failure, these patients have a significant dyslipidemia and a high cardiovascular mortality. They require careful lipid monitoring and aggressive treatment. The use of aspirin for similar reasons is also advisable.

Further reading

Ahmad J, Siddiqui MA, Ahmad H (1997). Effective postponement of diabetic nephropathy in normotensive type 2 diabetic patients with microalbuminuria. *Diabet Care* 20:1576–1581.

Diabetes Control and Complications Trial Research Group (1993). The effect of intensive treatment of diabetes on the development of microvascular complications of DM. *N Engl J Med* 329:304–309.

Diabetes Control and Complications Trial Research Group (1995). Effect of intensive therapy on the development and progression of diabetic nephropathy in the DCCT. *Kidney Int* 42:1703–1720.

EUCLID Study Group (1997). Randomized placebo-controlled trial of lisinopril in normotensive patients with insulin-dependent diabetes and normoalbuminuria or microalbuminuria. *Lancet* 349:1787–1792.

Laffel LMB, McGill JB, Dans DJ, for the North American Microalbuminuria Studsy Group (1995). The beneficial effect of angiotensin converting enzyme inhibition with captopril on diabetic nephropathy in normotensive IDDM patients with microalbuminuria. *Am J Med* 99:497–504.

Lewis EJ, Hunsicker LG, Bain RP, et al. (1993). The effect of angiotensin converting enzyme inhibition on diabetic nephropathy. *N Engl J Med* 329:1456–1462.

Microalbuminuria Captopril Study Group (1996). Captopril reduces the risk of nephropathy in IDDM patients with microalbuminuria. *Diabetologia* 39:587–593.

NICE (2002). Type 2 diabetes—renal disease. Clinical guidelines. http://www.nice.org.uk

NICE (2002). Type 2 diabetes—management of blood pressure and blood lipids. Clinical guidelines. http://www.nice.org.uk

Ravid M, Brosch D, Levi Z, et al. (1998). Use of enalapril to attenuate decline in renal function in normotensive, normalbuminuric patients with type 2 DM. *Ann Intern Med* 128:982–988.

UK Prospective Diabetes Study Group (1998). Intensive blood glucose control with sulphonylureas or insulin compared with conventional treatment and risk of complications in patients with type 2 diabetes (UKPDS 33). *Lancet* 352:837–853.

UK Prospective Diabetes Study Group (1998). Tight blood pressure control and risk of macrovascular and microvascular complications in type 2 diabetes: UKPDS 38. *BMJ* 317:703–713.

UK Prospective Diabetes Study Group (1998). Efficacy of atenolol and captopril in reducing risk of macrovascular and microvascular complications in type 2 diabetes: UKPDS 39. *BMJ* 317:713–720.

Diabetic neuropathy

Definition

Involvement of cranial, peripheral, and autonomic nerves may be found in patients with diabetes and is termed *diabetic neuropathy*. This usually suggests a diffuse, predominantly sensory peripheral neuropathy. The effects on nerve function can be acute or chronic as well as transient or permanent. The consequences of neuropathy include the following:

- Neuropathic ulcers, usually on the feet
- Charcot arthropathy
- Altered sensation (both pain and ↑ sensitivity to normal sensation)
- Impotence (with autonomic neuropathy)

📖 See box 107.1 for classification.

Box 107.1 Classification of diabetic neuropathies

- Sensory neuropathy
  - Acute
  - Chronic
- Autonomic neuropathy
- Mononeuropathy
  - Entrapment neuropathy
  - External pressure palsies
  - Spontaneous mononeuropathy
- Proximal motor neuropathy (diabetic amyotrophy)

Pathology

Diabetic neuropathy is one of the microvascular complications of diabetes. Pathologically, distal axonal loss occurs with focal demyelination and attempts at nerve regeneration.

The vasa nervorum often shows basement membrane thickening, endothelial cell changes, and some occlusion of its lumen. This results in slowing of nerve conduction velocities or a complete loss of nerve function. Both metabolic and vascular changes have been implicated in its etiology.

Pathogenesis

Hyperglycemia is probably the underlying cause of the histological and functional changes. Several possible mechanisms have been suggested:

- Overloading of the normal pathways for glucose metabolism resulting in ↑ use of the polyol pathway, which leads to ↑ levels of sorbitol and fructose and ↓ levels of myoinositol and glutathione. This may result in more free radical damage and lowers nitric oxide levels, thus altering nerve blood flow. Experimental models using aldose reductase inhibitors, which can improve some aspects of diabetic neuropathy, add some weight to this theory.
- Possible accumulation of AGE (via nonenzymatic glycation) may also have a role to play, as could the hypercoagulable state and altered blood rheology known to occur in all patients with diabetes. When used in animal studies, aminoguanidine, which blocks AGE formation, can increase nerve conduction velocities and nerve blood flow in diabetic subjects, strengthening the role of AGE accumulation in this process.
- In the more acute neuropathies, acute ischemia of the nerves due to vascular abnormalities has been suggested as the cause, but again the underlying reason for this is still unclear. Insulin-induced neuritis may occur when insulin therapy is started and blood glucose levels fall.

Other potential etiological factors include changes in local growth factor production and oxidative stress.

Further work is needed to clarify the exact role of each of the above mechanisms. In the meantime, studies showing improvements in neuropathy associated with good diabetic control strengthen the argument for the role of hyperglycemia and offer us a treatment option while we await other therapies.

Peripheral sensorimotor neuropathy

Although hyperglycemia can alter nerve function and often gives some sensory symptoms at diagnosis, correcting the hyperglycemia can often resolve these. Chronic sensorimotor neuropathy, however, is the most common feature of peripheral nerve involvement seen in patients with diabetes (see Box 107.2).

The exact prevalence of diabetic neuropathy varies in most studies because of the different definitions and examination techniques used. For example, sensitive nerve conduction studies can show up to 80% of patients having abnormal results.

In more normal practice, however, 20–30% of unselected patients can be expected to have either symptomatic neuropathy or abnormalities on examination that are clinically significant. At least 50% of these patients are asymptomatic. This figure will increase with longer duration of diabetes, so although 7–8% of type 2 patients may have abnormalities at diagnosis, 50% can be expected to have them 25 years later.

Mononeuropathies

Peripheral mononeuropathies and cranial mononeuropathies are not uncommon. These may be spontaneous or due to entrapment or external pressure. Of the peripheral mononeuropathies, median nerve involvement

---

Box 107.2 Features of peripheral sensorimotor neuropathy

- Usually insidious onset with numbness or paresthesia, often found on screening rather than as a presenting problem
- Starts in the toes and on the soles of the feet, then spreads up to mid-shin level, mostly in a symmetrical fashion. Less often, it also involves the fingers and hands.
- Affects all sensory modalities and results in reduced vibration perception thresholds, pinprick, fine touch, and temperature sensations.
- ↓ Vibration sensation and absent ankle reflexes are often the first features found. Another risk factor for ulceration is the inability to feel a 10 g monofilament.
- Less often, the skin is tender or sensitive to touch (hyperesthesia), or frank pain can occur.
- Painful neuropathy affects up to 5% of a general clinic population. This pain may be sharp, stabbing, or burning in nature and at times very severe.
- There may also be some wasting of the intrinsic muscles of the foot with clawing of the toes.

and carpal tunnel syndrome may be found in up to 10% of patients and require nerve conduction studies and then surgical decompression.

Entrapment of the lateral cutaneous nerve of the thigh is also seen more commonly in those with diabetes, producing pain over the lateral aspect of the thigh. Common peroneal nerve involvement causing foot drop and tarsal tunnel syndrome are also recognized but less common.

Cranial mononeuropathies usually occur suddenly and have a good prognosis. Palsies of cranial nerves III and VI are the most common ones seen, although these are not a common problem in patients with diabetes. In the third nerve palsy, sparing of the pupillary responses is usual.

Spontaneous recovery is slow over several months and no treatment apart from symptomatic help such as an eye patch is needed. Unlike entrapment neuropathies, where decompression may help, no effective treatment is currently available in most of these cases with spontaneous mononeuropathies.

Proximal motor neuropathy (diabetic amyotrophy)

This is an uncommon but disturbing condition that mostly affects men in their 50s with type 2 diabetes. It presents with severe pain and paresthesia in the upper legs and is felt as a deep, aching pain that may be burning in nature and can keep patients awake at night, prevent them from eating, and result in marked cachexia.

This neuropathy, with proximal muscle weakness and wasting of the quadriceps in particular, can be very debilitating. The lumbar sacral plexus lower motor neurons are affected, and improvement is usually spontaneous over 3–4 months. Before making this diagnosis, however, consider other causes, such as malignancies and lumbar disc disease.

Oral antidiabetic agents may play a part in the etiology of this problem. Conversion to insulin therapy is advised, although the anorexia experienced when the pain is severe can make this difficult. Although recovery happens over a few months, only 50% recover fully. No other treatment is currently known to improve on this rate.

Examination

- Mandatory at diagnosis and at least yearly in all asymptomatic patients
- Test vibration, fine touch (with a 10 g monofilament), and reflexes as a minimum. Use of a neurothesiometer or biosthesiometer gives a more quantitative measure of vibration than a 128 Hz tuning fork. Inability to feel the vibrating head at >25 V in the toes is associated with a significant risk of neuropathic ulceration and should be considered a sign of at-risk feet.

Differential diagnoses

- Uremia
- Vitamin B_{12} deficiency
- Infections (e.g., HIV and leprosy)
- Toxins (e.g., alcohol, lead, mercury)
- Malignancy

Treatment

For all patients

All patients should be reviewed by a podiatrist and, if indicated, an orthotist to give them education on foot care and suitable footwear. If followed by regular chiropody review, this can help prevent some problems from developing.

Asymptomatic patients

No drugs are currently available. In the past, aldose reductase inhibitors, such as *tolrestat,* were advocated by some for this indication, but a recent Cochrane review suggests no benefit over placebo.

Painful neuropathy

Initially, try capsaicin 0.075% topically to the affected area, being careful to avoid normal skin because this chili pepper extract, which depletes sensory nerve terminals of substance P, can be uncomfortable when applied to normal skin. It can take several weeks to be effective and may induce tingling and thus worsening of symptoms initially.

In some patients, simple analgesics have been shown to help. In more severe cases, tricyclic antidepressants (TCAs) are the first-line treatment of choice, with *imipramine* 20–100 mg at night being less sedative than *amitriptyline* 25–75 mg.

Although agents such as *carbamazepine*, *phenytoin*, and *paroxetine* have less anticholinergic effects, they are also not as effective and are therefore used as second-line treatment.

Gabapentin and *pregabalin* are well tolerated and more effective and thus are usually used before other anticonvulsants and antidepressants.

If the pain is severe and like an electric shock, anticonvulsants such as *carbamazepine* and *phenytoin* may be effective.

A more recent addition to the therapy for painful neuropathy is *duloxetine*, a combined serotonin and noradrenaline reuptake inhibitor. Comparative trials against other agents are currently not available, but it is effective compared to placebo in over half of people who have tried it.

For *hyperesthesia,* occlusive dressings such as Opsite® may prove helpful. For more severe pain, oral agents are needed.

More recent studies with agents such as the protein kinase C inhibitors show more encouraging results, and treatment with these agents may soon be available.

General treatments

While specific treatments are available for each form of neuropathy, there is some evidence for more general therapies.

Poor diabetic control appears to be associated with worsening neuropathy. Improving glycemic control is advocated in any patient, especially if neuropathy is present.

Results from the use of evening primrose oil in rats and in preliminary human studies suggest that this may improve some aspects of diabetic neuropathy. The mechanism by which this works is not certain, but it does increase production of cyclooxygenase-mediated prostanoids such as prostacyclin, which could act as a vasodilator and thus improve nerve blood supply.

Other more specific vasodilators have also been examined, with blockers and ACE inhibitors showing particularly useful results in experimental settings.

An alternative approach is not to try to improve the underlying problem but to alter the body's response to it. Nerve growth factor (NGF) and IGF-I have been examined for their ability to cause nerve regeneration and growth; NGF in particular may be promising in this role.

Other such agents are also under investigation, such as the protein kinase C β inhibitors. Study results of these are encouraging.

Autonomic neuropathy

The most common effect of autonomic neuropathy is erectile dysfunction, which affects 40% of males with diabetes. Only a small number develop severe GI and bladder dysfunction.

The recent interest in *sildenafil* has highlighted this effect. Abnormal autonomic function tests can be expected in 20–40% of a general diabetic clinic population.

The increased problems during surgery from cardiac involvement should also be remembered.

Clinical features
- Impotence
- Postural hypotension, giving dizziness and syncope in up to 12%
- Resting tachycardia or fixed heart rate/loss of sinus arrhythmia in up to 20%
- Gustatory sweating—sweating after tasting food
- Dysphagia with delayed gastric emptying, nausea/vomiting
- Constipation or diarrhea
- Urinary retention or overflow incontinence
- Anhidrosis—absent sweating on the feet is especially problematic as it increases the risk of ulceration
- Abnormal pupillary reflexes

Assessment
At least annually check the following:
- Lying and standing BP (measure systolic BP 2 minutes after standing; normal is <10 mmHg drop, >30 mmHg is abnormal)
- Pupillary responses to light

Other less commonly performed tests to consider if the diagnosis is uncertain or in high-risk patients include the following:
- *Loss of sinus arrhythmia:* Measure inspiratory and expiratory heart rates after 5 seconds of each (<10 beats/min difference is abnormal, >15 is normal).

- *Loss of heart rate response to Valsalva maneuver:* Look at the ratio of the shortest R–R interval during forced expiration against a closed glottis compared to the longest R–R interval after it (<1.2 is abnormal).
- *BP response to sustained hand-grip:* Diastolic BP prior to the test is compared to diastolic BP after 5 minutes of sustaining a grip equivalent to 30% of maximal grip. A diastolic BP rise >16 mmHg is normal, <10 mmHg is abnormal. A rolled-up BP cuff to achieve the required hand-grip may be used.
- For *gastric symptoms* consider a radioisotope test meal to look for delayed gastric emptying.

Treatment

This is based on the specific symptom and is usually symptomatic only. In all patients, improvement in diabetic control is advocated in case any of it is reversible, although this is not usually very helpful or effective.

Postural hypotension

- May be exacerbated by drugs such as diuretics, vasodilators, and TCAs
- Mechanical measures such as sleeping with the head elevated and wearing support stockings may help.
- Ensure an adequate salt intake.
- *Fludrocortisone* 100 mcg once daily initially and ↑ as required up to 400 mcg may be helpful, but watch for hypertension or edema.
- *Desmopressin* and *octreotide* have also been used.

Impotence (📖 see Erectile dysfunction, p. 306)

Libido is not normally affected and pain is also unusual, so look for hypogonadism and Peyronie's disease if these conditions are present. Autonomic neuropathy is the likely cause, but many drugs, especially thiazides and β-blockers, can also cause it, as can alcohol, tobacco, cannabis, and stress. These agents should be assessed by direct questioning.

Examination should include the following:
- Genitalia and secondary sexual characteristics
- Peripheral pulses, as vascular insufficiency may play a part
- Lower limb reflexes and vibration thresholds to confirm that neuropathy is present

Biochemical screening should at least include the following:
- Prolactin
- Testosterone
- Gonadotrophins (LH/FSH)

Exacerbating factors such as alcohol and antihypertensive drugs should be modified. The main therapies are as follows:
- Oral therapies include *sildenafil* (start at 25–50 mg, increase to 100 mg if needed and taken 1 hour prior to sexual intercourse), *vardenafil* (start at 10 mg, ↑ to 20 mg if needed and taken 25–60 minutes prior to sexual intercourse), and *tadalafil* (start at 10 mg ↑ to 20 mg if needed and taken 30 minutes to 12 hours prior to sexual intercourse).

- Intraurethral *alprostadil* (start at 125 mcg, increase to 250 or 500 mcg if needed)
- Intracavernosal *alprostadil* (trial dose is 2.5 mcg, treatment is 5–40 mcg)
- Vacuum devices

None of these therapies is ideal. Sildenafil, although an oral therapy, is effective in only 60% of those with diabetes and is contraindicated in those with severe heart disease and those on nitrates, which rules out many individuals.

Gastroparesis

Delayed gastric emptying can cause recurrent hypoglycemic episodes. Promotilic agents can also help. Treatment options are as follows:
- *Metoclopramide* (5–10 mg pre-meals/3 × day)
- *Domperidone* (10–20 mg pre-meals)
- *Erythromycin* acts as a motilin agonist to increase gastric emptying but may make patients feel nauseated so it is of limited use.
- *Surgery*—gastric drainage procedures should not be undertaken lightly.

Large bowel involvement

Constipation is treated with standard bulking and softening laxatives. The episodic diarrhea is more troublesome. Treatment for this may include
- *Loperamide* (2 mg 4 × day) or codeine phosphate (30 mg 4 × day)
- Antibiotics in case of bacterial overgrowth, such as *erythromycin* 250 mg 4 × day for 7 days, or tetracycline 250 mg 2 × day for 7 days

Neuropathic bladder

Sacral nerve involvement can cause bladder abnormalities with reduced sensations of bladder fullness and ↑ residual volume after micturition. Regular toileting initially may help, but intermittent self-catheterization or a long-term catheter may be required.

Anhidrosis

Dry feet can cause cracks in the skin and act as a site for infection. Use of emollient creams may help prevent this.

Further reading

Boulton AJM, Gries FA, Jervell LA (1998). Guidelines for the diagnosis and outpatient management of diabetic peripheral neuropathy. *Diabet Med* 15(6):508–514.

NICE (2004). Type 1 diabetes. Diagnosis and management of type 1 diabetes in adults Clinical guideline. http:// www.nice.org.uk

NICE (2004). Type 2 diabetes. Prevention and management of foot problems Clinical guideline. http://www.nice.org.uk

Macrovascular disease

People with diabetes have a significantly greater risk of coronary heart disease, cerebrovascular disease, and peripheral vascular disease than that of the nondiabetic population.

Most people with diabetes will die from one of these conditions (75% of patients with type 2). It has been suggested that a diagnosis of type 2 diabetes equates to a cardiovascular risk equivalent to aging 15 years.

Epidemiology

The exact prevalence and incidence of macrovascular disease and its outcomes vary depending on the age, sex, and ethnic mix of patients being assessed. In general, cardiovascular disease accounts for 75% of deaths in type 2 patients and 35% in type 1 patients.

Although the atheroma seen is histologically the same as that in a nondiabetic population, it tends to be more diffuse and progresses more rapidly. It also occurs at an earlier age and affects both sexes equally. Women, therefore, seem to lose their natural premenopausal advantage.

Overall, peripheral vascular disease occurs in up to 10% of patients and they have up to 15-fold greater risk of needing a nontraumatic amputation than that of the nondiabetic population.

Thromboembolic cerebrovascular events occur in up to 8%, which is a 2- to 4-fold ↑ risk compared to that of the nondiabetic population, and accounts for 15% of deaths in type 2 patients.

The risk of having a myocardial infarction is also ↑ 2–4 times. Women seem particularly at risk of cardiovascular disease compared to the nondiabetic population.

Patients with type 1 diabetes have half the rate of coronary heart disease, 1/3 the rate of cerebrovascular disease, and 2/3 the rate of peripheral vascular disease compared to rates for type 2 patients, but their incidence rate for all of these conditions is greater than that of the nondiabetic population.

Males and females are equally affected, with the incidence rates for ischemic heart disease being about 6 times that of both cerebrovascular and peripheral vascular disease.

Secondary prevention
- Stop smoking
- Aspirin
- β-blockers
- Lipid-lowering drugs

Pathogenesis

Atherosclerosis has a well-known set of risk factors, such as smoking and family history, all of which still apply in a diabetic population. Some factors, however, are more common in those with diabetes and may also confer a greater risk to the diabetic population. These include the following:

- *Glycemic control.* In patients with type 1 diabetes, worsening levels of hyperglycemia, as suggested by higher average HbA1c levels, are said to relate to the degree of disease present. In those with type 2 diabetes, this association is less clear-cut, although the UKPDS does suggest that this is the case, as better glycemic control was associated with a trend for fewer myocardial infarctions.

- *Hypertension* is more common in both type 1 and type 2 patients and results in vascular endothelial injury, thus predisposing to atheroma formation. The UKPDS suggests that BP control may be a more important individual risk factor than glycemic control.

- *Hyperlipidemia* is common—e.g., hyperinsulinemia in insulin-resistant type 2 patients causes reduced HDL cholesterol, elevated triglycerides (and VLDL), and smaller, denser, and, therefore, more atherogenic LDL cholesterol.

- *Obesity* is an independent risk factor, being more common in type 2 patients. Central obesity in particular is more atherogenic.

- *Insulin resistance* or elevated circulating insulin/proinsulin-like molecule levels are known to increase the risk of atherosclerosis in both diabetic and nondiabetic populations. This may be linked to impaired endothelial function.

- *Altered coagulability.* Circulating fibrinogen, platelet activator inhibitor (PAI)-1, and von Willebrand factor levels are ↑ and platelets are less deformable. This alteration may be more prothrombotic, but the exact significance remains uncertain.

The UKPDS has shown the major risk factors for coronary heart disease in type 2 patients to be elevated LDL cholesterol, ↓ HDL cholesterol, hypertension, hyperglycemia, and smoking. Exactly why these risk factors are commonly seen or linked in the same patient, particularly type 2 diabetic patients, is uncertain.

Several hypotheses have been put forward, but none as yet explains them all adequately. However, each suggests an element of genetic susceptibility mixed with environmental effects. A genetic predisposition to insulin resistance, for example, may combine with poor intrauterine nutrition to produce a low–birth weight infant with a susceptibility to vascular disease and diabetes later in life.

But other factors must be involved, as not all those who later develop diabetes and vascular disease were small at birth.

Lipid abnormalities found in patients with diabetes

Hyperlipidemia in a patient with diabetes, at any level of cholesterol, is associated with a greater risk of macrovascular disease than that for a nondiabetic population. Patients with diabetes may have altered activity of insulin-dependent enzymes such as lipoprotein lipase that results in delayed systemic clearance of certain lipids. This, combined with altered hepatic production of apoprotein-B-containing lipoproteins, gives a more atherogenic profile.

Usual findings are ↑ triglyceride-containing lipoproteins, chylomicrons, and VLDL. Although more common in insulin-resistant type 2 patients, this can also be seen in type 1 patients, as can a low HDL cholesterol level (HDL$_2$ especially).

Other atherogenic changes include a tendency to develop small, dense LDL cholesterol particles and a greater tendency toward oxidative damage, which renders patients even more atherogenic. Lipoprotein (Lpa) levels are also often raised.

Even so, other common primary causes of hyperlipidemia, such as familial hypercholesterolemia or familial combined hyperlipidemia, should not be missed. Screening for secondary causes of hyperlipidemia such as hypothyroidism or drug-induced causes (alcohol, thiazides, and β-blockers in particular) is also strongly advised.

Management

In all patients, the first treatment is dietary modification. In a patient who is actually following a good diabetic diet, however, there is often not much room for improvement.

Other standard advice should also be given:
- Stop smoking—this reduces risk of death by about 50% over a 15-year period.
- Reduce weight if overweight or obese.
- Increase physical activity.

While the reductions in mortality, reinfarction, and stroke in the major lipid-lowering trials such as the 4S study (Scandinavian Simvastatin Survival Study), CARE (Cholesterol and Recurrent Events Trial), LIPID (Long-term Intervention with Pravastatin in Ischemic Disease), and WOSCOPS (West of Scotland Coronary Prevention Study) are all very impressive, the diabetic subgroups show as good if not better reductions, although the numbers in each were relatively small (☐ see Table 108.1).

In the 4S study, for example, the simvastatin-treated diabetic subgroup (4.5% of those in the study) had a 23% rate of major coronary events compared to 45% in the diabetic placebo group; the nondiabetic simvastatin group had a rate of 19% and the placebo nondiabetic group, 27%.

On the basis of these results, it is suggested that if 100 patients with diabetes who have angina or are post–myocardial infarction are treated with simvastatin for 6 years, 24 of the 46 expected coronary deaths and nonfatal myocardial infarctions can be prevented.

More recent lipid-lowering trials including larger numbers of people with diabetes such as CARDS (Collaborative Atorvastatin Diabetes Study)

Table 108.1 Lipid reduction studies

Type of study	4S	WOSCOPS	CARE	LIPID
	2 prevention of CHD	1 prevention of CHD	2 prevention of CHD	2 prevention of CHD
Duration of study (years)	6	5	5	6
Number studied	4444	6595	4159	9014
Mean total cholesterol (mmol/L) (range)	6.8 (5.5–8.0)	7.0(>6.5)	5.4 (<6.2)	(4.0–7.0)
Age range (years)	35–70	45–64	21–75	31–75
% Men	81	100	86	83
% With diabetes	4.5	1	17	8.6
Treatment	Simvastatin 20–40 mg daily	Pravastatin 40 mg daily	Pravastatin 40 mg daily	Pravastatin 40 mg daily
Event reduction for	34% for nondiabetics 55% for diabetics	31% overall	23% for nondiabetics 25% for diabetics	23% overall

1, primary; 2, secondary; 4S, Scandinavian Simvastatin Survival Study; CARE, Cholesterol and Recurrent Event; LIPID, Long-term Intervention with Pravastatin in Ischemic Disease; WOSCOPS, West of Scotland Coronary Prevention Study;

and ASPEN (Atorvastatin Study for the Prevention of Endpoints in Non-insulin dependent diabetes) again show significant benefit, but the Anglo-Scandinavian Cardiac Outcomes Trial lipid-lowering arm (ASCOT-LLA) was not quite so encouraging.

Once lifestyle measures have been implemented, drug therapy should be considered. In the past, the Sheffield tables, New Zealand tables, Joint British Societies Coronary Risk Prediction Chart, and the Framingham Risk Score calculations (🕮 see Tables 113.1, pp. 664–665, and 113.2, pp. 666–667) were used to determine risk in primary prevention, but now any person with diabetes is thought of as being at such a high risk that secondary prevention targets of a total cholesterol <150 mg/dL, an LDL <80 mg/dL, and an HDL >38 mg/dL are now advocated.

A fit patient with diabetes has a similar risk to that of a nondiabetic of the same age and sex who has also had a coronary event. Other targets are advocated by many, especially for those patients post–coronary artery bypass grafting or post-angioplasty. Triglycerides should be brought to <140 mg/dL, as above this level atherogenic lipoprotein changes are said to occur.

In those with mixed hyperlipidemia, a fibrate or statin licensed for this indication should be considered. A fibrate will reduce triglycerides by 30–40% and LDL cholesterol by 20%, while a statin would reduce triglycerides slightly less (10–15%) and LDL cholesterol slightly more (25–35%). Fibrates also alter LDL cholesterol to its less atherogenic form. The choice of agent must be tailored to the individual patient.

For hypercholesterolemia alone, a statin is first choice, as in the nondiabetic patient, and in severely resistant patients combination therapy with statins, ezetimibe, fibrates, and, less often, resins may be required. Combination statin and ezetimibe may reduce LDL more effectively than increasing the statin dose alone.

Treatment aims for lipids

- Total cholesterol <4.0 mmol/l
- LDL cholesterol <2.0 mmol/L
- Aim to have triglycerides <1.5 mmol/L

Box 108.1 Investigations of lipid abnormalities

Take a full history and carefully examine the patient. In all patients, then check the following:

- Dip test urine for protein
- Serum urea, electrolytes, and creatinine (and creatinine clearance if creatinine is raised)
- Fasting lipids
- ECG (for left ventricular hypertrophy and signs of ischemia)

Also consider the following:

- The need for a chest X-ray for signs of heart failure or cardiomegaly
- An echocardiogram
- Cortisol + dexamethasone suppression test
- Catecholamines
- Renin/aldosterone

Hypertension

Epidemiology

Hypertension is twice as common in the diabetic population as in the nondiabetic population, and standard ethnic differences in the prevalence of hypertension still hold true. Hypertension worsens the severity and increases the risk of developing both microvascular and macrovascular disease. With a cutoff of >160/90 mmHg, hypertension occurs in

- 10–30% of patients with type 1 diabetes
- 20–30% of microalbuminuric type 1 patients
- 80–90% of macroalbuminuric type 1 patients
- 30–50% of Caucasians with type 2 diabetes

With suggested targets of 130/80, hypertension is even more common.

Pathogenesis

Type 1 diabetes

Hypertension is strongly associated with diabetic nephropathy and microalbuminuria and occurs at an earlier stage than that seen in many other causes of renal disease.

This may in part be linked to a genetic predisposition toward ↑ activity in red blood cell sodium–lithium countertransport activity, which leads to ↑ peripheral vascular resistance. Insulin may also have a suppressive effect on renin release, producing hyporeninemic hypoaldosteronism.

Type 2 diabetes

Hypertension is associated with insulin resistance and hyperinsulinemia; again, this may be genetically mediated. Hyperinsulinemia can directly cause hypertension through ↑ sympathetic nervous system activity, ↑ proximal tubule sodium resorption, and stimulating vascular smooth muscle cell proliferation.

Hyperglycemia also has an antinatriuretic effect, which, along with hyper-insulinemia leading to hypokalemia, results in both glucose and sodium reabsorption being increased. All of these factors increase the potential for hypertension.

Management

Treatment aim

The current recommendation is for all patients with diabetes to have a blood pressure <140/80 mmHg. The hypertension study in the UKPDS highlights the benefits for type 2 patients of this treatment level on mortality, diabetes-related end points, and microvascular end points. In this study, a 10/5 mmHg difference in BP was associated with a 34% risk reduction in macrovascular end points, a 37% risk reduction in microvascular end points, and a 44% risk reduction in stroke.

The Hypertension Optimum Treatment (HOT) study again suggests a target of <140/80 mmHg, although in those who already have significant end-organ damage a lower target (<130/80) is advocated by some.

The Anglo-Scandinavian Cardiac Outcomes Trial–Blood Pressure Lowering Arm (ALLHAT–BPLA) reinforced the beneficial role of calcium channel blockers and ACE inhibitors in combination.

Predisposing conditions

Other conditions that can cause both hypertension and hyperglycemia should be considered, e.g., Cushing's syndrome, acromegaly, and pheochromocytoma.

End-organ damage

Look for evidence of end-organ damage (eyes, heart, kidneys, and peripheral vascular tree in particular).

Assessment of cardiac risk factors

Look for associated risk factors for coronary heart disease.

Treatment

General

Once this initial assessment is complete, modify other risk factors such as glycemic control, smoking, and dyslipidemia. Then look at the following:
- Weight reduction if obese
- Reduced salt intake (<6 g/day)
- Reduced alcohol intake (<21 units/week in males, <14 in females)
- Exercise (20–40 minutes of moderate exertion 3–5×/week)

Pharmacological

After modifying risk factors, drug therapy should be started for the hypertension. Most agents currently available will drop systolic BP by no more than 20 mmHg. In the UKPDS BP study, 1/3 of those achieving the tight BP targets now aimed for required three or more drugs to do so.

Recently, the National Institute for Health and Clinical Excellence (NICE) guidelines for BP treatment were updated and now advocate an "A/CD" approach: starting with an ACE inhibitor (or an angiotensin II receptor blocker/antagonist if the ACE inhibitor is not tolerated) and then adding in either a calcium channel blocker or a thiazide-type diuretic with an α-blocker, a β-blocker, or further diuretic therapy if this fails to reduce BP adequately.

In the presence of microalbuminuria or frank proteinuria, an ACE inhibitor should always be considered first line, or an angiotensin II receptor antagonist if ACE inhibitors are not tolerated.

In Afro-Caribbean diabetics, a diuretic may also be needed to improve the efficacy of ACE inhibitors, as these and β-blockers are less effective than calcium channel blockers and diuretics in these patients.

Several agents, such as high-dose thiazides and β-blockers, can worsen diabetic control, mask hypoglycemia, and exacerbate dyslipidemia. Thus the drugs chosen need to be tailored to each patient.

A recent review of data from the Nurses Health Study (NHS I and II) and the Health Professionals Follow-up Study (HPFS) suggested that while these agents may increase the risk of developing diabetes, they may not be

Box 108.2 Management of acute myocardial infarction

Patients with diabetes are more likely to have a myocardial infarction (MI) and more likely to die from it than the nondiabetic population. This may be due to a greater likelihood of myocardial pump failure. Several studies highlight this:

Trial and outcome examined	Nondiabetic subgroup	Diabetic subgroup
ISSI-2		
Non-streptokinase	27%	41%
4-year mortality		
GUSTO		
In-hospital mortality	6.2%	10.6%
GISSI-2		
Reinfarction rates	14%	30%

In those with angina, a β-blocker has added benefits.

In those with peripheral vascular disease, vasodilators such as the calcium channel blockers may be beneficial.

Up to 20–40% of patients admitted to the hospital with an MI will have hyperglycemia, many of whom not previously diagnosed with diabetes.

As in the nondiabetic population, streptokinase, aspirin, and acute angioplasty have proven benefits. The previous contraindication for thrombolysis in those with proliferative diabetic retinopathy has been questioned by many investigators.

Tight glycemic control (blood glucose 120–180 mg/dL) using IV glucose and insulin for at least 24 hours followed by SC insulin, as used in the DIGAMI study, also has benefits. In this study, patients with an admission blood glucose >200 mg/dL who were treated with this regimen had a 7.5% absolute risk reduction in mortality at 1 year and an 11% risk reduction at 3.5 years compared to the control group (i.e., 33% mortality with treatment vs. 44% in controls at 3.5 years). This equates to 1 life saved for every 9 treated with this regimen. The exact reason for this outcome is unclear.

It is suggested that all patients with a blood glucose >200 mg/dL benefit from such treatment whether previously known to have diabetes or not. Using an admission HbA1c to detect those with undiagnosed or stress-related hyperglycemia can be useful, but should not result in withholding acute treatment of this hyperglycemia in such patients. It may, however, help to identify those who may be troubled by hypoglycemia and may not therefore be suitable for SC insulin or sulfonylureas in the intermediate or long term.

Box 108.2 (Contd.)

Use of ACE inhibitors early after an MI gives a 0.5% absolute risk reduction in 30-day mortality and a 4–8% risk reduction over 15–50 months in the general population.

Analysis of the diabetic subgroup in the GISSI-3 study showed a 30% relative risk reduction in 6-week mortality for the diabetics (8.7% vs. 12.4%) compared to a 5% reduction for nondiabetics. In view of the greater proportion of diabetics with poor left ventricular function after MI than that of the nondiabetic population, this difference is very important.

associated with an ↑ risk of cardiovascular or total mortality, which may be related to BP control, although this is not certain.

Further reading

Hanssen L, Zanchetti A, Carruthers SG, et al. (1998). Effects of intensive blood pressure lowering and low dose aspirin in patients with hypertension: principal results of the Hypertension Optimun Treatment (HOT) randomised trial. *Lancet* 351:1755–1762.

Malmberg K, for the DIGAMI (DM, Insulin Glucose Infusion in Acute Myocardial Infarction) study group (1997). Prospective randomized study of intensive insulin treatment on long-term survival after acute myocardial infarction in patients with DM. *BMJ* 314:1512–1515.

NICE (2006). Hypertension: management of hypertension in adults in primary care. NICE clinical guidelines 34 (partial update of NICE clinical guideline 18). http://www.nice.org.uk

NICE (2008). Type 2 diabetes: the management of type 2 diabetes. Management of blood pressure and lipids. Clinical guideline CG 66. http://www.nice.org.uk

Pyorala K, Pedersen TR, Kjekshus J, et al. (1997). Cholesterol lowering with simvastatin improves prognosis of diabetic patients with coronary heart disease. *Diabetes Care* 20:614–620.

Taylor EN Hu FB, Curhan GC (2006). Antihypertensive medications and the risk of incident type 2 diabetes. *Diabetes Care* 29:1065–1070.

UKPDS Group (1998). Tight blood pressure control and risk of macrovascular and microvascular complications in type 2 diabetes: UKPDS 38. *BMJ* 317:703–713.

UKPDS Group (1998). Efficacy of atenolol and captopril in reducing the risk of acrovascular and microvascular complications in type 2 diabetes; UKPDS 39. *BMJ* 317:713–720.

Zuanetti G, Latini R, Maggioni AP, et al. (1997). Effect of the ACE inhibitor lisinopril in diabetic patients with acute myocardial infarction. Data from GISSI-3 Study. *Circulation* 96:4239–4245.

Diabetic foot

📖 See Boxes 109.1 and 109.2.

Box 109.1 Clinical features of diabetic feet

Neuropathic feet

- Warm
- Dry skin
- Palpable foot pulses
- No discomfort with ulcer
- Callus present

Ischemic feet

- Cold/cool.
- Atrophic/often hairless.
- No palpable foot pulses
- More often tender/painful.
- Claudication/rest pain
- Skin blanches on elevation and reddens on dependency.

Box 109.2 Wagner's classification of diabetic foot lesions[1]

- Grade 0—high-risk foot, no ulcer present
- Grade 1—superficial ulcer, not infected
- Grade 2—deep ulcer with or without cellulitis but no abscess or bone involvement
- Grade 3—deep ulcer with bone involvement or abscess formation
- Grade 4—localized gangrene (toe, forefoot, heel)
- Grade 5—gangrene of the whole foot

1. Reprinted with permission from Wagner FW, O'Neal LW. Algorithms of diabetic foot care. In Levin ME, O'Neil LW (1983). *The Diabetic Foot*, 2nd ed., pp. 291–302. Copyright 1983, Elsevier.

Risk factors for foot ulcer development

Several features and factors are thought to predispose to ulcer formation. Awareness of these may help in identifying at-risk patients for education and other preventive strategies.

These ulcers can occur anywhere on the foot, but the tips of claw toes and hammertoes and over the metatarsal heads are the most frequent sites. The risk factors and features include the following:

- *Peripheral neuropathy* (seen in up to 80% of diabetic patients with foot ulcers) reduces awareness of pain and trauma caused by footwear and foreign bodies in shoes. Look for reduced monofilament sensation (e.g., reduced to a 10 g monofilament) and reduced vibration perception thresholds (e.g., reduced sensation to a 128 Hz tuning fork for <10 seconds or >25 V with a biosthesiometer), which suggest at-risk feet.

- *Autonomic neuropathy* leading to anhidrosis can dry out the skin and cause it to crack, thus allowing a portal of entry for infection. These feet are often warm and dry with distended veins.

- *Motor neuropathy* can result in altered foot muscle tone, wasting of small muscles, raising of the medial longitudinal arch, and clawing of the toes. This can produce more pressure on the metatarsal heads and heels, thus predisposing them to callus and ulcer formation. Electrophysiology can help in examining this condition but is too invasive for widespread routine use.

- *Peripheral vascular disease* (seen in up to 10% of patients) and *microvascular circulatory disease* lead to local ischemia, increasing the potential for ulcer formation, and can delay wound healing when ulceration occurs. Always examine peripheral pulses and consider getting Doppler studies if they are abnormal. An ankle/brachial artery ratio of >1.1 suggests arterial disease (a ratio of the BP in the ankle and the arm measured while at rest).

- *Duration of diabetes* relates to the presence of the above factors but is often quoted as an independent risk factor, as is ↑ age. But type 2 diabetes may be present and have gone undiagnosed for some time.

- The presence of *other microvascular complications,* such as nephropathy and retinopathy, is also a risk factor for foot ulcer development.

- *Previous ulceration* is another important risk factor. Anyone with previous problems deserves very careful monitoring and follow-up.

- *Lack of diabetes monitoring* and lack of previous examinations of the feet are also recognized risk factors.

- *Mechanical, chemical, or thermal trauma or injury* is often the predisposing factor. Any profession or pastime that increases the risk of any of these is a risk factor.

Treatment

This is a multidisciplinary problem requiring collaboration among diabetologists, podiatrists, orthtopedic, and vascular and plastic surgeons. Treatment is aimed at several distinct areas:

- At-risk feet with no current ulceration
- Treating existing ulcers
- Treating infected ulcers
- Treating osteomyelitis
- Treating vascular insufficiency

At-risk feet with no current ulceration

When at-risk feet are identified in any patient with diabetes, standard advice should be given. This will need to be repeated and reinforced regularly. Such advice would usually include the following:

- General advice on nail care, hygiene, and care with footwear
- Reinforce the need for regular daily examination of the feet by the patient or caregiver.
- Consider regular podiatry review and self-monitoring. Also reinforce the need for more urgent review if the patient discovers problems.
- Consider the need for modification of footwear or special footwear if there are abnormalities with foot posture or problems with pressure loading on certain parts of the foot. Padded socks can also reduce trauma. Advise patients to examine shoes before putting them on, wear lace-ups or shoes with lots of room for toes, and avoid ill-fitting shoes. For some people, protective toecaps can prove useful.
- Avoid walking barefoot.

Currently, no other therapy is advocated in this group of patients. As discussed in Chapter 107 (Diabetic neuropathy), good diabetic control is important and other agents may be useful in the future, such as aldose reductase inhibitors, inhibitors of nonenzymatic glycation, and various growth factors.

Existing ulcers

All ulcers should be considered deep and involving bone until proven otherwise. The following factors are also important:

- Optimize diabetic control.
- Reduction of edema is important to aid healing.
- Regular debridement of callus and dead tissue and skin is important for both neuropathic and ischemic ulcers.

Debridement is usually best done with a scalpel and forceps, although chemical agents (such as varidase, which contains streptokinase) can occasionally help. Because these agents can also damage healthy tissue, they should be used under careful supervision.

After debridement, dressings should be applied, and changed regularly. Be careful that tight dressings do not further impair a poor circulation and that thick dressings or quantities of sticky tape holding them on do not cause their own skin trauma or pressure effects.

Infection control

Infection may be localized, but any evidence of deeper infection or sinus formation raises the possibility of osteomyelitis. Systemic symptoms of an infection may be minimal, as may pain and tenderness in the foot itself, so be suspicious of more severe infection than those usually seen.

The organisms may be ordinary skin commensals that have found a port of entry. Send swabs for culture and think of *Staphylococcus aureus* or streptococci as likely organisms.

If a sinus is present, probe it and if down to bone, assume there is osteomyelitis. Culture anything you get out. Plain radiographs may show bone erosion or destruction with osteomyelitis; radioisotope scans with technetium can show ↑ uptake with both infection and Charcot arthropathy. MRI scanning can be useful to differentiate the two.

If infection is present, use triple therapy with *flucloxacillin* (500 mg 4× daily), *ampicillin/amoxicillin* (500 mg 3× daily), and *metronidazole* (200mg 3× daily) or consider using *amoxicillin/clavulanic acid* (250/125 mg 3× daily) or *ciprofloxacin* (500–750 mg 2× daily) and *clindamycin* (300–450 mg 2× daily) depending on the organisms grown and patient tolerability. This will need to be given IV initially if the infection is severe. For deeper infections, several months of therapy may be needed.

If osteomyelitis is present, consider using *ciprofloxacin* or *sodium fusidate*, both of which have better bone penetration. Use for several months.

Linezolid is also useful as a second- or third-line agent, but requires extra caution used in those with hepatic and renal impairment. This caveat and the need to monitor for potential thrombocytopenia, anemia, or pancytopenia may limit its use.

In some patients, this approach fails to control osteomyelitis adequately and resection or amputation is required. Regular consultation with a capable surgeon is imperative.

Reducing trauma and pressure relief

For treatment of neuropathic ulcers, padded socks can reduce sheer stress and trauma. Suitable shoes and insoles can help relieve pressure to enable healing, as long as unnecessary walking is minimized.

If these measures are not enough, a pneumatic or Aircast boot or a total contact cast may be needed. These allow the patient to be mobile while taking the weight away from the ulcerated area or foot. Instead, all of the weight and pressure is directed through to the calf. The involvement of podiatrists and orthotists is essential.

Revascularization

Always consider coexistent vascular disease in a neuropathic foot or predominantly ischemic ulcers and feet. Vascular bypass grafting and reconstruction or angioplasty can give excellent results, with a 70–95% limb salvage rate often quoted. The improved blood supply will also help healing of existing ulcers and may negate the need for amputation or minimize the area requiring resection.

If vascular intervention is unsuccessful or not possible, then amputation is required, preferably as a below-knee procedure, to give a better mobilization potential postoperatively.

Box 109.3 The Charcot foot

Epidemiology
This is a relatively rare complication of diabetes: an average general hospital clinic will have 3–10 patients with this problem.

Pathogenesis
Blood flow increases from sympathetic nerve loss. This causes osteoclast activity and bone turnover to increase, thus making the bones of the foot more susceptible to damage. Even minor trauma can result in destructive changes in this susceptible bone.

Clinical features
The most likely site is the tarsal–metatarsal region or the metatarsophalangeal joints. Initially, the foot is warm or hot, swollen, and often uncomfortable, features that may be indistinguishable from cellulitis and gout. Peripheral pulses are invariably present, and peripheral neuropathy is evident clinically.

Plain radiographs will be normal initially and later show fractures with osteolysis and joint reorganization with subluxation of the metatarsophalangeal joints and dislocation of the large joints of the foot.

Isotope scans with technetium are abnormal from early on; differentiation from infective or other inflammatory causes can be difficult. MRI scanning may prove more useful for this, as may ^{111}indium-labeled white cell studies if infection is suspected.

Eventually, in the untreated patient, two classic deformities are seen:
- A "rocker bottom" deformity due to displacement and subluxation of the tarsus downward
- Medial convexity due to displacement of the talonavicular joint or tarsometatarsal dislocation

Management
If diagnosed early, immobilization may help prevent joint destruction. While the best means of doing this is not agreed on, use of a nonwalking plaster cast or an Aircast type of boot is needed for at least 2–3 months while bone repair or remodeling is taking place.

Some clinicians advocate immobilization for up to a year. The recent use of bisphosphates to speed up the repair process by reducing osteoclast activity is interesting and under further evaluation.

Further reading

Boulton AJM (2003). Foot problems in patients with DM. In Williams G, Pickup JC (Eds.), *Textbook of Diabetes*, 3rd ed. Oxford, UK: Blackwell Science.

NICE (2004). NICE clinical guideline. Type 2 diabetes—foot care. http://www.nice.org.uk

Scottish Intercollegiate Network (SIGN) (1997). National Clinical Guideline (recommended for use in Scotland). Management of diabetic foot disease. Available from SIGN Secretariat, 9 Queen Street, Edinburgh, EH2 1JQ. http://www.sign.ac.uk/guidelines/

Wagner FW (1983). Algorithms of diabetic foot care. In Levin ME, O'Neil LW (Eds), *The Diabetic Foot*, 2nd ed. St. Louis: Mosby Yearbook, pp. 291–302.

Diabetes and pregnancy

Background

Of women who become pregnant, 0.27% have previously diagnosed diabetes and account for 0.10% of live births, and 2–3% of pregnant women have a diagnosis of gestational diabetes made during their pregnancy. In both cases, there are risks to both the mother and the fetus. These fetuses have a historical fetal abnormality rate of up to 30%, or 12 × that of the background population.

Given the increasing proportion of women with type 2 diabetes, these pregnancies should also be looked for.

Risks

Fetal

With greater emphasis on improving glycemic control, a 2.5- to 3-fold ↑ in congenital malformation rate in mothers with previously known diabetes and a 1.8-fold increase in those without it being known, compared to rates in the nondiabetic population, is more realistic now. Cardiac, renal, and neural tube defects occur, particularly sacral agenesis.

Hyperglycemia in the first 8 weeks of fetal life, during organogenesis, is thought to be the underlying cause. This explains the lower rate in those with gestational diabetes, which classically occurs later, but not completely. Alterations in oxygen free radicals, myoinositol, and arachidonic acid metabolism and alterations in zinc metabolism are also implicated.

The most common problem seen in the infant is macrosomia (in 8–50%), which can result in birth trauma and an ↑ intervention rate. As well as causing obesity, fetal hyperinsulinemia also accelerates skeletal maturation, delays pulmonary maturation, and causes ↑ growth of insulin-sensitive tissues producing hypertrophy of the liver and heart.

These infants also have an ↑ risk of hypoglycemia, seen transiently in up to 50%, and jaundice, with rates of 6–50% quoted. Up to 50% of these infants require phototherapy. Polycythemia is also seen.

Maternal

Maternal problems include an ↑ risk of infection and of pre-eclampsia, which is 2–3 times as likely to occur as in a nondiabetic mother. Women with type 1 diabetes have a 3-fold ↑ prevalence of thyroid dysfunction during the pregnancy and postpartum, so this needs to be screened for.

Inheritance of diabetes

If the background rate of diabetes is 0.15%, the infant of a diabetic mother has a 2% risk and the infant of a diabetic father a 6% risk of developing diabetes. The risk of type 2 diabetes in a child of a type 2 mother is much higher, at 15–30%, and rises to 50–60% if both parents have type 2 diabetes.

Known diabetes and pregnancy

Most women with diabetes have normal deliveries and normal babies. In most instances, these are women with type 1 diabetes, although in some ethnic groups type 2 patients may make up a sizable group. In both groups it is of utmost importance to have pre-conception glycemic control optimized, e.g., preferably an HbA1c level in the nondiabetic range or <7.0% if that is not possible.

The congenital malformation and spontaneous abortion rates are significantly higher when the HbA1c is elevated. Once the HbA1c is 4–6 standard deviations above the normal nondiabetic range, there is a 4-fold increase in the malformation rate; at over 6 standard deviations above normal, this rises to a 12-fold risk.

In type 2 patients, converting from oral agents to insulin is important. If this is not possible prior to conception, it should be done as soon as a woman is found to be pregnant.

Pre-conception management

Pre-conception and post-conception advice to diabetic women is similar to that given to nondiabetic women: stop smoking, reduce alcohol intake, avoid unpasteurized dairy products, and add oral folate supplements (5 mg/day). Any potentially teratogenic drugs they may be taking (e.g., antihypertensive agents) also need to be reviewed.

Ideally, all patients who have diabetes and are pregnant should be managed in a combined clinic by an obstetrician and a diabetologist. Reviews are initially every 2–4 weeks then every 1–2 weeks in the last 1/3 of pregnancy. Screening and monitoring for conditions such as associated thyroid disease at these reviews is also advisable.

Maintaining good glycemic control

This is important not just because of the risk of ketoacidosis, which occurs in <1 % of diabetic pregnancies and is associated with fetal loss in 20% of episodes, but also because of macrosomia in the fetus and the ↑ fetal mortality (up to 2.2% of births in diabetic mothers) and ↑ intervention rate at delivery.

The aim is to keep the glucose and HbA1c levels in the nondiabetic range, to reduce the morbidity and mortality associated with pregnancy and diabetes (Box 110.1). Even with perfect control, however, there is a small but significant excess of major congenital malformations in these children and an unexplained risk of late stillbirths.

Box 110.1 Monitoring during pregnancy
- Capillary blood glucose monitoring is performed at least 4× per day.
- Monitor thyroid function.

Target glycemic control
- Fasting glucoses of <90 mg/dL
- Postprandial glucoses of <126 mg/dL
- Keep the HbA1c level in the nondiabetic range.

Treatment regimen

A basal bolus regimen gives the greatest flexibility and is commonly used to achieve this target. In type 1 patients, insulin requirements often fall in the first trimester, increase slightly in the second, then continue to rise until about 36 weeks, falling back to pre-pregnancy levels after delivery.

In type 1 women, early pregnancy is a cause of falling insulin requirements and recurrent hypoglycemia. It has been suggested that up to 40% of women with type 1 diabetes will experience significant hypoglycemic episodes when pregnant and hypoglycemic awareness may alter. Advice regarding care with driving and other potentially hazardous pursuits is therefore needed early in pregnancy, if not before conception.

Type 2 women requiring insulin usually need 0.9 units/kg/day initially and 1.6 units/kg/day later in the pregnancy.

Monitoring of diabetic complications during pregnancy

Certain diabetic complications are known to worsen during pregnancy. Screening for nephropathy and retinopathy in particular is advised at least each trimester.

Fetal monitoring

Scanning of the fetus is performed at 10–12 weeks to look for congenital abnormalities and to confirm dates.

Repeat scanning is used to check for excessive growth or macrosomia at 18–20 weeks, 28 weeks, 32 weeks, and 36 weeks, although the exact timing and frequency can vary between centers.

Management of delivery

At delivery, most units have set protocols (see Box 110.2). In general, induction soon after 38 weeks' gestation (or not later than the expected delivery date) and use of a continuous insulin infusion with a separate dextrose and potassium infusion to maintain stable blood glucose levels are advisable.

This infusion is important, as maternal hyperglycemia during delivery can be associated with neonatal hypoglycemia and an adverse neurological outcome in the infant. The infant responds to a hyperglycemic environment in utero by increasing its own insulin production.

After delivery

Monitoring of the infant's capillary blood glucose levels post-delivery is also often performed. The ↑ potential for hypoglycemia in the mother

---

Box 110.2 Treatment regimen for labor and delivery

- If labor is induced, omit the previous evening's long-acting insulin.
- Infuse 10% glucose at 75–125 mL/h (with 20 mmol potassium per 500 mL bag). Infuse via syringe driver 2–4 units/h of soluble insulin initially (usually made as 50 mL soluble insulin in 50 mL of 0.9% saline in a 50 mL syringe).
- Monitor capillary blood glucose levels hourly and adjust infusion rate of the insulin to keep blood glucose levels in the 110–150 mg/dL range.
- Monitor fluid balance carefully (especially if oxytocin is also being given).
- Check serum sodium if labor lasts over 24 hours (or 8 hours with oxytocin)

---

and the baby if breast-feeding also needs to be watched for. Extra carbohydrate snacks for the mother are often needed, along with a 20–25% reduction in pre-conception insulin requirements.

One day's worth of breast milk contains about 50 g of carbohydrate.

Also consider monitoring thyroid function at 3 and 6 months post-delivery.

After delivery

- Halve the IV insulin infusion rate.
- Continue to monitor capillary blood glucose hourly for at least 4 hours then every 2–4 hours until the mother is eating normally.
- Return to the pre-pregnancy regimen when the mother is eating normally, but be careful, as insulin requirements can be low for the first 24 hours.

Gestational diabetes

Epidemiology

Pregnancy induces a state of insulin resistance with increases in the levels of growth hormone, placental growth hormone, progesterone, placental lactogen, and cortisol. This can result in altered glucose handling.

Impaired glucose tolerance during pregnancy occurs in up to 2–3% of pregnant women and may be associated with an ↑ risk of subsequent type 2 diabetes in 20–50% of patients. Worsening maternal insulin resistance and associated hyperglycemia usually becomes evident from the second trimester on if it is going to occur.

As with women previously known to have diabetes, there is an association with worsening carbohydrate intolerance and a worse maternal and fetal outcome.

Untreated gestational diabetes has a perinatal mortality of 4.4–6.4% compared to 0.5–1.5% in a similar ethnic normoglycemic population. Intensive insulin treatment has been shown to reduce such complications. This is the rationale for careful multidisciplinary care of these patients.

Treatment

Initial treatment is with dietary advice; in 10–30%, insulin is also required. Insulin therapy should be considered if fasting blood glucoses are >110 mg/dL or postprandial levels are >150 mg/dL.

Obesity is not uncommon in these patients. The importance of post-delivery dietary modification and weight reduction, to reduce the risk of future type 2 diabetes, should also be reinforced.

The varying insulin requirements during pregnancy occur as in those with previously known diabetes, and most (but not all) patients will not need insulin treatment following delivery. Monitoring is with home capillary blood glucose measurements, daily if on diet alone and more frequently if on insulin therapy.

The frequency needed depends on the results obtained, with the aim of keeping all readings <126 mg/dL. If diet alone fails, a basal bolus insulin regimen as used in the known diabetic is usually required. The total initial daily dose is determined on the basis of the degree of hyperglycemia present; 4–6 units per bolus is usual.

As with the previously known diabetic mother, the aim is to have a normal delivery, more often at 38 weeks to term, depending on fetal growth. An oral glucose tolerance test (OGTT) should be performed 6 weeks after delivery in all patients not requiring insulin post-delivery, to confirm a return to normal glucose metabolism. A further reinforcement of diet and weight advice at this time is also usual practice.

Whether these patients should be followed up because of their ↑ risk of diabetes is unclear, although annual fasting blood glucose levels in asymptomatic women with a normal 6-week postpartum OGTT is often advised. More careful review is suggested for those with abnormal OGTTs.

High-risk groups

Most women with gestational diabetes are found on routine screening at about 30 weeks, but certain high-risk groups should be screened earlier (see Box 110.3 for screening methods).

These risk factors include the following:
- Previous gestational diabetes
- A large baby in their last pregnancy, e.g., >4.0 kg at term
- A previous unexplained stillbirth or perinatal death
- Maternal obesity
- Family history of diabetes (first-degree relatives)
- Polyhydramnios

Contraception and diabetes

Oral contraceptives

The early combined oral contraceptive pills (OCP) impaired glucose tolerance and so were not advised in patients with diabetes. The use of third-generation low-dose estrogen-containing combined OCPs (e.g., 20 mcg ethinylestradiol) is safe in women <35 years of age. Third-generation OCPs are advised, as they have a better risk profile for arterial disease and only occasionally increase insulin requirements.

Box 110.3 Methods of screening

• Urine dip testing for glucose should be performed on every pregnant woman at every antenatal visit.
• If glycosuria is found, a fasting glucose test is performed, and if >110 mg/dL, a 75 g OGTT is needed (see Table 110.1).
• Routine screening at 28–32 weeks is also often done, either with random blood glucose tests or a fasting blood glucose level. If a fasting level is >110 mg/dL or a postprandial level is >126 mg/dL, an OGTT is required.
• The diagnostic criteria for diabetes are no different from those in the nonpregnant population. A diagnosis of gestational diabetes or gestational IGT is made if the fasting glucose is 110–140 mg/dL and/or the 2-hour postprandial level is 160–200 mg/dL by St. Vincent definition. The WHO definition has a fasting level of 140 mg/dL and/or a 2-hour postprandial level of 140–200 mg/dL.

Table 110.1 Interpretation of 75 g oral glucose tolerance test during pregnancy

	Plasma glucose (mg/dL)	
Diabetes	Fasting >126	2-hour postprandial level >200
Gestational IGT	110–140	160–199
Normal	<109	160

As in the nondiabetic population, standard advice regarding the pill should be given. Its use should be avoided in at-risk groups such as overweight smokers with a family history of thromboembolism and coronary heart disease. There is an ↑ risk of cerebral thromboembolism in type 1 patients, but the OCP dose not increase this.

In those with microvascular disease or coronary risk factors, the progesterone-only "mini-pill" (POP) is safer than the combined OCP, as it has no significant adverse effects on lipid metabolism, clotting, platelet aggregation, or fibrinolytic activity.

It has been suggested that levonorgestrel- and norethisterone-containing POPs may reduce HDL$_2$ cholesterol subfractions. The avoidance of POPs in those with established arterial disease is advised.

Barrier methods
The condom and the diaphragm were historically the contraceptive method of choice in people with diabetes and do not have the metabolic risks of the oral contraceptives described above.

But both are less effective forms of contraception with a failure rate of 0.7–3.6/100 couple years for the condom and 2/100 couple years for the diaphragm, compared to nearly 0.2/100 female years with the combined

OCP. In a population in which pregnancy carries significant risks, other forms of contraception are now more often advocated.

Intrauterine contraceptive devices (IUD)
There is concern that diabetes might make a pelvic infection associated with an IUD more severe and render both copper-containing and inert IUDs less effective, but not all studies have confirmed these worries.

Nevertheless, if an IUD is used in a woman with diabetes, a progestagen-releasing variety or a small copper device with regular use of spermicides are the current favorite options.

Hormone replacement therapy (HRT)
As with the OCP, diabetes itself is not a contraindication to the use of HRT. The estrogens in HRT differ from those in the OCP and may actually reduce insulin resistance and also protect against coronary disease, although they may not actually reduce cardiovascular events in those with established coronary artery disease.

Further reading

Dornhorst A, Chan SP (1998). The elusive diagnosis of gestational diabetes. *Diabet Med* 15:7–10.Garner P (1995). Type 1 DM and pregnancy. *Lancet* 346:157–161.

Iikova H (1995). Screening for gestational diabetes. *Diabet Rev Int* 3(3):1–2.

NICE (2008). Interpartum care. Clinical guideline CG63. Diabetes in pregnancy. http://www.nice.org.uk /guidanceNICE (2008).

NICE guidelines. Diabetes in pregnancy. http://www.nice.org.uk/guidance

Intercurrent events or disease

Surgery

Preoperative assessment

Careful preoperative assessment is essential because of an ↑ risk of death and complications such as fluid overload from coronary heart disease and diabetic nephropathy. Any preoperative assessment in a patient with known diabetes should therefore include the following:

- An adequate history of diabetic complications
- A full examination looking for evidence of peripheral vascular disease, peripheral neuropathy, and lying or standing BPs in case of autonomic neuropathy
- Assessment of current and overall diabetic control using blood glucose measurements in all patients and glycated hemoglobin
- General investigations should include serum urea + electrolytes/creatinine, FBC, urine dip testing for protein, and an ECG (in anyone >45 years old).

Any further investigation will be based on problems found in the history or examination, such as foot ulceration and potential osteomyelitis, which may give a source for infection such as an MRSA.

Attempts should be made to improve diabetic control, either on the ward or in a diabetic clinic, for any patient undergoing an elective procedure whose control is inadequate. An HbA1c <7.2% is considered good control, but an acceptable levels for most procedures would be <9%.

Even with a good HbA1c level, the preoperative glucose level (and if >200 mg/dL, the urine ketones) should always be measured, as the perioperative treatment is based on this and some stabilization before administration of an anesthetic may be required, particularly in an emergency situation.

Perioperative management

Ideally, patients with diabetes are best operated on in the morning at the start of the list.

Patients normally on diet alone should have their capillary blood glucose levels checked hourly. IV dextrose, should be avoided in these patients. Often no other modification to their treatment is needed.

Patients taking oral agents should stop metformin for at least 48 hours preoperatively and miss their other agents on the morning of the procedure. Capillary blood glucose levels are again monitored regularly (every 1–2 hours) and insulin IV infusion may be started if necessary.

In patients taking insulin who are undergoing a morning operation, from 0 to one-half of the morning insulin dose might be given and IV insulin infusion may be started. The aim is to keep the blood glucose in the 120–180 mg/dL range.

Every hospital in the United States has developed insulin infusion protocols used in the intensive care unit (ICU) in pre-, peri- and postoperative patients as well as in patients on enteral and parenteral nutrition.

Skin, connective tissue, or joint disease

Skin

Diabetes results in an ↑ occurrence of infections such as vaginal candida, *Candida balanitis*, and *Staphylococcus aureus* folliculitis. Ulceration in the feet due to neuropathy and peripheral vascular disease should also be considered. Other skin features to look for include the following.

Conditions specific to diabetes
- Pretibial diabetic dermopathy—shin spots
- Diabetic bullae—bullosis diabeticorum, very rare tense blistering on feet and lower legs classically
- Diabetic thick skin—cleroderma of diabetes seen in 2.5% with type 2 diabetes
- Periungual telangectasia—venous capillary dilatation at the nail fold seen in up to 50% of people with diabetes

The most common skin lesion in diabetes is shin spots, or diabetic dermopathy. These occur more commonly in males than in females and affect up to 50% of people with diabetes. Their etiology is uncertain.

They present initially as red papules and progress to give well-circumscribed atrophic areas that are brownish in color. Usually seen on the shins, they can also be found on the forearms and thighs.

There is no effective treatment of these; they usually resolve spontaneously over 1–2 years.

Conditions seen more commonly in those with diabetes
- Necrobiosis lipoidica
- Vitiligo (seen in 2% with type 1 diabetes)
- Granuloma annulare (although this association is not proven conclusively)

Necrobiosis lipoidica is seen in 0.3–1% of people with diabetes, and 40–60% of those with necrobiosis also have diabetes. It is more common in females than in males.

Classically seen on the shins, it has an atrophic centre with telangectasia around the edge of an oval or irregular lesion, although early lesions can be dull red plaques or papules.

Treatment with topical or injectable steroids may help improve these lesions; skin grafting and cosmetic camouflage have also been used.

*Conditions associated with the other biochemical features
seen in diabetes*
- Acanthosis nigricans—with insulin resistance
- Eruptive xanthomata—with hypertriglyceridemia

When looking at the skin do not forget to check injection sites for lipohypertrophy or lipoatrophy as these are often much more amenable to treatment or correction. In the past, an insulin allergy rash was also commonly seen, but more recently a transient local reaction, thought to be an IgE-mediated reaction, is more often seen.

Connective tissue and joint disease

Diabetes is associated with an ↑ incidence of pseudogout and osteoarthritis, but the classical condition to consider is the "stiff hand syndrome," or *diabetic cheiroarthropathy*.

In this disorder, the skin thickens and tightens, which, in association with sclerosis of the tendon sheaths, results in limited joint mobility in the hands and, less commonly, the feet. This reduced joint mobility leads to an inability to place the palms of the hand flat together and make the "prayer sign." No specific treatment for this currently exists.

Emergencies in diabetes

Diabetic ketoacidosis

Diabetic ketoacidosis has a mortality of 2–5%. Many deaths occur from delays in presentation and initiation of treatment. It has a mortality rate of up to 50% in the elderly.

Diagnosis

This is usually based on a collection of biochemical abnormalities:

- Hyperglycemia >200 mg/dL
- Acidosis arterial pH <7.3, serum bicarbonate <15 mmol/L, base excess <–10
- Ketonuria. Some dip testing methods only check for acetoacetate and acetone but not β-hydroxybutyrate. Captopril can also give a false-positive test for urinary acetone. Ketones may interfere with some creatinine assays and give falsely high readings.

There is an uncommon condition of *euglycemic ketoacidosis* (in 1–3% of cases at most) when ketones are produced early on in patients with a reduced carbohydrate intake. Blood glucose is <300 mg/dL, acidosis is marked, and dehydration is not usually severe. Clinical features are listed in Box 112.1.

Box 112.1 Clinical features of diabetic ketoacidosis

Polyuria, polydypsia, and weight loss are often seen. Muscle cramps, abdominal pain, and shortness of breath (air hunger or Kussmaul's breathing, with deep, regular, rapid breaths, suggesting acidosis) can also occur. Subsequent nausea and vomiting can worsen both the dehydration and electrolyte losses that often precede the onset of coma (occurring in about 10% of cases).

Consider other causes of coma and a raised blood glucose level, such as head injury, alcohol, and drug overdose.

On examination, the breath can smell of ketones (like nail-varnish remover). Postural hypotension (exacerbated by peripheral vasodilatation due to acidosis) and hypothermia are also frequently seen. Infection and trauma can precipitate this problem and should be carefully looked for, especially in the unconscious patient.

Hypovolemia at presentation is usually at least 5 L, along with electrolyte losses of 300–700 mmol of sodium, 200–700 mmol of potassium, and 350–500 mmol of chloride. The daily intake of both sodium and potassium is 60 mmol, so the severity of this condition is apparent

Initial treatment is to start oral carbohydrate intake and monitor the need for IV insulin/fluids as in full-blown hyperglycemic ketoacidosis.

Epidemiology

Diabetic ketoacidosis is common in patients with type 1 diabetes. The incidence is 5–8/1000 diabetic patients per year, usually patients with type 1 diabetes. Up to 25% of cases are patients with newly diagnosed or presenting diabetes, some of whom subsequently obtain adequate control with oral agents or diet alone.

In up to 50% of cases an infection is the precipitant, and in 10–30% of cases it is their first presentation with diabetes.

Pathogenesis

Diabetic ketoacidosis occurs as a result of insulin deficiency and counterregulatory hormone excess. Insulin deficiency results in excess mobilization of free fatty acids from adipose tissue. This provides the substrate for ketone production from the liver. Ketones (β-hydroxy-butyrate, acetoacetate, and acetone) are excreted by the kidneys and buffered in the blood initially, but once this system fails, acidosis develops.

Hyperglycemia also occurs, as the liver produces glucose from lactate and alanine generated by muscle proteinolysis. The reduced peripheral glucose utilization associated with insulin deficiency exacerbates this.

Hyperglycemia and ketonuria cause an osmotic diuresis and hypovolemia with both intracellular and extracellular dehydration. Glomerular filtration is reduced and blood glucose levels thus rise even further, as do the levels of counterregulatory hormones such as glucagon.

The metabolic acidosis due to ketone accumulation leads to widespread cell death that, combined with hypovolemia, is fatal if untreated.

Management

Having first assessed the need for immediate resuscitation and started a 0.9% saline IV infusion, take a history and examine the patient to look for obvious precipitants, such as surgery, trauma, sites of infection, or myocardial infarction (Box 112.2). While initial investigations will be modified by the history and examination and suggested site of infection, they should include at least the following:

- Blood for urea/electrolytes (note ketone/creatinine assay interaction)
- CBC (a leukocytosis can occur without infection)
- Arterial blood gases (P_aCO_2 will be low due to hyperventilation with a metabolic acidosis; check pH and bicarbonate)
- Cultures of blood and urine
- Chest X-rays and ECG
- In the older patient (>40 years), also include an ECG and cardiac enzymes, even if asymptomatic.

Replacement of fluids, electrolytes, and insulin is the mainstay of treatment, along with treatment of any precipitant, such as infection. To monitor this treatment, central venous access and urinary catheterization are often necessary and an NG tube may be useful, especially in the unconscious patient.

Box 112.2 Precipitants of diabetic ketoacidosis

- Infection   30–40%
- Noncompliance with treatment   25%
- Inappropriate alterations in insulin   13%
  (i.e., errors by patient or doctor)
- Newly diagnosed diabetes   10–20%
- Myocardial infarction   1%

In elderly people, those with a cardiac history, or those with autonomic neuropathy, central venous access is imperative.

Monitoring

Once treatment has commenced, monitor fluid balance carefully and avoid fluid overload. Check capillary blood glucose hourly, serum potassium, sodium, and glucose every 2 hours, and arterial blood gases every 2–4 hours depending on response.

Reduce the frequency of tests once the patient is stabilized, but check electrolytes at least daily for the first 72 hours. Continuous ECG monitoring will aid in detection of hypo- and hyperkalemia in the acute phase.

Magnesium and phosphate levels should also be checked, as these can occasionally require replacement therapy.

Additional therapies

IV bicarbonate is only rarely indicated, as it can cause hypokalemia and paradoxically worsen intracellular acidosis. If used, give only when the pH is <6.9 using 250 mL of 1.26% bicarbonate given over 30–60 minutes initially. Monitor arterial blood gases to assess response, aiming for pH no greater than 7.1.

This should probably only be used in an intensive care setting. Do not use 8.4% bicarbonate, as its high sodium load can too rapidly alter electrolyte levels and precipitate pulmonary edema as well as cause local tissue necrosis if it extravasates.

In severe hypotension unresponsive to colloids and crystalloids, inotropes may be required, but agents such as *dopamine*, *dobutamine*, and *adrenaline* will all exacerbate insulin resistance, necessitating a more aggressive sliding-scale regime.

Heparin in SC prophylactic doses can be given in the unconscious or immobile patent.

Cover with *IV broad-spectrum antibiotics* should be used if no obvious precipitant is found and appropriate antibiotics used if a site of infection is found.

Cerebral edema typically presents 8–24 hours after starting IV fluids with a declining conscious level and can have a mortality rate as high as 90%. If this occurs, *dexamethasone* (12–16 mg/day) and *mannitol* (1–2 g/kg body weight) may be given.

Subsequent treatment
Once the blood glucose is stable in the 180–270 mg/dL range, the ketoacidosis has settled, and the patient is eating and drinking normally, consider switching to a SC insulin regimen, but overlap the IV and the first SC dose by 2 hours. Stabilize the patient on this therapy before discharge from the hospital.

Once the IV potassium supplements have been stopped, give oral supplements for at least 48 hours with regular serum monitoring.

Patient education on determining the cause and avoiding a further occurrence, or on earlier presentation if it does occur, should also ideally be given before discharge.

Initial treatment of ketoacidosis

IV 0.9% saline
- 2 L in 2 hours, then 1 L over 2 hours, 2 L in next 8 hours, and 4 L/ day thereafter until blood glucose is <200 mg/dL. Then convert to dextrose saline or 5% dextrose.

If the patient is profoundly shocked (e.g., systolic BP <80 mmHg with severe dehydration or sepsis) or oliguric, this dosage may need to be given more rapidly and colloids may also be needed. If the patient is elderly or there are signs of heart failure or cerebral edema, it may need to be given more slowly.

Potassium
Once the serum potassium is known, potassium is added to the 0.9% saline. The dose of potassium is adjusted on the basis of hourly serum potassium measurements until the patient is stable, and measured every 2–4 hours over the next 12–24 hours. Add the following:
- 40 mmol/L if K^+ <3.0 mmol/L
- 30 mmol/L if K^+ 3.0–4.0 mmol/L
- 20 mmol/L if K^+ 4.1–5.0 mmol/L
- 10 mmol/L if K^+ 5.1–6.0 mmol/L
- None if K^+>6.0 mmol/L

Insulin (via continuous IV infusion)
Every hospital in the United States has developed IV insulin infusion protocols. Following these protocols is mandatory and the safest way of administering insulin IV.

Hyperosmolar, nonketotic hyperglycemia

This is a more sinister complication than ketoacidosis with a mortality rate as high as 50%. It is found in 11–30% of adult hyperglycemic emergencies. It affects an older population than that with ketoacidosis (middle-aged or elderly), 2/3 of cases are in patients with previously undiagnosed diabetes, and its insidious onset can be mistaken for many other conditions, including stroke. See Box 112.3 for clinical features.

Diagnosis

This is again a biochemical diagnosis:

- *Hyperglycemia* (usually 30–70 mmol/L)
- Serum osmolality is *high* (>350 mmol/kg)
- *No acidosis* arterial pH 7.35–7.45, serum bicarbonate >18 mmol/L, but lactic acidosis with infection or a myocardial infarction may alter this.
- *No ketonuria* + on urine dip testing can occur with starvation and vomiting.

Serum osmolality (in mosmol/kg) can be calculated if not available from the laboratory using the following equation:

Osmolality = 2(sodium + potassium) + glucose + urea

Epidemiology

This condition occurs in an older age group of insulin-producing type 2 patients, a large proportion of whom will not previously be known to have diabetes.

Ingestion of high-sugar-containing drinks, intercurrent infection, and myocardial infarction are all commonly seen as precipitants of this condition. Drugs such as glucocorticoids, cimetidine, phenytoin, thiazide, and loop diuretics are all implicated in the pathogenesis of this problem.

Pathogenesis

This condition results from a combination of insulin deficiency and counterregulatory hormone excess. The insulin present stops ketone production but in insufficient quantities to prevent worsening hyperglycemia.

Box 112.3 Clinical features of hyperosmolar, nonketotic hyperglycemia

There is normally an insidious onset with several days of ill health and profound dehydration at presentation (equivalent to a 9–10 L deficit). Confusion is not uncommon, nor is coma (especially once serum osmolality >440). Occasionally, fits occur.

Gastroparesis and associated vomiting with gastric erosions and subsequent hematemesis can occur. These patients are also hypercoagulable, and venous thromboses and cerebrovascular events are important to exclude.

Management

Initial investigation and treatment are the same as for ketoacidosis, with fluid, electrolyte, and insulin replacement, although there are a few important exceptions as these are older patients:

- The fluid regimen should be less rapid and vigorous. Central venous access for monitoring is more often required, e.g., 1 L of 0.9% saline over the first hour, 1 L q2h for the next 2 hours, then 1 L q4–6h.
- If hypernatremic (serum sodium >155 mmol/L) consider 0.45% saline, rather than 0.9%, although this may increase the risk of cerebral edema if serum sodium or osmolality is altered too rapidly, which has a mortality as high as 70%.
- Prophylactic SC heparin should be considered, although recent evidence suggests more formal anticoagulation carries a high risk of upper gastrointestinal bleeding.
- A gentler insulin regimen is needed, with 3–6 units/hour of soluble insulin IV, aiming to reduce the blood glucose by a maximum of 5 mmol/h to avoid precipitating cerebral edema.
- A more aggressive use of IV antibiotics is encouraged.

Subsequent treatment

Continue IV fluids and insulin for at least 24 hours after initial stabilization and then convert to maintenance therapy such as SC insulin or oral hypoglycemic agents. Patient education on how to avoid further episodes is also advisable.

Hypoglycemia

This complication of the treatment of diabetes should be excluded in any unconscious or relevant patient. If prolonged it can result in death. Most insulin-treated patients can expect to experience hypoglycemic episodes at some time, with up to 1/7 having a more severe episode each year and 3% suffering recurrent episodes. The 25% of people on long-term insulin who lose their hypoglycemic awareness are of particular concern.

Nocturnal hypoglycemic episodes with a hyperglycemic response the next morning (due to ↑ counterregulatory hormones—the Somogyi phenomenon), which tend to occur in younger insulin-treated patients, should be assessed for and may only present with morning headaches or a drunken feeling.

Diagnosis

This is a biochemical diagnosis from a blood glucose <50 mg/dL, but is often first picked up by the patient, their family, or their doctor from the clinical features listed in Box 112.4.

Saving serum before treatment for blood glucose, insulin, and C-peptide levels will confirm the diagnosis and may help determine the cause.

Box 112.4 Clinical features

The features of hypoglycemia can be divided into two main groups: *autonomic* symptoms and *neuroglycopenic* symptoms, as shown in Box 112.5.

The autonomic symptoms usually occur first (when the blood glucose is <65 mg/dL), but some drugs, such as the nonselective β-blockers, and alcohol may mask these with neuroglycopenia (at blood glucose <46 mg/dL), causing confusion with no warning. Some patients lose these predominantly autonomic warning symptoms and are therefore at higher risk of injury.

Box 112.5 Signs and symptoms of hypoglycemia

Autonomic
- Sweating
- Pallor
- Anxiety
- Nausea
- Tremor
- Shivering
- Palpitations
- Tachycardia

Neuroglycopenia
- Confusion
- Tiredness
- Lack of concentration
- Headache
- Dizziness
- Altered speech
- Incoordination
- Drowsiness
- Aggression
- Coma

Pathogenesis

Hypoglycemia results from an imbalance between glucose supply, glucose utilization, and Insulin levels that results in more insulin than is needed at that time.

A reduced glucose supply occurs when a meal or snack is missed, or as a late effect of alcohol. It can also be due to delayed gastric emptying with autonomic neuropathy or be associated with celiac disease, Addison's disease, or an acute illness, such as gastroenteritis.

Increased utilization occurs with exercise and high insulin levels mostly with sulfonylurea or exogenous insulin therapy. The net result of this imbalance is hypoglycemia.

Human insulins have a slightly faster onset of action and a shorter duration of action than their animal predecessors, and a lot of patients report alterations in hypoglycemic awareness when they switch from one form to the other. Even so, no definite evidence of specific hypoglycemic alterations due to human insulin itself has been reported.

Sulfonylurea therapy can cause hypoglycemia due to β-cell stimulation. This is most commonly seen from *glibenclamide*, especially in the elderly and those with reduced renal excreting ability, but can occur in anyone who takes this therapy and fasts.

The biguanide *metformin* and the α-glucosidase inhibitor *acarbose* are unlikely to precipitate hypoglycemia.

Management

In the conscious patient, oral carbohydrate (20–30 g) is often sufficient to resolve the problem. This can be given as 5–6 glucose tablets or as a glass of milk or orange juice. Having raised the sugar rapidly, the patient should then eat something to maintain a normal blood glucose.

In the confused patient, a buccal gel (e.g., GlucoGel®, a 30% glucose gel) is an alternative, although this should not be used in the unconscious patient as there is a risk of aspiration.

In the unconscious patient, once a blood sample has been taken for glucose estimation, treat with 25–50 mL of 50% glucose IV or 1 mg of IM or deep SC glucagon. Glucagon mobilizes glycogen from the liver and will not work if given repeatedly or in starved patients with no glycogen stores. In this situation or if prolonged treatment is needed, IV glucose is better (50% initially then 10%).

The worry with 50% glucose is tissue necrosis if extravasation occurs.

Subsequent management

Having corrected the acute event, determine why it happened and, if possible, alter treatment or lifestyle to prevent recurrance. Extreme exercise may require an alteration in insulin doses for 24 hours, and alcohol causes not only initial hyperglycemia but also a degree of hypoglycemia 3–6 hours after ingestion, and may alter insulin requirements the next morning.

Education on how to avoid precipitating hypoglycemic episodes in these situations is advisable. Recurrent hypoglycemic events may also herald deterioration in renal or liver function; these conditions should be excluded.

Patients on long-acting sulfonylureas who experience hypoglycemia will need careful monitoring, as the drug may last longer than the glucose or glycogen given to correct it and repeated hypoglycemic episodes may occur. A continuous IV glucose infusion is therefore often needed in this situation, particularly in overdose with these agents.

Further reading

Amiel SA, Tamborlane WV, Sherwin RS (1987). Defective glucose counterregulation after strict glycemic control of insulin-dependent DM. *N Engl J Med* 316:1376–1384.

Cranston ICP, Amiel SA (1995). Hypoglycaemia. In Leslie RDG, Robbins DC (Eds). *Diabetes: Clinical Science and Practice.* Cambridge, UK: Cambridge University Press, pp. 375–391.

Hepburn D, Deary IJ, Frier BM, et al. (1991). Symptoms of acute insulin induced hypoglycaemia in humans with and without IDDM. *Diabetes Care* 14:949–957.

Krentz AJ, Nattrass M (1997). Acute metabolic complications of DM: diabetic ketoacidosis, hyperosmolar non-ketotic syndrome and lactic acidosis. In Pickup J, Williams G (Eds.), *Textbook of Diabetes*, 2nd ed. Oxford, UK: Blackwell Science, pp. 1–23.

Lebovitz HE (1995). Diabetic ketoacidosis. *Lancet* 345:767–772.

Pickup JC, Williams G (Eds.) (2003). Hypoglycaemia in diabetes. In *Textbook of Diabetes*, 3rd ed. Oxford, UK: Wiley-Blackwell.

Part 12

Lipids and hyperlipidemia

Barrie Weinstein and Dina Green

Lipids and coronary heart disease

Physiology

The two main circulating lipids, triglycerides and cholesterol, are bound with phospholipid and lipoproteins to make them more water soluble for transportation throughout the body. The apoproteins on the surface of these soluble masses help the body to recognize each of the different transport complexes.

Chylomicrons

These contain 85% triglycerides and 4% cholesterol. Made in the mucosa of the small intestine, they are broken down in the liver and peripheral tissues by lipoprotein lipase. Initially they contain apoprotein B-48 (apo B-48) but also acquire apo E and apo C-II from circulating HDL.

Following metabolism by lipoprotein lipase in capillary endothelial cells, which is activated by apo C-II, chylomicron remnants are then removed by specific apo B and apo E receptors in the liver.

Very low–density lipoproteins (VLDLs)

VLDLs contain 50% triglyceride, 15% cholesterol, and 18% phospholipid. They are the main carrier of triglycerides in circulation. Made with triglycerides synthesized in the liver, they also contain apo B-100 and apo E.

VLDLs are broken down by lipoprotein lipase in peripheral tissue to give IDLs, or other remnants that are removed by the liver.

Intermediate-density lipoproteins (IDLs)

These VLDL remnants contain mostly cholesterol and phospholipid and are either removed by the liver or metabolized to form LDLs.

Low-density lipoproteins (LDLs)

LDLs contain 45% cholesterol, 10% triglycerides, and 20% phospholipid. LDL has apo B-100 in its surface and transports most of the cholesterol in circulation.

The liver has specific LDL receptors to extract it from the circulation. Half of the body's circulating LDL is removed from the plasma each day, mostly by the liver. Small dense or oxidized LDL (usually only 15% of the LDL pool) is not so easily recognized by these receptors and a scavenger pathway in macrophages and liver sinusoidal endothelial cells removes these via an acetyl-LDL receptor.

Accumulation of oxidized LDL in macrophages produces the foam cells seen in atheromatous plaques.

High-density lipoproteins (HDLs)

HDLs are made in the liver and gut and contain 17% cholesterol, 4% triglycerides, and 24% phospholipid. HDL transports 20–50% of circulating cholesterol.

In practice, patients are managed by their levels of cholesterol (total [TC], LDL, HDL) and triglycerides. Elevated total or LDL cholesterol with normal triglycerides is hypercholesterolemia. Isolated elevation of triglycerides is hypertriglyceridemia; both together is combined or mixed hyperlipidemia.

There is a direct linear relationship between hypercholesterolemia and coronary heart disease (CHD). A man with a TC of 250 mg/dL has double the risk of CHD of a man with a TC of 201 mg/dL and half the risk of a man with a cholesterol of 302 mg/dL. Intervention studies show that reductions in total and LDL cholesterol reduce coronary and cerebrovascular events, as well as mortality.

HDL cholesterol has an inverse relationship with CHD, i.e., increased levels are beneficial. A low HDL cholesterol may be due to lack of physical exercise, obesity, or the presence of hypertriglyceridemia and occurs in smokers and the metabolic syndrome.[1] Whether isolated hypertriglyceridemia causes vascular disease is still debated.

Mixed hyperlipidemia is clearly associated with CHD. The Helsinki Heart Study[2] showed a 4-fold greater risk of cardiac events if the LDL:HDL ratio was >5.0 and the triglycerides >203 mg/dL compared to the rate for those with lower levels of triglycerides.

Hypertriglyceridemia is associated with a low HDL cholesterol level as well as small, dense LDL particles. The aim of keeping triglycerides <132 mg/dL is to indirectly increase the HDL cholesterol as well as for the small, dense LDL to revert to the more benign, less dense LDL.

Small, dense LDL has a lower binding affinity for the LDL receptor, resulting in a longer t½ as well as greater susceptibility to oxidation.

Pathogenesis

Hyperlipidemia is due to a combination of genetic factors and dietary intake and is secondary to other conditions. It is a major risk factor for atherosclerosis.

• Primary hyperlipidemias are usually genetically determined.
• Secondary hyperlipidemias are due to a combination of other diseases, drugs, and dietary anomalies.

1 American Heart Association (2009). Harmonizing the metabolic syndrome. *Circulation* 120:1640–1645.

2 Frick MH, Elo O, Haapa K, et al (1987). Helsinki Heart Study: primary-prevention trial with gemfibrozil in middle-aged men with dyslipidemia. Safety of treatment, changes in risk factors, and incidence of coronary heart disease. *N Engl J Med.* 317:1237-45.

Atherosclerosis

In atherosclerosis, subintimal plaques start in medium-sized blood vessel walls when LDL cholesterol accumulates. A cholesterol-rich necrotic core surrounded by smooth muscle cells and fibrous tissue then develops. These plaques can calcify. If the surface of the plaque ulcerates, thrombosis occurs, which can obliterate the lumen of a blood vessel.

Plaques may result from diffusion of elevated LDL cholesterol, a qualitative abnormality of LDL cholesterol, endothelial cell damage, or a combination of these. Endothelial cell damage may be due to the following:

- Physical trauma, e.g., with hypertension
- Toxins, e.g., tobacco or alcohol
- Low-grade infection or inflammation, e.g., *Chlamydia*
- Immune complex damage

CHD/atherosclerosis risk factors

Male sex, ↑age, and a positive family history are all linked with a greater risk for atherosclerosis, but these factors are beyond our control. Several modifiable risk factors are, however, recognized:

- *Cigarette smoking* >10 cigarettes/day increase the CHD odds ratio by 6.7-fold, while stopping smoking reduces risk of myocardial infarction (MI) by 50–70% within 5 years.
- *Hypertension* increases the CHD odds ratio by 2.7-fold. Each 1 mmHg drop in diastolic blood pressure reduces the MI risk by 2–3%. Aspirin reduces MI risk by 33%.
- *Diabetes mellitus* (📖 see Epidemiology, p. 605)
- *Hyperlipidemia:* A 10% fall in total cholesterol results in a 25% decrease in CHD risk, and plaque regression with reducing lipids is well documented.
- *Other:* Less strongly associated factors include type A personality, hyperuricemia, lack of exercise or sedentary lifestyle, and obesity.

Assessment of CHD risk

According to the Adult Treatment Panel (ATP) III guidelines, lipid-lowering therapy should be based on a person's absolute risk for CHD. This risk for CHD is divided into three categories: established CHD and CHD risk equivalents, multiple (2+) risk factors, and 0–1 risk factor.

Risk factors include cigarette smoking, hypertension (BP >140/90 mmHg or on antihypertensive therapy), HDL <40 mg/dL, family history of premature CHD (<55 years for males and <65 years for females, and age (men ≥45 years and women ≥55 years old).

One risk factor is subtracted from the count for an HDL >60 mg/dL.

CHD risk equivalents include diabetes and clinical atherosclerotic diseases such as peripheral arterial disease and carotid artery disease.

If an individual is noted to have multiple (2+) risk factors for CHD, a 10-year risk assessment for CHD should be carried out using Framingham risk scoring (see Tables 113.1 for men and 113.2 for women). The number of points for each risk factor is first calculated (risk factors include age, smoking, TC, HDL, and systolic BP), then management is determined on the basis of risk (see Chapter 116, p. 677).

Lipid measurements

Measurements should not be taken during an acute illness or during periods of rapid weight loss as these artificially lower the results. It is therefore recommended to measure a full lipid profile 8–12 weeks after the acute event.

However, according to the ATP III guidelines, a lipid analysis should be measured within 24 hours of an acute coronary event. This analysis is to serve as a guideline for initiating therapy in these individuals in which LDL lowering is crucial.

Pregnancy or recent weight gain will increase lipid levels. Following rapid weight gain or weight loss, at least one month should pass before reassessing lipid levels.

Full lipid profile
This gives the following:
- TC
- HDL cholesterol
- LDL cholesterol
- Triglycerides

Table 113.1 Estimate of 10-year risk for men (Framingham point scores).
Reprinted with permission from the Third Report of the National Cholesterol Education Program (NCEP) Expert Panel on Detection, Evaluation, and Treatment of High Blood Cholesterol in Adults (Adult Treatment Panel III) Final Report. *Circulation* 2002; 106(25):3143–3421.

Age	Points	Total Cholesterol	Points at Ages 20–39	Points at Ages 40–49	Points at Ages 50–59	Points at Ages 60–69	Points at Ages 70–79
20–34	−9	<160	0	0	0	0	0
35–39	−4	160–199	4	3	2	1	0
40–44	0	200–239	7	5	3	1	0
45–49	3	240–279	9	6	4	2	1
50–54	6	>280	11	8	5	3	1
55–59	8						
60–64	10	Nonsmoker	0	0	0	0	0
65–69	11	Smoker	8	5	3	1	1
70–74	12						
75–79	13						

HDL	Points
≥60	-1
50-59	0
40-49	1
<40	2

Systolic BP	If Untreated	If Treated
<120	0	0
120-129	0	1
130-139	1	2
140-159	1	2
≥160	2	3

Point Total	10-Year Risk
<0	<1%
0	1%
1	1%
2	1%
3	1%
4	1%
5	2%
6	2%
7	3%
8	4%
9	5%
10	6%

Point Total	10-Year Risk
11	8%
12	10%
13	12%
14	16%
15	20%
16	25%
≥17	≥30%

Table 113.2 The 10-year risk estimates for women (Framingham point scores). Reprinted with permission from the Third Report of the National Cholesterol Education Program (NCEP) Expert Panel on Detection, Evaluation, and Treatment of High Blood Cholesterol in Adults (Adult Treatment Panel III) Final Report. *Circulation* 2002; 106(25):3143–3421.

Age	Points	Total Cholesterol	Points at Ages 20–39	Points at Ages 40–49	Points at Ages 50–59	Points at Ages 60–69	Points at Ages 70–79
20–34	−7	<160	0	0	0	0	0
35–39	−3	160–199	4	3	2	1	1
40–44	0	200–239	8	6	4	2	1
45–49	3	240–279	11	8	5	3	2
50–54	6	≥280	13	10	7	4	2
55–59	8						
60–64	10	Nonsmoker	0	0	0	0	0
65–69	12	Smoker	9	7	4	2	1
70–74	14						
75–79	16						

HDL	Points
≥60	−1
50–59	0
40–49	1
<40	2

Systolic BP	If Untreated	If Treated
<120	0	0
120–129	1	3
130–139	2	4
140–159	3	5
≥160	4	6

Point Total	10-Year Risk	Point Total	10-Year Risk
<9	<1%	20	11%
9	1%	21	14%
10	1%	22	17%
11	1%	23	22%
12	1%	24	27%
13	2%	≥25	≥30%
14	2%		
15	3%		
16	4%		
17	5%		
18	6%		
19	8%		

This should be a fasting sample, preferably after a 9- to 12-hour[1] overnight fast (water is allowed). If nonfasting, only TC and HDL cholesterol measurements are accurate. Triglycerides rise postprandially and LDL is usually calculated with the formula below, so is inaccurate if not fasting. It is also invalid if triglycerides are >400 mg/dL:

LDL (in mg/dL) = TC − HDL − (TG/5)

ATP III introduced a new secondary target for patients with elevated triglycerides ≥200 mg/dL, non-HDL-C:

TC-HDL = LDL + VLDL= non-HDL-C

The goal for non-HDL-C is 30 mg/dL above the LDL goal.[1]

1 Third Report of the National Cholesterol Education Program (NCEP) Expert Panel on Detection, Evaluation, and Treatment of High Blood Cholesterol in Adults (Adult Treatment Panel III) final report. *Circulation* 2002; 106(25):3143–3421.

Primary hyperlipidemias

Background

There are two distinct elements in the diagnosis of primary hyperlipidemias: the genotype and the phenotype. The family history and the phenotypic findings in other family members are used as a surrogate for a genetic diagnosis. DNA-based technology currently employed in research can be clinically useful, not just for initial diagnosis but also for family screening.

Polygenic hypercholesterolemia

This is the most common cause of isolated hypercholesterolemia. LDL clearance appears to be reduced by a variety of mechanisms, and the E4 allele of apo E is a common association. Patients do not have the characteristic xanthelasmata or extensor tendon deposits (xanthomata) seen in familial hyperlipidemia.

It is usually diagnosed by primary screening programs or when investigating some manifestation of atherosclerosis.

Familial hypercholesterolemia (FH)

FH is an autosomal dominant disorder. Its gene frequency is 1 in 500 in Western Europe and North America.

In FH, hypercholesterolemia is mainly (>95%) due to an increase in LDL cholesterol because of an LDL receptor mutation (on the short arm of chromosome 19) reducing the number of high-affinity LDL receptors by up to 50%, so reducing LDL clearance and thus prolonging the circulating time before catabolism from the normal 2.5 days to >4.5 days.

More than 1000 mutations have so far been described. Less commonly, FH is due to familial defective apolipoprotein B-100 (3–4%) and proprotein convertase subtilisin/kexin 9 gene (*PCSK9*) mutation (<1%).

These can lead to several situations causing elevation of circulating LDL cholesterol by
- Not producing any LDL receptors.
- Failure of LDL receptors to move to the cell surface.
- Abnormal binding of the receptor to LDL.
- Inability to adequately internalize LDL for metabolism.

Patients with FH have premature CHD (i.e., men <55 years old, women <65 years old) and must be treated vigorously, as their standardized mortality ratio is at least $9\times$ greater than normal.

Clinical characterization

- TC >300 mg/dL (>481 mg/dL in homozygotes), LDL is high from birth.
- Normal triglycerides
- *Clinical stigmata:* xanthelasmic deposits around the eyes and on the tendons (i.e., fingers, hands, elbow, knee, and the Achilles tendon)

Tendon xanthoma is more specific for FH than corneal arcus or xanthelasma. 7% of heterozygote FH patients (aged >19 years of age) have tendon xanthomas, although 75% of their parents exhibit this feature. Separate studies suggest 75% of males and 72% of females with homozygous FH have tendon xanthomas. It is important to note that tendon xanthomata may not be present until after 40 years of age.

Early onset of a *corneal arcus* (in the 30- to 40-year age group) may occur.

Achilles tendonitis in childhood may be the first clue to the presence of FH.

Homozygotes can have CHD presenting in childhood and certainly before the age of 30. Heterozygotes usually present after 30 years of age.

A strong case can be made for FH where there may not be clinical stigmata but there is a strong family history and first-degree relatives with early-onset CHD, e.g., before 50 years of age.

It is estimated that >50% of heterozygous FH patients will die from CHD before reaching 60 years of age if left untreated. One in 20 patients under 60 years old surviving an MI are FH heterozygotes.

FH patients need to have their families investigated and the homozygous FH may need nonpharmacological therapies, such as plasmapheresis, or surgical procedures such as ileal bypass, portocaval shunts, or liver transplantation. These treatments are not readily available and, along with pharmacological treatments, may be superseded by gene therapy in the future.

Screening is by measurement of blood lipids and looking for clinical stigmata or signs. It should involve immediate family members and can be done at any age.

In newborn infants, cord blood has been used to look at LDL cholesterol levels, but this screening method may be unreliable, especially in heterozygote FH.

Screening children is best carried out before 10 years of age, and then again at adolescence and early childhood. Between the ages of 1 and 16 years, heterozygotes will have a 2-fold higher cholesterol level than that of unaffected siblings, so standard lipid profiles can be used.

Over 16 years of age, a full fasting lipid profile and clinical examination should be used.

Familial defective apolipoprotein B-100 (FDB)

FDB is an autosomal dominant trait in which a genetic defect of apo B-100 results in the delayed clearance of cholesterol. It is due to a single point mutation on apo B (e.g., Arg 3500 → Gln). This condition affects about 1/600 people.

All lipids originating from the liver are bound to apo B-100. Two different mutations have also been described that result in ↑ levels of an LDL more prone to oxidation, causing delayed receptor pathway clearance of LDL, which overloads the scavenger pathways, thereby increasing circulating cholesterol levels.

The diagnosis is made on slowly rising cholesterol levels and DNA studies for the point mutation. The management is similar to that of FH. 2% of cases previously described as FH are estimated to be due to FDB. Protease inhibitors have been reported to exacerbate this condition, which may present with eruptive xanthomata.

Familial hypertriglyceridemia

This affects up to 1/300 people, often as an autosomal dominant trait with elevated VLDL levels, and is frequently accompanied by hypercholesterolemia.

Eruptive xanthomata (red and painful) and lipemia retinalis can accompany massive triglyceridemia, as can pancreatitis.

Exacerbating factors include alcohol and drugs such as thiazide diuretics, glucocorticoids, and the oral contraceptive pill.

Adherence to a low-fat, alcohol-free diet with weight reduction usually helps.

Rare genetic hypertriglyceridemias

Two rare but important familial causes of gross hypertriglyceridemia are lipoprotein lipase deficiency and apolipoprotien C-II deficiency. Both are autosomal recessive conditions that present in childhood and are characterized by the presence of hyperchylomicronemia.

Lipoprotein lipase is the enzyme needed to metabolize chylomicrons; complete absence of this enzyme and production of an inactive form are both recognized defects. A usually heterozygous, but much rarer and more severe homozygous form is also seen.

Apo C-II is needed for the activation of lipoprotein lipase, and its deficiency results in hyperchylomicronemia. Patients do not have premature CHD but can have recurrent abdominal pain due to pancreatitis.

Familial combined hyperlipidemia (FCHL)

FCHL is a definite risk factor for CHD. It occurs in 1/250 people.

Patients usually present around 10 years later than those with FH. The etiology is not known.

It is the most common type of inherited dyslipidemia, estimated to cause 10% of cases of premature CHD.

It has no unique clinical manifestations and the diagnosis is based on raised lipids (>95th centile for age) and a family history of premature CHD in first-degree relatives.

Familial dysbetalipoproteinemia

This is also known as type III hyperlipidemia or broad beta disease. It is associated with early-onset CHD.

It is an uncommon disorder affecting 0.01–0.04% of people, with elevated IDL and chylomicron remnants.

A characteristic clinical feature is the presence of palmar striae xanthoma (orange-yellow discolorations of the palmar creases). Tuberous xanthomata, found over the tuberosities of the elbows and knees, may also be present. The xanthomata of this familial disease can also be found in pressure areas, e.g., heels.

Apo E is a constituent lipoprotein of IDL that has three genetically determined isoforms: E_2, E_3, and E_4.

- E_3/E_3 occurs in 55% of people, E_2/E_2 occurs in 1%.
- E_2 has the lowest binding affinity to the apo receptors and is therefore cleared from serum mostly slowly.
- Apo E_4 has the greatest affinity and is more rapidly cleared.
- Patients with familial dysbetalipoproteinemia are phenotype E_2/E_2.

Rare familial mixed dyslipidemias

These should be considered in any patient with unexplained neurological symptoms, organomegaly, or corneal opacities.

Two inborn metabolic disorders associated with atherosclerosis are as follows:

- *Apolipoprotein A1-CIII deficiency:* should be suspected if hyperlipidemia is corrected within 24 hours of infusing 500 mL of normal fresh frozen plasma
- *Familial lecithin:cholesterol acyltransferase (LCAT) deficiency:* In this recessively inherited disorder, an enzyme necessary for intravascular lipoprotein metabolism is deficient, resulting in elevated cholesterol and triglycerides. Clinically, corneal lipid deposits result in visual disturbances and renal deposits in glomerular damage, proteinuria, and, often, renal failure.

The following disorders are not linked to the occurrence of premature atheroma formation:

- *Tangier disease (analphalipoproteinemia or familial alphalipoprotein deficiency):* In this autosomal recessive condition, apo A-I, which is found on HDL, is deficient. HDL level is low (<5 mg/dL), as is TC, while triglycerides are normal or high. Cholesterol accumulation gives enlarged, orange tonsils, hepatosplenomegaly, polyneuropathy, and corneal opacities.
- *Fish eye disease:* a rare disorder from northern Sweden characterized by high VLDL levels, low HDL, fasting hypertriglyceridemia, and a triglyceride rich LDL. It is a variant of familial LCAT deficiency. Dense corneal opacities occur, resulting in visual impairment.
- *Abetalipoproteinemia:* results in fat accumulation due to failure of apo B-100 production. Cholesterol levels are low with, in many cases, no LDL and VLDL. This results in fat accumulation in the gut and nerves. Vitamin E injections may prevent some of the neurological abnormalities observed (ataxia, nystagmus, dysarthria, and motor plus sensory neuropathies), but usually not the retinitis pigmentosa and acanthocytes, which are also features.
- *Hypobetalipoproteinemia:* This autosomal dominantly inherited condition gives a TC of 38.5–154 mg/dL and can be associated with organomegaly and neurological changes in middle age due to fat deposition and abnormal red cells. The homozygous state is similar to abetalipoproteinemia.
- *Hyperalphalipoproteinemia or HDL hyperlipoproteinemia:* results in mildly elevated HDL and TC, and may be beneficial. No treatment is needed; raised HDL can also occur with exercise, exogenous estrogen, and phenytoin and phenobarbital use, or from alcohol.

Secondary hyperlipidemias

Background

Secondary dyslipidemias are relatively common, accounting for 10–20% of hyperlipidemic adults. These can give a mixed hyperlipidemia or a lone increase in cholesterol or triglycerides.

There are multiple causes, and treatment is based on managing the primary disease before making a further decision on the raised lipids. Often more than one cause is apparent in secondaryehyperlipidemias.

Causes

Causes include those described below and listed in Table 115.1.

Table 115.1 Potential causes of secondary hyperlipidemia

Elevated LDL cholesterol	Elevated triglycerides	Reduced HDL cholesterol
Diet (high saturated fats, high calories, anorexia)	Diet (weight gain + excess alcohol)	Diet (some low-fat diets)
Drugs (glucocorticoids, thiazide + loop diuretics, ciclosporin)	Drugs (glucocorticoids, β-blockers, estrogens, isotretinoin)	Drugs (anabolic steroids, tobacco, β-adrenergic blockers)
Hypothyroidism	Hypothyroidism	Type 2 diabetes
Nephrotic syndrome	Type 2 diabetes	Insulin resistance syndromes/obesity
Chronic liver disease	Insulin resistance syndromes	Chronic renal failure
Cholestasis + biliary obstruction	Cushing's syndrome	
Cholestasis + biliary obstruction	Cushing's syndrome	
Pregnancy	Chronic renal failure Peritoneal dialysis Pregnancy	

Diet
Excessive consumption of saturated fats and carbohydrate can contribute to this condition. Anorexia nervosa can also cause hypercholesterolemia, as a strict low-fat, low-calorie diet results in reduced cholesterol and bile acid turnover, thus increasing circulating levels.

Obesity
📖 See Clinical features (p. 528).

Diabetes mellitus
📖 See Lipid abnormalities found in patients with diabetes (p. 629).

Hypothyroidism
This is estimated to occur in 4% of those with hyperlipidemia, and compensated (subclinical) hypothyroidism in a further 10%. It usually results in hypercholesterolemia with a TC of 349–776 mg/dL. It also worsens genetic dyslipidemias through ↓ synthesis of hepatic LDL receptors.

Chronic renal disease
Increased creatinine clearance is accompanied by hypertriglyceridemia and a reduction in HDL cholesterol. Proteinuria in the nephrotic syndrome is associated with hypercholesterolemia. Peritoneal dialysis may increase gut glucose load and worsen hypertriglyceridemia. Remember—cyclosporine increases LDL cholesterol.

Liver disease
Cholestatic liver disease results in hypercholesterolemia. Primary biliary cirrhosis produces marked increases in LDL and may elevate TC to >462 mg/dL. Severe hepatocellular damage may lower LDL cholesterol by d production of its component parts and the enzymes that metabolize it.

Cushing's syndrome
Glucocorticoids increase VLDL production and thus hypertriglyceridemia. The associated weight gain and glucose intolerance can make this effect more pronounced.

Lipodystrophies
This is a very rare group of congenital or acquired disorders whose hallmark is regional, partial, or generalized fat loss associated with hyperlipidemia, especially unusually raised triglycerides. They are also associated with severe insulin resistance.

Glycogen storage diseases
Elevated lipids (triglycerides, cholesterol and mixed hyperlipidemia) are common, but usually only in type I (Von Gierke disease), type III (Forbes disease), and type IV (Hers disease).

Gout
Hypertriglyceridemia occurs in about one-third of those with gout. Alcohol excess plays a part but it is not the sole cause.

Drugs

Medications commonly implicated are as follows:

- β-blockers, especially the noncardioselective ones
- Thiazide diuretics
- Exogenous estrogens
- Anabolic steroids
- Glucocorticoids
- Isotretinoin
- Protease inhibitors (said to cause hyperlipidemia in 50% after 10 months of treatment)

Excessive alcohol consumption

There is a J-shaped relationship between alcohol consumption and CHD. The American Heart Association (AHA) recommends no more than 1 alcoholic drink per day for women, and 2 drinks per day for men.

Pregnancy

Cholesterol rises throughout pregnancy, mostly in the second trimester, with LDL-C levels peaking mid-third trimester. Triglyceride levels follow a similar pattern to that of LDL-C. Levels decrease by 6 weeks postpartum but may take up to 1 year to return to normal.

Management of dyslipidemia

Background

The emphasis will depend on the cause of the hyperlipidemia and is aimed at reducing cardiovascular, peripheral vascular, and cerebrovascular risk. There are now recommended target values when treating patients.

Primary and secondary prevention

It is universally accepted that tackling hypercholesterolemia in secondary prevention works. We now have solid evidence to support this, especially in the context of CHD, where a 10% fall in TC is estimated to result in a 25% decrease in CHD risk.

Fatty lesion regression has also been clearly demonstrated. The gain is within 2 years of lowering the cholesterol, whether by diet or a combination of diet and drugs.

Two groups need special mention: patients with type 2 diabetes mellitus and those with acute coronary syndrome. Both groups show early benefit with statin treatment (high-dose atorvastatin 80 mg).

In post-MI patients, omega-3 fatty acids are recommended as they reduce the incidence of sudden death due to arrhythmias.

Tackling cholesterol in primary prevention is controversial. There have been primary prevention trials showing benefit from lowering cholesterol. The financial burden of this has to be confronted.

Specific interventions

Dietary advice

All patients should see a dietitian. Total fat intake should constitute <35% of energy consumed (with the majority of fat intake being from polyunsaturated and monounsaturated fats) and saturated fats must be <30% of the total fat content. Vegetable and marine mono- and polyunsaturated fats should be ↑ in the diet. Total dietary cholesterol should not exceed 200 mg/day.

Foods advocated include fresh fruits and vegetables, which are also important sources of antioxidants. These foods should be tried for 3 months to see if dietary manipulation will work (monitor at 6-week intervals). It is unusual to see >15% fall in cholesterol from dietary measures; a reduction of 5% is more likely in free-living individuals on a diet.

Alcohol intake should be no more than 1 drink per day for a female and no more than 2 drinks per day for a male. At this level, alcohol intake confers CHD protection in men >40 years old and postmenopausal women.

Plant sterols and stanols, 2 g daily, can reduce blood cholesterol by 10–15%. They are available commercially in enriched margarine spreads, yogurt, and milky drinks.

Weight control

All overweight patients must be encouraged to lose weight. Weight reduction is closely attuned to dietary advice and physical exercise. Most weight is lost in the first 4 months of a regimen. A 10 kg weight loss in an obese subject can reduce LDL cholesterol by 7% and increases HDL cholesterol by 13%.

Physical activity

Physical activity, especially aerobic exercise, is recommended. This should involve moderate intensity exercise performed for a minimum of 30 minutes, at least 5 times per week.

Acute exercise will transiently change lipoprotein levels and increase lipoprotein lipase activity. These effects become more permanent with regular training.

Triglyceride levels fall, HDL cholesterol levels rise, especially the HDL_2 subfraction, with more vigorous exercise, and the LDL cholesterol is of the less-dense variety, which is not so atherogenic. The changes are dose dependent with ↑ exercise, and a 20% alteration in each variable is achievable after 6 weeks.

Modification of other risk factors

Other risk factors such as hypertension, smoking, and diabetes mellitus must also be addressed.

Drug therapy

Numerous agents can be used for both primary and secondary prevention in patients in whom diet has been ineffective.

HMG CoA reductase inhibitors (statins)

Indications

These include high LDL or VLDL, i.e., primary hypercholesterolemia, heterozygous + homozygous FH, mixed hyperlipidemia. Not all of these medications are licensed for use in children and should be used with caution in women of childbearing age because of insufficient safety data on pregnancy and of potential teratogenicity.

The medication should be stopped for at least 3 months before pregnancy is planned. Women must be warned about pregnancy when on these drugs.

Mechanism of action

There is competitive inhibition of 3-hydroxy-3-methylglutaryl coenzyme A (HMG CoA), which is the rate-limiting enzyme in cholesterol synthesis. Its activation increases hepatocyte LDL receptor numbers and reduces VLDL synthesis while enhancing its hepatic clearance.

📖 See Table 116.1 for a comparative lipid-lowering profile and Table 116.2 for dosage.

Table 116.1 Comparative lipid lowering profile of statins

Statin	% Fall in LDLc	% Fall in triglycerides	% Rise in HDLc
Atorvastatin	38–54	13–32	3–7
Fluvastatin	17–34	8–12	3–6
Pravastatin	18–34	5–13	5–8
Rosuvastatin	50–63	10–28	3–14
Simvastatin	26–48	12–38	8–12

Side effects

Statins are usually very well tolerated but are known to cause headaches, nausea, and some abdominal discomfort. The main concerns are a hepatitis-like picture and myopathy.

LFTs and creatine kinase should be measured before statins are prescribed. They should be used with caution in those with excessive alcohol intake. It is recommended that the medication be discontinued if liver enzymes aspartate transaminase (AST) and/or alanine transaminase (ALT) show >3-fold elevation above the upper limit of normal.

LFTs should be checked every 3–4 months initially and at least annually in the long term. Statin-associated myopathy is rare and tends to occur when prescribed with other medications, e.g., cyclosporine, fibrates, or macrolide antibiotics or when renal impairment or untreated hypothyroidism is present.

Clinically, there is a picture of swollen tender muscles and creatine kinase >10×the upper limit of normal. Rhabdomyolysis is even rarer.

Interactions

All statins can interact with cyclosporine and nicotinic acid and are used with caution with fibrates.

Warfarin interacts with atorvastatin, simvastatin, and rosuvastatin. Erythromycin interacts with all statins.

Digoxin interacts with atorvastatin and simvastatin. Rifampicin interacts with fluvastatin and pravastatin.

Atorvastatin and rosuvastatin may also interact with the oral contraceptive pill, antacids, and some antifungals.

Fibrates

Indications

These are high VLDL, triglycerides, or IDL, i.e., mixed hyperlipidemias that have not responded adequately to diet or other therapy. These medications are less effective than the statins at lowering cholesterol but better at ↑ HDL cholesterol and more effective in lowering triglycerides.

Reduce triglycerides by 20–60%, increase HDL by 15–30%, and reduce LDL by 5–25%.

Mechanism of action

Fibrates alter lipoprotein metabolism to reduce VLDL triglyceride synthesis by ↑ lipoprotein lipase activity and LDL-receptor-mediated LDL clearance while increasing HDL synthesis.

The effect on LDL cholesterol may vary in isolated hypertriglyceridemia to increase LDL cholesterol. 📖 See Table 116.2 for dosage.

Side effects

Occasionally, fibrates cause nausea, anorexia, or diarrhea and precipitate gallstones (mostly clofibrate, although this is not approved in the U.S.). Also, pruritus, rashes, hair loss, and impotence can occur.

They should not be used in patients with severe liver disease (AST/ALT >2–3× upper limit of normal) and renal dysfunction (creatinine >2 mg/dL), as they are conjugated in the liver prior to excretion by the kidney.

Myopathy, although rare, is the main concern, and the risk of this increases if fibrates are used with statins.

Table 116.2 Dosage of lipid-lowering drugs

Drug	Dose/day
Statins	
Atorvastatin	10–80 mg
Fluvastatin	20–80 mg
Pravastatin	10–40 mg
Rosuvastatin	10–40 mg (5–20 mg in patient of Asian origin)
Simvastatin	10–80 mg
Fibrates	
Clofibrate	50–65 kg, 1.5 g; >65 kg, 2 g
Fenofibrate	67–267 mg
Gemfibrozil	0.9–1.2 g
Anion-exchange resins	
Cholestyramine	12–36 g (in single dose or up to 4× day)
Colestipol hydrochloride	5 g 1–2×day (max 30 g/day)
Colesevelam	1.875 g (oral suspension or 3 tablets) twice daily with meals
Nicotinic acid group	
Niacin	1.5–6 g in divided doses
Niaspan®	500–2000 mg
Omega-3 fatty acids	
Omacor®	1–4 g
Lovaza®	1–4 g
Cholesterol absorption blocker	
Ezetimibe	10 mg

Interactions

Use with caution in combination with statins. Fibrates can enhance the effects of warfarin and antidiabetic agents and are contraindicated in those on orlistat.

Anion exchange resins (bile acid sequestrants)

Indications

These include high LDL, i.e., hypercholesterolemia. Although largely superseded by statins, these are now best used as adjuncts when LDL has not fallen enough with a statin alone. They are also the only drug licensed for use during pregnancy.

Mechanism of action

These agents bind to bile acids in the gut, thus reducing their enterohepatic circulation and increasing bile acid excretion. This increases hepatocyte cholesterol requirements, which increases LDL receptor production, thus reducing circulating LDL levels.

Under optimum conditions, LDL cholesterol can be reduced by 20–30%, triglycerides rise by 10–17%, and HDL increases by 3–5%.

Side effects

These agents remain in the gut, so constipation, bloating, nausea, and abdominal discomfort are not uncommon. Constipation, found in 35–40% of those on these agents, can be helped with bulking laxatives. Less often a bleeding tendency due to vitamin K malabsorption can be seen.

These agents can also exacerbate hypertriglyceridemia, but HDL cholesterol is often ↑ slightly. To reduce the side effects, patients should start with low doses and build up gradually over the next 3–4 weeks while maintaining a good fluid intake.

Interactions

These agents can reduce the absorption of warfarin, digoxin, β-blockers, pravastatin, fluvastatin, and hydrochlorothiazide. Many other agents such as simvastatin have not been checked, so to avoid any potential interaction, advise patients to take all other drugs 1 hour before or 4 hours after the resin.

Nicotinic acid

Indications

These include high LDL, VLDL, IDL, or triglycerides. Nicotinic acid is the most effective medication for ↑ HDL-cholesterol.

In practice, however, their use is limited by the side-effect profile, especially flushing. Niaspan®, a modified-release nicotinic acid product, is now available and does seem to cause fewer unwanted side effects and should be the first choice.

Mechanism of action

Nicotinic acid works by inhibiting lipolysis in adipocytes, thus altering fatty acid flux and reducing VLDL synthesis and HDL clearance. VLDL levels fall, as do those of triglycerides (by 20–50%) and LDL (by 5–25%), whereas HDL levels rise (by 10–50%).

Side effects
Side effects are common, with 30% of patients being unable to tolerate these agents. Vasodilatation giving cutaneous/facial flushing occurs in most patients but tends to improve after 2–3 weeks of therapy or if patients are given prostaglandin inhibitors such as aspirin in combination with nicotinic acid.

Patients should avoid taking it with hot drinks as these increase its absorption and worsen the flushing. Gastritis is also a common problem; the more severe hepatitis occurs in only 3%.

Tachycardias, dry skin, and exacerbations of gout and precipitation of acanthosis nigricans and retinal edema are also recognized side effects.

Nicotinic acid can adversely affect glucose control in diabetes mellitus.

Interactions
These agents potentiate the effects of antihypertensive therapies.

Omega-3 fatty acids (Omacor®, Lovaza®)
Indications
These include severe hypertriglyceridemia.

Mechanism of action
They inhibit the secretion of VLDL through ↑ intracellular apo B-100 destruction. Normal patients see both a fall in VLDL and LDL, but LDL may rise in the hypertriglyceridemic individual.

Side effects
As high doses are needed, this high-calorie load may increase obesity. More commonly it gives nausea and belching. Omacor® produces fewer unwanted effects and is less calorific, as it is used in a smaller dose.

Interactions
There are none that are significant.

Cholesterol absorption blocker
Presently only one preparation, ezetimibe, is available, and is now the second-line of treatment after a statin.

Indications
This agent is used for LDL cholesterol-lowering in patients who are intolerant of statins or in combination with a statin in those whose levels are not adequately controlled with a statin alone.

It is also used in the very rare condition of sitosterolemia, where there is an ↑ absorption of plant sterols.

Mechanism of action
Dietary and biliary cholesterol absorption is selectively inhibited. Ezetimibe (10 mg) monotherapy produces an 18% fall in LDL cholesterol, an increase in HDL cholesterol of 1–3%, and triglycerides are not affected. In combination therapy with a statin, ezetimibe reduces levels by an additional 22% to that obtained by statin alone.

Interactions
None are significant.

Which drug to use when (for diet-resistant dyslipidemias)

Elevated LDL cholesterol only

First choice
- Statins

Second choice
- Cholesterol absorption blocker

Then:
- Bile acid sequestrants
- Nicotinic acid
- Fibrates

Combination therapy if the above fail to reduce LDL adequately includes:
- Statin + bile acid sequestrant (can give 50% fall in LDL + 10–15% rise in HDL)
- Statin + cholesterol absorption blocker (can give an additional 22% fall in LDL + 3% rise in HDL)
- Statin + nicotinic acid (can give 50% fall in LDL + 25–50% rise in HDL)
- Nicotinic acid + bile acid sequestrants (can give 35% fall in LDL + 25–50% rise in HDL)
- Statin + bile acid sequestrant + nicotinic acid (can give 66% fall in LDL + 25–50% rise in HDL)

Elevated triglycerides only

First choice
- Fibrates

Second choice
- Omega-3 fatty acids

Third choice
- Nicotinic acid

All three groups can occasionally be used together if one or two of the above groups are insufficient.

Mixed hyperlipidemia

First choice
- Fibrate

Second choice
- Fibrate + statin (but needs close monitoring)
- Fibrate + nicotinic acid

As with elevated LDL alone, combination therapy may sometimes be useful with emphasis on avoiding side effects and interactions as above.

Aims of treatment

In the United States the decision to treat lipids is based on an assessment of any individual's cardiovascular risk:

- For individuals with 0–1 risk factor, the LDL goal is <160 mg/dL.
- For individuals with multiple (2+) risk factors, LDL goal is <130 mg/dL.

For patients with CHD and CHD risk equivalents, the primary treatment goal is as follows:

- LDL cholesterol <100 mg/dL with a therapeutic option for <70 mg/dL
- Although an optimal triglyceride value is <150 and an optimal HDL is >40 (men), the primary goal of treatment is LDL lowering.

An alternative to the above is to begin assessment with the Framingham risk scoring (10-year risk assessment) (see Tables 113.1, pp. 664–665 and 113.2, pp. 666–667) and use the associated goals listed in Table 116.3.

Table 116.3	
10-year risk	**LDL goal**
≥20%	<100 mg/dL
10–20%	<130 mg/dL
<10% with multiple (2+) risk factors	<130 mg/dL
<10% with 0–1 risk factor	<160 mg/dL

Further reading

American Diabetes Association (2004). Position statement, Dyslipidemia management in aduts with diabetes. *Diabetes Care Suppl* 21:s68–s71.

Bhatnagar D (2006). Diagnosis and screening for familial hypercholesterolaemia: finding the patient, finding the genes. *Ann Clin Biochem* 43:441–456.

Cannon CP, Braunwald E, McCabe CH, et al. (2004). Intensive versus moderate lipid lowering with statins after acute coronary syndromes. *N Engl J Med* 350:1495–1504.

Colhoun H, Betteridge DJ, Durrington PN, et al. (2005). Rapid emergence of effect of atorvastatin on cardiovascular outcomes in the collaborative atorvastatin diabetes study (CARDS). *Diabetelogia* 48:2482–2485.

De Backer G, Ambrosioni E, Borch-Johnsen K, et al. (2003). European guidelines on cardiovascular disease prevention in clinical practice. *Eur Heart J* 24, 1601–10.

Downs JR, Clearfield M, Wies S, et al. (1998). Primary prevention of acute coronary events with lovastatin in men and women with average cholesterol levels: results of AFCAP/TexCAPS. Air Force/Texas Coronary Atherosclerosis Prevention Study. *JAMA* 299:1615–1621.

Durrington P (2003). Dyslipidaemia. *Lancet* 362:717–731.

Dyslipidaemia Advisory Group, on behalf of the Scientific Committee of the National Heart Foundation of New Zealand (1996). 1996 National Heart Foundation guidelines for the assessment and management of dyslipidaemia. *N Z Med J* 109:224–232.

Hippisley-Cox J, Coupland C, Vinogradova Y, et al. (2007). Derivation and validation of QRISK, a new cardiovascular dis-ease score for United Kingdom: prospective open cohort study. *BMJ* 335:136–141.

International Atherosclerosis Society (1996). *Clinician's Manual on Hyperlipidaemia*, 4th ed. London: Science Press.

Joint British Society 2 (2005). Joint British Societies' Guidelines on prevention of cardiovascular disease in clinical practice. *Heart* 91 (Suppl 5):1–52.

National Institute for Health and Clinical Excellence (2006). Statins for the prevention of cardio-vascular events. *Technology Appraisal* 94. http://www.nice.org.uk/TA094

Reckless JPD (1996). Economic issues in coronary heart disease prevention. *Curr Opin Lipidol* 7:356–362.

Royal College of General Practitioners (1992). Guidelines for the management of hyperlipidaemia in general practice. *Occas Pap R Coll Gen Pract* 55:1-15.

Sacks FM, Pfeffer MA, Moye LA, et al. (1996). The effect of pravastatin on coronary events after myocardial infarction in patients with average cholesterol levels. *N Engl J Med* 335:1001–1009.

Scandinavian Simvastatin Survival Study Group (1994). Randomized trial of cholesterol lowering in 4444 patients with CHD: the Scandinavian Simvastatin Survival Study. *Lancet* 334:1383–1389.

Shepherd J, Cobbe SM, Ford I, et al. (1995). West of Scotland Coronary Prevention Study Group. Prevention of CHD with pravastatin in men with hypercholesterolemia. *N Engl J Med* 333:1301–1307.

Part 13

Laboratory endocrinology

E. Chester Ridgway

Pitfalls in laboratory endocrinology

Introduction

The previous issue of this Handbook contained a chapter entitled "Normal ranges" for endocrine-related laboratory tests. The purpose of this chapter is to explain why this compendium of data needs to be viewed with a degree of caution and why you, as a clinical endocrinologist, should be actively liaising with your laboratory service about the assays that they provide, their reference ranges, and the performance of these assays.

Laboratory methods are complex and are affected by a number of factors (Box 117.1) that can often only be considered and explored if information is shared by frequent liaison between clinicians and laboratory scientists. Uncritical use of numbers obtained from the literature may lead to errors and bad management decisions.

Box 117.1 Factors to be considered for laboratory investigations

Pre-analytical factors
- Sample timing
- Which tube?
- Sample transport factors
- Biological variation
- Which stimulation test?

Analytical factors
- Assay specificity
- Assay standardization
- Analytical performance
- Hook effects
- Antibody interference
- Particularly problematic assays

Post-analytical factors
- Reference ranges
- Units
- Interpretation

Pre-analytical factors

Half of all errors in the diagnostic process are due to pre-analytical factors (Box 117.2), and 20% of errors are related to sample collection. Even in hospitals where there is a heightened awareness of these problems, there is a prevalence of 1% pre-analytical errors.

These effects can be of sufficient magnitude to alter the analysis enough to create situations for clinical errors. Most problems can be prevented by clear instructions and documented policies for sampling.

Some issues are relatively straightforward, such as collecting the sample into the correct blood tube and ensuring that samples are transported to the laboratory fast enough at the correct temperature. A comprehensive list can be found at http://www.specimencare.com/.

In order to be certain whether two or more samples taken from an individual are different, it is important to consider the biological variation that naturally occurs (see Box 117.3). A comprehensive list can be found at http://www.westgard.com/intra-inter.htm.

In addition, the clearance t½ of each hormone should be considered: endogenous hormones and tumor markers are like pharmaceuticals and 90% of the change occurs after 4.5x t½.

Box 117.2 Examples of pre-analytical errors

- Incorrectly or unlabeled samples
- Undefined or inappropriate sample timing
- Wrong tubes
- Hemolysis
- Lipemia
- Delayed transport
- Incorrect transport temperature

Box 117.3 Examples of within-person (biological) variation

Aldosterone	29%
Androstenedione	16%
CA125	36%
CA153	5.7%
CEA	10.6%
DHAS	3.4%
Prolactin	24%
SHBG	9%
Testosterone (male)	10%
TSH	20%

Variation expressed as cv(%) [Coefficient of variation = (standard deviation/ mean)*100]

Many endocrine function tests require stimulation tests. What is the evidence for the one you plan to use? How much difference exists for different stimulation tests? For examples of the effects of different stimulants of GH see Rahim et al. (1996).[1]

Analytical factors

Most endocrine assays are immunoassays that rely on binding of a hormone or metabolite by a diagnostic antibody. The binding specificity will depend on the care and attention with which the manufacturer has chosen the reagents.

Typical interferences may be due to slightly different molecular forms such as occurs with steroid or thyroid hormones. Peptide hormones are more complex because so many differently glycosylated isoforms of those peptides exist.

Standards for pituitary hormones are generally derived from purified pituitary extracts that contain a mixture of peptides. This leads to different assays having quite marked biases between each other due to different binding affinities of the antibodies to the different isoforms. A similar situation exists with hCG, for which many multiple molecular forms co-exist.

Attempts to find international consensus for standards that can be used in diagnostic systems are being made, particularly for growth hormone and glycated hemoglobin.

Analytical performance or assay reproducibility is important in determining the critical differences between patient samples. A significant difference between consecutive samples at 95% confidence will require a difference of 1.96x the method standard deviation at the appropriate concentration.

The hook effect occurs when very high hormone concentrations flood the available antibody in vitro, leading to artifactually low results. It is less common as assays have larger dynamic ranges, but new cases continue to be reported, and there are published case reports for all hormones and tumor markers.

Antibody interference is a widespread problem that affects approximately 1% of immunoassays. It is insidious and due to endogenous antibodies that interfere with hormone binding in vitro. Most importantly, they cannot be detected by usual-quality control mechanisms. There are a number of laboratory techniques that can be used to clarify whether such interference is present, but it is inherent on the clinician to alert the laboratory to a potential clinical mismatch.

Some assays can only be classified as problem assays. These include thyroglobulin and low concentrations of estradiol (<300 pmol/L) and testosterone (<5 nmol/L). The former is due to the high prevalence of endogenous antithyroglobulin antibodies, which are particularly prevalent in patients with thyroid disease. The latter are due to antibody specificity; however, it is hoped that this will be resolved with the introduction of mass spectrometry into routine clinical practice.

1 Rahim A, Toogood AA, Shalet SM (1996). The assessment of growth hormone status in normal young adult males using a variety of provocative agents. *Clin Endocrinol* 45:557–562.

Post-analytical factors

Interpretation of assay results is made in relation to reference ranges provided by the laboratory. These usually represent the 95th percentiles of a population of healthy individuals. However, the definition of *normality* is subjective, and reference ranges are affected by such factors as age, gender, and, in some cases, ethnicity.

Moreover, for hormones, time of day, month, and season are important. For some hormones, it is difficult to obtain appropriate samples to construct ranges, such as in children, and in circumstances that make it difficult to obtain samples in health, e.g., following pharmacological stimulation or samples of CSF.

If the central 95th percentile reference ranges are used, there is a 5% chance that a result will be out of range due to chance. As the number of tests taken are ↑, so will the risk of a chance abnormality. The increase will be x% (where $x = 1 - 0.95^a$, and a is the number of tests performed).

Literature from U.S. and European journals may use different units—beware! SI units use molar or mass (g) and volumes are reported in liters.

Most assays are standardized with international preparations. These are usually the molecular forms that are most prevalent when basal samples are taken. However, following stimulation, nonstandard molecules are released into the circulation that have different clearance rates and different binding characteristics to the diagnostic antibodies in vitro.

This can lead to marked differences between methods. For example, following stimulation by ACTH, corticosteroid precursors are released that will compete with cortisol for binding in the assay. Similarly, following stimulation of GH release, different isoforms of GH are secreted and the most abundant 20 and 22kDa isoforms clear at different rates, leading to variations in recognition by the diagnostic antibodies at different times during the test.

Box 117.4 Disastrous outcomes

Assay interference

A series of patients has been described in whom aggressive therapy for choriocarcinoma was instituted for diagnoses based on assays affected by in vitro artifacts.

Antibody specificity

A patient has been described who had prolactin measured by three different assays, giving three different answers. The solution awaited a clinical answer when the hyperprolactinemia resolved after the offending medication was stopped.

Interference by insulin autoantibodies

A patient has been described with recurrent hypoglycemia due to insulin autoantibodies caused by myeloma. This patient demonstrated in vivo interference by endogenous antibodies as well as in vitro interference.

Hook effect

A patient presents with a large pituitary tumor that appears nonfunctioning; prolactin is normal and the patient is treated surgically. The next day, the blood sample is reassayed after dilution, and high prolactin is uncovered when the antibody is no longer flooded by excess prolactin.

Reference intervals

Introduction

> **Box 118.1 Definitions**
>
> - *Serum* A serum sample is collected in a plain tube, left to permit clotting, then centrifuged and separated.
> - *Plasma* A plasma specimen is collected in a tube containing EDTA or lithium heparin, centrifuged immediately, and separated.
>
> All values are for serum unless specified otherwise.

Thyroid function

Table 118.1 Thyroid Function Tests

Hormone	SI Units	Traditional units	Conversion factor
TSH	0.35–4.50 mU/L	0.35–4.50 mU/L	1
Total T$_4$	60–140 nmol/L	4.5–11.0 mcg/dL	12.9
Free T$_4$	10.3–22.7 pmol/L	0.8–1.8 ng/dL	12.9
Total T$_3$	1.2–2.8 nmol/L	80–180 ng/dL	0.0154
Free T$_3$	3.5–6.5 pmol/L	2.3–4.3 pg/mL	1.54
Thyroglobulin	1.0–30 mcg/L	1.0–30 ng/mL	1

Acid-containing container (20 mL 6M HCl).

Adrenal and gonadal function

Table 118.2 Adrenal and gonadal function tests

Hormone		SI units	Traditional units	Conversion factor
Cortisol (9 A.M.)		140–635 nmol/L	5–23 mcg/dL	27.6
Aldosterone	Supine	0.8–3.0 nmol/L	3–10 ng/dL	0.0277
	Erect	1.4–8.0 nmol/L	5–30 ng/dL	0.0277
Plasma renin activity	Supine		0.6–3 mcg/L/hr	
	Erect		3–10.8 mcg/L/hr	
DHEAS	Women	6–10 micromol/L	22–380 mcg/dL	0.0027
	Men	6–17 micromol/L	22–640 mcg/dL	0.0027
Androstene-dione	Women	0.3–7.4 nmol/L	0.1–2.1 ng/mL	3.49
	Men	1.0–4.6 nmol/L	0.3–1.3 ng/mL	3.49
17–hydroxy-progesterone	Women	0.3–10 nmol/L	0.1–2.9 ng/mL	3.3
	Men	0.3–4.6 nmol/L	0.1–1.4 ng/mL	3.3
Estradiol	Women			
	Pre-M	110–1468 pmol/L	30–400 pg/mL	3.6
	Post-M	0–110 pmol/L	0–30 pg/mL	3.6
	Men	36–185 pmol/L	10–50 pg/mL	3.6
Progesterone	Follicular	<3 nmol/L	<1.0 ng/mL	3.2
	Luteal	6.5–80 nmol/L	2.0–25 ng/mL	3.2
	Men	<3 nmol/L	<1.0 ng/mL	3.2
Testosterone	Men	6.9–38 nmol/L	200–1080 ng/dL	0.035
	Women	0.35–2.45 nmol/L	10–70 ng/dL	0.035
Dihydro-testosterone	Men	1–2.6 nmol/L	29–76 ng/dL	0.034
	Women	0.3–0.8 nmol/L	8.7–23 ng/dL	0.034
Sex hormone binding globulin	Women	18–114 nmol/L	18–114 nmol/L	1
	Men	13–71 nmol/L	13–71 nmol/L	1

*A variety of different units are used by non-UN labs.

Pituitary hormones

Table 118.3 Pituitary hormones

Hormone		SI units	Traditional units	Conversion factor
FSH	Follicular	0.5–5 IU/L	0.5–5 mU/mL	1
	Mid-cycle	8–33 IU/L	8–33 mU/mL	1
	Luteal	2–8 IU/L	2–8 mU/mL	1
	Post-menopausal	>30 IU/L	>30 mU/mL	1
	Men	1.0–18 IU/L	1.0–18 mU/mL	1
LH	Follicular	1–10 IU/L	1–10 mU/mL	1
	Mid-cycle	20–80 IU/L	20–80 mU/mL	1
	Luteal	3–16 IU/L	3–16 mU/mL	1
	Post-menopausal	>30 IU/L	>30 mU/mL	1
	Men	3–8 IU/L	3–8 mU/mL	1
Prolactin	Women	0–25 mcg/L	0–25 ng/mL	1
	Men	0–20 mcg/L	0–20 ng/mL	1
Growth Hormone		0–20 mU/L	0–10 ng/mL	3
IGF-1	20 years	16–115 nmol/L	120–885 ng/mL	0.13
	40 years	14–46 nmol/L	105–353 ng/mL	
	60 years	10–35 nmol/L	79–263 ng/mL	
	>60 years	7–28 nmol/L	52–210 ng/mL	
ACTH*		2–18 pmol/L	10–80 pg/mL	0.22
Antidiuretic hormone			0–4.7 pg/mL	

*Lithium heparin tube is cold spun immediately.

Bone biochemistry

Table 118.4 Bone biochemistry tests

Hormone	SI units	Traditional units	Conversion factor
Parathyroid hormone*	1.0–6.0 pmol/L	10–60 pg/mL	0.1
Total 25-hydroxy-cholecalciferol*	75–200 nmol/L	30–80 ng/mL	2.5
1, 25-dihydroxy-cholecalciferol*	35–180 pmol/L	15–75 pg/mL	2.4
Calcitonin†		0–7.5 pg/mL	

*Serum, cold spun, flash frozen.
†Lithium heparin tube is cold spun immediately.

Plasma gastrointestinal and pancreatic hormones

Table 118.5 Plasma GI and pancreatic hormones

Hormone	SI units	Traditional units	Conversion factor
Insulin (fasting)*	21–133 pmol/L	3–19 mU/L	6.9
C-peptide (fasting)	0.25–1.2 nmol/L	0.8–3.5 ng/mL	0.33
Gastrin*	0–45 pmol/L	0–100 pg/mL	0.45
Glucagon*	11–36 pmol/L	40–130 pg/mL	0.28
Vasoactive intestinal polypeptide (VIP)*	0–25 pmol/L	0–60 pg/mL	0.42
Pancreatic polypeptide*	0–104 pmol/L	0–435 pg/mL	0.24
Somatostatin*	0–150 pmol/L		
Chromogranin A*	0–50 pmol/L		
Vasopressin		0–4.7 pg/ml	

*Fasting, Trasylol® tube, lithium heparin, cold spun and flash frozen.

Tumor markers

Table 118.6 Tumor markers

Tumor marker	Traditional units
BhCG	0
Carcinoembryonic antigen (CEA)	0–3.0 ng/mL
Prostate-specific antigen (PSA)	0–4 ng/mL
α-Fetoprotein	0–15 ng/mL
Thyroglobulin	0-30 ng/ml

Urinary collections

Table 118.7 Urinary collections: hormones

Urine hormone	Traditional units (mcg/24 hours)
Norepinephrine	0–100 mcg/24 hours
Epinephrine	0–25 mcg/24 hours
Dopamine	60–440 mcg/24 hours
Cortisol, free	0–60 mcg/24 hours
5-hydroxyindoleacetic acid	2–8 mg/24 hours

Table 118.8 Urinary collections: analytes

Urinary analyte	Traditional units (mg or mmol/24 hours)
Calcium	100–250 mg/24 hours
Phosphate	400–1300 mg/24 hours
Potassium	25–125 mmol/24 hours
Sodium	50–285 mmol/24 hours

Index